**Congenital dysplasia
and dislocation of the hip**

Congenital dysplasia and dislocation of the hip

SHERMAN S. COLEMAN, M.D.

Professor of Orthopaedic Surgery
Department of Surgery
University of Utah Medical Center
Salt Lake City, Utah

with 363 illustrations

THE C. V. MOSBY COMPANY

Saint Louis   1978

Copyright © 1978 by The C. V. Mosby Company

All rights reserved. No part of this book may be reproduced in any manner without written permission of the publisher.

Printed in the United States of America

The C. V. Mosby Company
11830 Westline Industrial Drive, St. Louis, Missouri 63141

Library of Congress Cataloging in Publication Data

Coleman, Sherman S   1922-
    Congenital dysplasia and dislocation of the hip.

    Bibliography: p.
    Includes index.
    1. Hip joint—Dislocation. 2. Hip joint—Abnormalities. 3. Pediatric orthopedia. I. Title.
[DNLM: 1. Hip dislocation, Congenital. WE860 C692c]
RD772.C64   617′.376   78-59669
ISBN 0-8016-1018-4

CB/CB/B 9 8 7 6 5 4 3 2 1

to JANE

FOREWORD

It is my good fortune to contribute a foreword to this book written by Dr. Sherman Coleman. I hold high the author's qualifications. He has had a long and continuing interest in congenital dysplasia and dislocation of the hip, and few have the knowledge and expertise that he possesses in this area.

The excellence that one expects of Dr. Coleman is apparent in his approach to this complex subject. He has attempted to cover every conceivable phase and has established fairly definite guidelines. Indeed, almost every abnormality related to congenital dysplasia and dislocation of the hip in infants and adults is discussed in detail.

Many significant changes have occurred in the past two decades in the treatment of the unfortunate child who is born with this condition. In recent years we have seen the introduction of the innominate osteotomy of Salter as well as the pericapsular osteotomy of Pemberton. Other osteotomies that have been developed during the past two decades include the triple innominate osteotomy of Steel, the double innominate osteotomy of Sutherland and Greenfield, and the dial osteotomy proposed by Eppright and Wagner. The role of each of these osteotomies is described in detail. The author also clearly delineates the indications for salvage procedures such as the Chiari osteotomy, the shelf procedure of Wilson, and the Colonna arthroplasty.

There has existed for a great many years a compelling need for a textbook such as this. I confidently anticipate that this book will meet this need and serve as a guide for everyone interested in the subject of congenital dysplasia and dislocation of the hip.

Wood W. Lovell, M.D.
Medical Director,
Scottish Rite Hospital
for Crippled Children,
Atlanta, Georgia

PREFACE

Over the past 30 years the perplexing and often distressing problems encountered in the diagnosis and treatment of congenital dislocation of the hip have become better defined and as a consequence more clearly understood. Correspondingly, the treatment of the condition has undergone major changes. The principles of diagnosis and treatment and the technical solutions to the many problems posed by this condition are better established now than at any time in the past. Our understanding of the clinical expressions of hip dysplasia in the infant, both during the newborn period and in the early weeks of infancy, and our improved programs for early detection have greatly reduced the number of problems caused by late diagnosis. It has been demonstrated that if hip dysplasia is recognized early and is appropriately treated, many of its worrisome sequelae are preventable. However, given the capricious nature of dysplasia and dislocation, there will always be the patient who has an atypical prenatal dislocation, a hip that does not respond favorably to conventional treatment, or a complex problem of iatrogenic origin that will challenge the expertise of any surgeon experienced in children's hip disorders.

The need for a book that discusses the early diagnostic features of this condition so that early recognition and treatment can be provided has become evident. The need for an extension of such a text to respond to the problems posed by the more complicated hip dislocation or by the ineffectively treated hip dislocation is equally obvious. The inevitable and uncontrollable variations in the disease process, as well as the unpredictable responses of patients to the various treatment modalities, suggest that the major problems associated with hip dysplasia and its sequelae will always exist. Thus an analysis of these issues and a logical synthesis of their solutions will continue to be necessary.

Because the clinical manifestations of congenital dislocation of the hip encompass not only the newborn period but also all ages from infancy through old age, I believe that it is appropriate to include the many ways in which the condition affects patients of all ages. The syndrome presents a complex though logical series of problems. Furthermore, each problem has its own unique set of characteristics, depending on the age of the patient, the past treatment history, the specific pathology of the hip, and many other highly individualized factors.

Ideally, the need for surgical treatment of congenital dislocation of the hip should eventually become a rarity, except for occasional difficult antenatal and teratologic dislocations, which will always remain a challenge. However, the complete prevention of all sequelae of a problem that is both genetically and environmentally caused is unrealistic, even in the most medically sophisticated setting. The first and most important goal of this text is to deal with the diagnostic and therapeutic criteria of the neonate and infant with hip dysplasia and dislocation. Second, the scope and complexity of the condition, including the variations in which congenital hip disease may be present, are described. A review of the current surgical and nonsurgical approaches that are now available for treatment is covered next. Finally, some of the problems and complications that are unique to this condition are discussed, with suggestions of how to deal with such untoward occurrences.

This book is sufficiently broad in scope that it should provide a practical guide to the diagnosis and care of common problems in congenital hip disease that are encountered by pediatricians, general family physicians, and orthopedic surgeons from other areas of expertise. It is not primarily directed to the attention of the experienced hip surgeon who is already familiar with much that I have written. Nor do I expect that all will fully agree with the principles presented or the experiences on which they are based, for each builds on his or her own experience, which very possibly will differ.

Any effort that is designed to satisfy such broad objectives requires more than simple factual knowledge and clinical experience; it requires the selfless participation of the several hundred patients afflicted with congenital dislocation who have entrusted me with their care. These people have provided me with an irreplaceable source of clinical and factual information. This includes the cooperation and continuing support of the many medical and paramedical personnel who are involved in their care. Such a volume is also built on the invaluable exchange of ideas that has taken place among my teachers, colleagues, and students. But even more, it requires the tolerance and devotion of my understanding and patient wife and family, whose personal lives were often inconvenienced by the demands made to produce this book. To all these individuals I want to extend my deep gratitude. Special thanks are due my son, Dr. S. Michael Coleman, and some of my residents, including Drs. Howard A. King, Kenneth D. Johnson, and Peter M. Stevens, for their research efforts on several of the chapters. I also want to thank Mrs. Ruth C. Henson, Mrs. Kathryn A. Morton, and Mrs. Tarza L. Peterson for their editorial assistance in composition, bibliography, and secretarial support. Thanks are also due Mr. Julian Maack, who was responsible for producing all of the original illustrations as well as adaptations.

Sherman S. Coleman

CONTENTS

1. Embryology and anatomy of the hip joint, 1
2. Etiology and pathogenesis, 27
3. Diagnosis and treatment in the newborn, neonate, and young infant, 40
4. Diagnosis and treatment of congenital dislocation in the child under 18 months of age, 72
5. Diagnosis and treatment of congenital dislocation in the child 18 months to 4 years of age, 95
6. Diagnosis and treatment of residual dysplasia in the older child or adolescent, 155
7. Problems and complications in treatment, 175
8. Salvage procedures, 209
9. "Teratologic" congenital dislocation, 249
10. Implant hip reconstruction, 257

**Congenital dysplasia
and dislocation of the hip**

CHAPTER 1

Embryology and anatomy of the hip joint

Embryology
    General considerations
    Clinical considerations relating to the development of the hip joint
Gross and functional anatomy
    General considerations
    Clinical correlations

EMBRYOLOGY

To comprehend the etiology and pathogenesis of congenital hip dislocation, it is necessary to understand the development of the human hip joint. Many detailed and comprehensive studies of the developing hip have been reported. Bardeen's[4] investigations, beginning in 1901, represent some of the early, more sophisticated studies on this subject. Subsequently, the contributions of Strayer,[28] Badgley,[1] Laurenson,[17] Gardner and Gray,[12] Watanabe,[32] and others have helped to expand and further our understanding of hip joint development. With these concepts about the normal development we can better envisage some of the problems and conditions that result from the pathologic development of the hip. In this chapter only a synopsis of the embryogenesis and morphogenesis of the hip will be described; more detailed information can be obtained by referring to the references at the end of the chapter.

General considerations

The prenatal development of the hip has been arbitrarily divided into the embryonic and fetal periods. The *embryonic period* involves the first 2 months after fertilization. At 2 months of gestation the embryo measures about 30 mm in crown-rump length; it is during this period that the limb buds are formed by differentiation from a blastemal mass. The limb buds ultimately become the definitive appendages. During the embryonic period the circulation to the limb is established and the hip joint becomes completely formed in cartilage, with an identifiable femoral head, acetabulum, capsule, synovial membrane, and ligamentum teres.

The *fetal period* begins at the conclusion of the embryonic stage and continues through the final prenatal development at term. It is during this time that the complex developmental characteristics of the human hip take place and the features of the hip that relate to antenatal dysplasia and dislocation are established.

Embryonic development of the hip. Early investigators* demonstrated that the anlage of the skeleton consists of un-

---

*See references 2 to 4, 8, 14, and 15.

differentiated cell masses. Bardeen[2,4] showed that during the third week of embryonic life the limb buds become filled with mesenchyme, the origin of which is uncertain but was thought to be from the parietal layers of the unsegmented mesoderm. Strayer[29] later believed that this mesenchymal tissue possesses multipotential characteristics and contains all the elements necessary for the development and growth of the joint, with the exception of the blood vessels and nerves, which appear later. These concepts, although not universally accepted, seem to have the support of the majority of investigators.

At 4 weeks of gestation the embryo is about 5 mm in crown-rump length and the limb buds, which consist of densely packed cells with multipotential capacity, can be seen as folds along the ventrolateral aspect of the body. At this stage the hip shows little differentiation; however, the knee joint, feet, and toes already show some early evidence of development.[32]

When the length of the fetus is 10 mm (5 to 6 weeks), the os innominatum blastema begins to separate into three masses, representing the ilium, ischium, and pubis. At the 12-mm stage (6 weeks) the femoral shaft begins to show precartilage cells and assumes a somewhat "club-shaped" appearance (Fig. 1-1). Centrally, the cartilage of the femur grows by interstitial cell proliferation, and, at the periphery, the growth is appositional, as the cells and matrices are laid down in successive layers. At 6 weeks of gestation the femoral shaft is composed of the most differentiated cartilage cells,

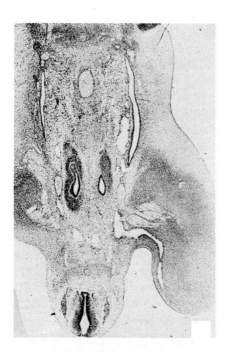

Fig. 1-1. At 6 weeks of gestation (fetal length, 12 mm) the lower limb appendage has developed precartilage cells in the region of the acetabulum and the femur. (From Strayer, L. M.: The embryology of the human hip joint, Yale J. Biol. Med. **16:**13, 1943.)

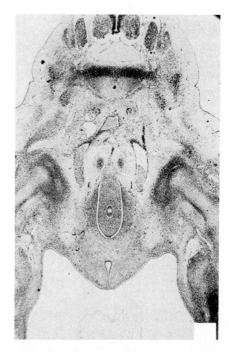

Fig. 1-2. At 7 weeks of gestation (length, 15 mm) the femur and acetabulum become better defined and the femoral head assumes a globular shape. (From Strayer, L. M.: The embryology of the human hip joint, Yale J. Biol. Med. **16:**13, 1943.)

with the head of the femur, the distal femur, and the trochanters appearing progressively less differentiated in that order.

Strayer[29] observed that, after the 12-mm blastemal stage previously described, each skeletal primordium (that is, the femur and os innominatum) passes through three or more stages of development. These are called the blastema, the precartilage, the cartilage, and the fetal bone stages. He found the femur of a 17- to 20-mm embryo to be a typical example of this developmental process. In this primitive stage the femoral shaft is composed of cartilage cells, the ends are made up of precartilage cells, and the greater trochanter is composed of cells resembling blastema.

Bardeen[4] and Strayer[28] both found that the initial skeletal primordium of the hip joint consists of densely packed, multipotential, primitive mesenchymal cells. Gardner and Gray[12] in 1950 concurred with these observations and also added evidence that showed that the general form and major components of the hip are present before the joint space actually develops. In Bardeen's[3] detailed studies of the embryogenesis and morphogenesis of the hip, he concluded that the development of the acetabulum takes place by means of the fusion of the cartilaginous primordia of the ilium and ischium and that these in turn fuse with the smaller and the more slowly developing pubic primordium. He observed that the proportional amounts of each pelvic cartilage contributing to development of the acetabulum were the same as for those ultimately contributed by the corresponding portions of the innominate bone in the adult; namely, two fifths ischium, two fifths ilium, and one fifth pubis. During this acetabular formation, which can be observed as early as 6 to 7 weeks of gestation (length, 15 mm), the femoral head can be seen to develop in situ as a globular structure within the primitive cartilage of the hip joint.

When the fetus is 15 mm long, or at approximately 6 to 7 weeks of gestation, the femoral head and acetabulum show further signs of differentiation. The femoral head becomes globular in shape and the femoral shaft also begins to acquire a slightly convex shape (Fig. 1-2). At length 17 mm (7 weeks of gestation) a definite interzone develops between the femoral head and the acetabulum, and when the fetus has reached 20 mm in length (7½ weeks of gestation) this interzone differentiates into three layers. The middle layer or zone represents the first evidence of the synovial membrane, and the outer layers represent the perichondrium of the acetabulum and femoral head.[12] Also, at 20 mm of length the muscle groups are outlined and the femoral neck has formed a recognizable angle of inclination with the shaft of the femur.[32] This angle varies from 130 to 160 degrees.

When the length of the fetus is about 30 mm (8 weeks), at the conclusion of the embryonic stage, there is noticeable deepening of the acetabulum and the greater trochanter becomes evident. By this stage the cartilage has become hyaline in nature. Also, the ligamentum teres and other capsular structures have become vascularized; the labrum glenoidale (limbus) also shows signs of development at the periphery of the acetabulum (Fig. 1-3).

Fetal development of the hip. The *fetal period* begins at 8 weeks of gestation when the fetus measures approximately 30 mm in crown-rump length; it is during this time that all the definitive development of the hip joint occurs, leading to the final fetal or prenatal development at term.

When the length of the fetus is about 30 mm (8 weeks) the hip joint space begins to form as a small, slitlike cavity lined by flattened cells. Strayer[28] postulated

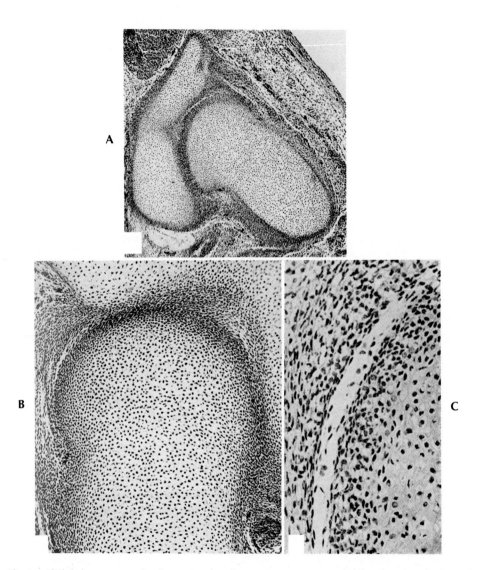

Fig. 1-3. Slightly later, at 8 weeks of gestation (length, 30 mm), an interzone develops between the femoral head and acetabulum, **A.** The perichondrium of these two structures is defined, the labrum glenoidale is beginning to develop, **B,** and the cartilage becomes slightly hyaline in character, **C.** (From Gardner, E., and Gray, D. J.: Prenatal development of the human hip joint, Am. J. Anat. **87:**163, 1950).

that the joint cavity develops as a degenerative and mechanical process because he observed degeneration and cell splitting along the joint margins as the embryo grew from 37 to 45 mm (8 to 9 weeks) in size. He also proposed that the developing neuromuscular mechanism had a significant effect on the joint development and that abnormalities in the neuromuscular system could cause adverse changes in hip growth and development. At 30 to 40 mm an ingrowth of blood vessels invades the deepened acetabular fossa, and synovial-like tissue develops around the reflection of the developing labrum glenoidale or limbus. The acetabulum more clearly shows the iliac, pubic, and ischial cartilages entering into the formation of the acetabulum.[12] The femoral head also reveals a definite fovea capitis femoris, and the ligamentum teres is well defined (Fig. 1-4).

Strayer[29] observed that the development of the acetabular elements is accompanied by lateral growth and proliferation of the labrum. He believed the growth of the limbus to be "the most important mechanism concerned with deepening of the acetabulum." Hence he believed that the labrum and its normal growth are critical in lending stability to the hip during its fetal development.

At 11 weeks the fetus is approximately 50 mm in length. The hip joint has been completely formed, and the femoral head presents a spherical contour; it is approximately 2 mm in diameter.[32] The head shows signs of vascularization, predomi-

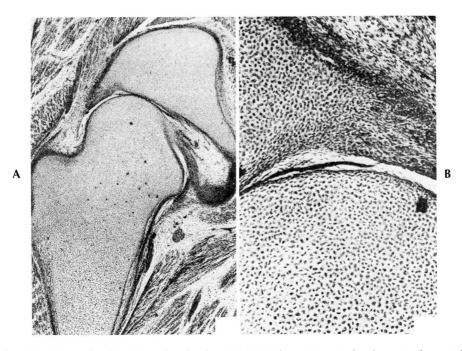

Fig. 1-4. At 9 weeks of gestation (length, about 40 mm), the joint cavity has begun to form, with synovial-like tissue reflected about the limbus, and the ligamentum teres becomes defined, **A.** The cartilage has become hyaline in nature and the perichondrium is well developed on both sides of the joint, **B.** (From Strayer, L. M.: The embryology of the human hip joint, Yale J. Biol. Med. **16**:13, 1943.)

6 *Congenital dysplasia and dislocation of the hip*

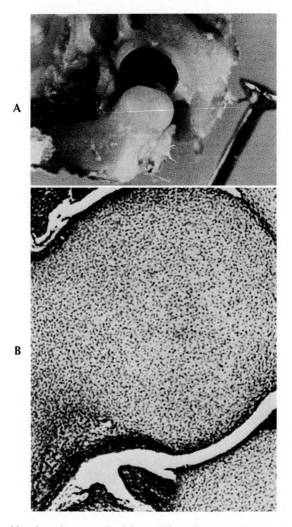

Fig. 1-5. The femoral head can be manually dislocated from the acetabulum at about 11 or 12 weeks of gestation (length, 50 mm). This is shown well in **A.** The size of the femoral head is shown in relationship to the head of a pin. The joint space at this time is completely formed, **B.** (From Watanabe, R. S.: Embryology of the human hip, Clin. Orthop. **98:**8, 1974.)

nantly by vessels from the perichondrium of the neck and also by a few vessels entering from the trochanteric fossa and the ligamentum teres.[12] The lines of cleavage have now formed at the joint, and, at this time, the head is covered by well-defined hyaline cartilage. Also at this point, because the femoral head is now separate from the acetabulum, it is possible for the head to be manually dislocated from the acetabulum (Fig. 1-5).[32]

At this same 50-mm stage, Badgley[1] reported that femoral anteversion measures approximately 5 to 10 degrees and that the acetabular inclination averages 40 degrees in the sagittal and 70 degrees in the vertical plane. These values have subsequently been affirmed by Wata-

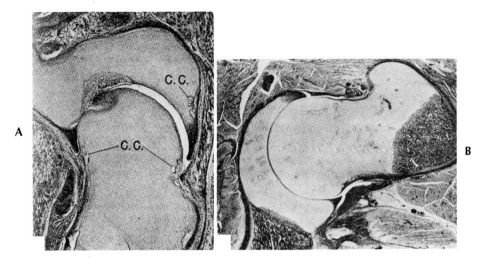

Fig. 1-6. At 13 weeks of gestation (length, 70 mm), the capsular structures become better defined and the acetabular roof more completely covers the femoral head, **A.** The zona orbicularis is also evident, and the cartilage of the head and neck and trochanters, along with the acetabulum, are well vascularized, **B.** (From Gardner, E., and Gray, D. J.: Prenatal development of the human hip joint, Am. J. Anat. 87:163, 1950.)

nabe.[32] However, these fetal calculations of the various directional planes of the acetabulum appear subject to considerable uncertainty from the standpoint of accuracy because of difficulty in establishing a critical point of reference. I believe, therefore, that this particular aspect of hip joint development does not deserve further discussion. The vasculature of the capsule and the synovial membrane have also become well developed at the 50 mm stage, and the pattern now largely resembles that of the adult hip.

When the length of the fetus is 70 mm, the roof of the acetabulum extends over the femoral head and the vascularity of the entire hip becomes more pronounced. Also at the 70-mm stage of development (12 to 13 weeks of gestation), the fibrous capsule becomes thickened as a result of the further development of collagenous fibers, which help form a well-defined zona orbicularis (Fig. 1-6). By 14 weeks of development, the crown-rump length of the fetus is approximately 90 mm. Because of the increasing length of the limbs, the hips and knees seem to become forced into greater flexion and the left lower limb usually overlaps the right.

At the sixteenth week of gestation (length, 120 mm), a demonstrable enlargement of the femoral head and the trochanters is evident. At this stage the musculature about the hip is fully developed and active hip motion can be observed. The vasculature has matured and the main source of supply to the femoral head is by way of the epiphyseal and metaphyseal vessels. The vessels of the ligamentum teres, which contribute to the femoral head, are very small and insignificant at this age. Moreover, as Gardner and Gray[12] have shown, the arteries of the round ligament contribute very little to the blood supply of the developing femoral head until late in childhood.

At 20 weeks of gestation the fetus averages 170 mm in length and has completed one half of its prenatal development.

Also at this point, the fetus is completely formed and morphologically resembles a newborn infant. The shaft of the femur and the acetabulum have become progressively more ossified. The femoral head, however, shows no evidence of ossification and ordinarily does not ossify until approximately 3 to 6 months *after* birth. The vasculature of the hip continues to mature and the capsular ligaments become better defined and appear as localized thickenings of the capsule. The iliofemoral ligament is especially prominent and contains many bundles of collagenous fibers. At this same age, the ischiocapsular and pubocapsular thickenings are also distinguishable as ligaments (Fig. 1-7).

As the fetus develops to 250 mm in length (28 to 29 weeks) the vasculature becomes very complex and numerous sources of blood supply to the head are evident. By 285 mm of length (32 weeks) the ischium and ilium are almost completely ossified and the femoral shaft has ossified to a level proximal to the trochanters. The trochanters, however, are still cartilaginous at this stage and will remain so until after birth. When the fetal length has reached 308 mm (35 weeks) the hip has developed to a point where the changes that take place before term are only those of increasing size.

One of the more controversial issues involved in the morphogenesis of the human hip has to do with the depth of the acetabulum during the later months of intrauterine development. In 1912 LeDamany[18] and later Morville[19] believed that the depth of the acetabulum actually decreased during the last 3 months of gestation. LeDamany, therefore, postulated

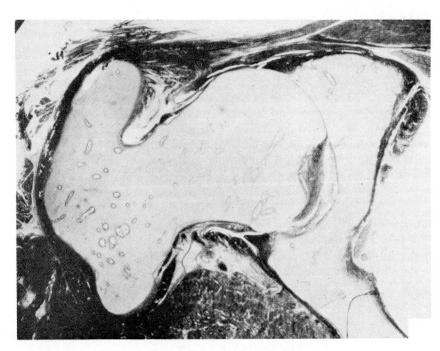

Fig. 1-7. Halfway through the fetal development at 20 weeks of gestation (length, 170 mm), the vasculature and ligamentous structures are even better defined. Most changes from this point until term are those only of increasing size. (From Strayer, L. M.: The embryology of the human hip joint, Yale J. Biol. Med. **16:**13, 1943.)

Embryology and anatomy of the hip joint   9

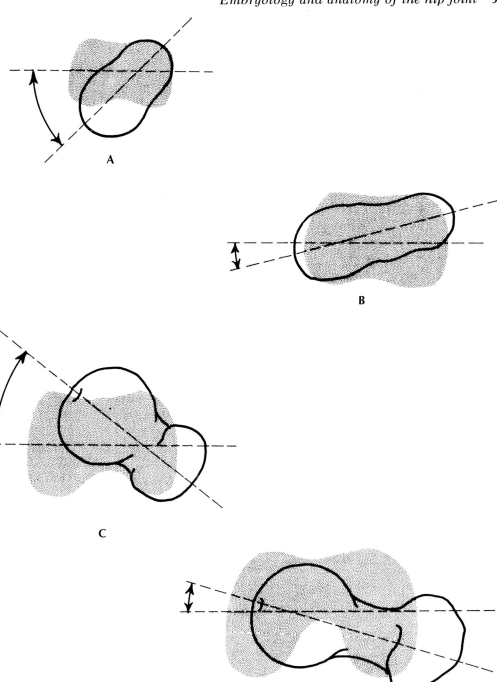

Fig. 1-8. Diagrammatic representation of the developing changes in anteversion of the femoral neck occurring in **A,** the embryo, **B,** early fetal period, **C,** late fetal period or at term, and **D,** adult. (From Gardner, E.: Prenatal development of the human hip joint, femur, and hip bone. In American Academy of Orthopaedic Surgeons: AAOS Instructional Course Lectures, vol. 21, St. Louis, 1972, The C. V. Mosby Co., p. 150.)

that this may be a factor in the etiology of congenital dislocation of the hip. This conclusion was derived from some very carefully performed anthropomorphic studies. More recently, Ralis and McKibbin[21] confirmed these observations of LeDamany and concluded that the acetabulum at birth is more shallow than at any time during its development. On the other hand, Gardner and Gray[12] have shown that the acetabulum continues to deepen during this period by means of the continued growth of the limbus over the femoral head.

Throughout the development of the hip joint, the acetabulum and the proximal femur undergo certain alterations in their configuration. The neckshaft angle of the femur (the angle of inclination) was measured by Strayer[28] at 150 to 155 degrees at length 23 mm (8 weeks of gestation). This angle gradually decreases to 130 degrees at birth. The angle of declination is in retroversion early in fetal life; this gradually reverses to varying degrees of anteversion throughout subsequent prenatal growth (Fig. 1-8). Although it has been suggested that these changes in anteversion are related to limb bud rotation, Gardner[11] believes that this unusual reversal of the angle has no specific relationship to limb bud rotation but rather is a remodeling process that occurs after the rotation of the limb buds has started. During this process of proximal femoral development, Watanabe[32] showed that there is a wide range in the angles of declination seen from one fetus to another at different stages of gestation. These angles varied in Wantanabe's studies from -30 to +40 degrees. Stanisavljevic and Mitchell found that at birth the average angle of anteversion is from 25 to 30 degrees.[27] The fetal acetabulum shows similar alterations with growth; however, as noted earlier, these are very much more difficult to measure and document because of the effect that pelvic tilt and pelvic obliquity can have on the determination of these data.

Clinical considerations relating to the development of the hip joint

Etiologically there appears to be no intrinsic defect in the development of the hip joint that can readily or consistently explain dislocation of the hip. Gardner and Gray,[12] for example, studied fifty-two fetuses and were unable to demonstrate any evidence to show that defective development of the hip joint could be incriminated as a *prima facie* cause of dislocation. Because the femoral head develops inside the joint, there must be several other factors that are ultimately responsible for the dislocation. Some appear to be antenatal and some postnatal.

The principal antenatal and underlying factors that may have a bearing on the abnormal development of the joint and its eventual dislocation are the postural attitudes adopted by the fetus. Badgley,[1] Watanabe,[32] and others have pointed out that either anteversion, retroversion, or both may be related to the intrauterine position, and Dunn[9] has suggested that the increased incidence of abnormalities occurring on the left side is similarly related to the intrauterine position. Furthermore, the striking and consistent observation that congenital dislocation of the hip (CDH) has a much higher incidence in breech births, especially in instances of frank breech presentations, can only be explained by intrauterine position. The observations of LeDamany[18] and Ralis and McKibbin[21] offer some evidence to support that the acetabulum is more shallow and that there is therefore greater instability of the hip at birth than at any other time. This, coupled with ligamentous laxity, may render the hip most vulnerable to dislocation at this age.

Strayer's[29] observations on the response of the developing hip joint to the integrity of the neuromuscular mechanism essentially parallels the observations commonly seen in postnatal situations. The normal configuration of the proximal femur and the proper development of the acetabulum are very much affected by abnormalities in the neuromuscular mechanism that functions around the hip joint. This is especially seen in patients with cerebral palsy, poliomyelitis, myelodysplasia, and similar conditions. However, in true congenital dysplasia and dislocation of the hip, abnormalities of the neurologic system are not present.

As observed by Strayer[29] and Watanabe,[32] the earliest possible time that an actual dislocation of the femoral head can occur is after the joint cavity has become fully formed. This occurs at 11 weeks of gestation (length, 50 mm) (Fig. 1-5). Despite the capability for dislocation at this early age, the youngest fetus ever to exhibit an antenatal dislocation was recorded during the third trimester,[11] at an age in which positional factors are known to play a very significant role in the etiology of many congenital abnormalities. These and other factors will be discussed in greater detail in Chapter 2.

GROSS AND FUNCTIONAL ANATOMY
General considerations

Anatomically, the hip is a diarthrodial joint of the ball-and-socket type. This means that it has a spherical head that articulates with a reciprocally shaped acetabulum, it possesses a joint cavity that is lined with synovial membrane, and it is supported by ligaments. It is basically a stable joint by virtue of its bony configuration and surrounding musculature. Furthermore, it has a considerable range of

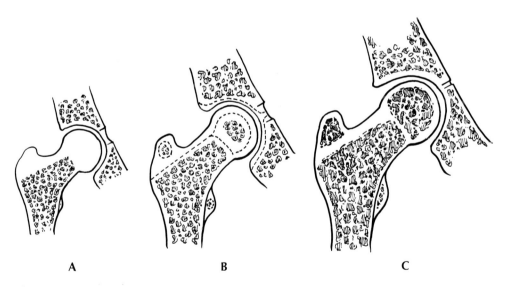

Fig. 1-9. Diagrammatic representation of growth and ossification of proximal femur. At birth neither the femoral head nor the trochanter are ossified, yet the cartilage anlagen are fully formed, **A.** The iliac and ischial ossification centers are separated by a generous synchondrosis, representing the triradiate cartilage. In **B** the femoral head and greater trochanter have begun to ossify. The line of dots represents germinal cartilage cells, which are proliferating new cartilage (which is replaced by bone) and then move away from the underlying bone that they have produced. By age 6 or 7 years the femoral head and the trochanters have become further ossified, and the triradiate cartilage remains open, **C.** Any insult to the capital epiphysis and its cartilage growth center may result in growth arrest with resulting deformities caused by disturbed and asymmetric growth of these centers. (Adapted from Dr. R. S. Siffert.)

12 *Congenital dysplasia and dislocation of the hip*

motion in all directions, not only because of the spherical nature of the head but also because the diameter of the neck is significantly narrower than that of the head.

Femoral head. The femoral head is not a perfect sphere, being slightly flattened on its superior weight-bearing surface, but from a practical point of view it can be considered a sphere. It is covered by hyaline articular cartilage, which serves not only as a "shock absorber" but also as an important growth center of the capital femoral epiphysis during the prenatal and postnatal development of the hip joint. Most of the femoral head articular cartilage opposes the articular cartilage of the acetabulum; however, in the upright, biped (extended) position of the hip, a generous portion of the femoral head's articular surface is not covered by the acetabulum, but rather articulates directly with the iliofemoral "Y" ligament of Bigelow. In the approximate center of the medial articulating portion of the femoral head, there is a fovea or depression where the ligamentum teres is attached. In this area there is no articular cartilage.

During the first 6 months of postnatal life, the cartilaginous head of the femur is invaded by osteogenic cells and a secondary center of ossification forms, which then in turn creates the physis or epiphyseal plate. This physis remains open until about age 13 to 15 years. Prior to that time it serves, along with the articular car-

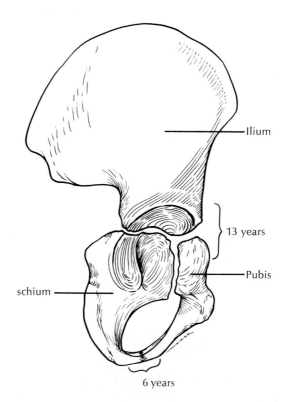

Fig. 1-10. An illustration of the triradiate synchondrosis that separates and serves as a growth center for the ilium, pubis, and ischium. The age at which fusion of each portion of the triradiate cartilage takes place is illustrated. (Reproduced by permission from J. C. B. Grant's An atlas of anatomy, ed. 7. Copyright © 1978, The Williams & Wilkins Co.)

Embryology and anatomy of the hip joint 13

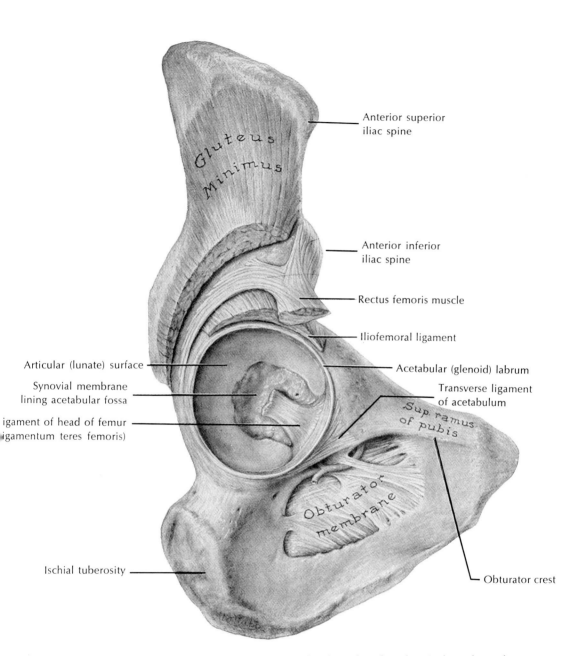

Fig. 1-11. Lateral view of pelvis and acetabulum showing the "horseshoe-shaped" articular surfaces of acetabulum, acetabular fossa (filled with fat), and ligamentum teres attached to transverse acetabular ligament. The labrum (or limbus) encompasses the entire periphery of the acetabular rim. (Reproduced by permission from J. C. B. Grant's An atlas of anatomy, ed. 7. Copyright © 1978, The Williams & Wilkins Co.)

tilage of the femoral head, as the major growth center of the proximal femur[24] (Fig. 1-9). From birth to skeletal maturity these growth centers of the proximal femur contribute approximately 30% to the total length of the femur. It appears that most of this growth occurs during the first 5 or 6 years of life and that thereafter this contribution slows down. Thus any noxious insult to these growth centers that occurs during the first 3 to 4 years of life will have a much greater effect on growth than if it occurred later. Correspondingly, it appears that the proximal femur has a much greater capacity to remodel prior to age 5 years than after 5 years of age. These impressions are based on considerable circumstantial and archeologic evidence, such as the downward "migration" of internal fixation devices in the proximal femur[25] and natural markers, such as those observed in the growth lines as a result of high-dose phosphorous ingestion.[22]

Acetabulum. The acetabulum (vinegar cup) is reciprocally shaped to receive the spherical femoral head. Developmentally, it is formed by the ischium, ilium, and pubis, each being separated during postnatal growth by a cartilaginous growth center that forms a "Y" configuration. It is thus known as the triradiate cartilage. It ossifies at puberty, between 12 and 15 years of age (earlier in girls) (Fig. 1-10). Residual evidence of these growth centers is identifiable in the adult in two locations; namely the iliopectineal eminence anteriorly and at the posterior junction of the ischium and the pubis.[16] Prior to puberty the ischiopubic synchondrosis (which ossifies earlier at age 5 to 7 years) often becomes enlarged and has been associated (erroneously) with the osteochondritides. It has been called the Van Neck disease in these circumstances.

The articular cartilage of the acetabulum assumes a horseshoe shape, resembling an inverted "U" (Fig. 1-11). The

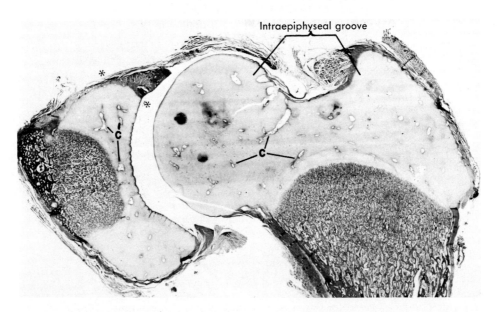

Fig. 1-12. Photomicrograph of hip joint in 2-month-old infant. Blood vessels enter from intraepiphyseal groove and distribute within proximal femoral epiphysis in canals, **C.** Similar canals are present in acetabulum. Differences of hyaline and fibrocartilage (*) of acetabular rim are evident. (From Proceedings of the second open scientific meeting of The Hip Society, St. Louis, 1974, The C. V. Mosby Co.)

central noncartilaginous portion of the acetabulum is a depression, called the acetabular fossa, which is occupied by the ligamentum teres and a large pad of fat often called the haversian gland. This fat pad has also been called the "pulvinar" in the past. Some have believed that it becomes hypertrophied after dislocation occurs and as a result may become an obstruction to relocation. The two limbs of the U-shaped articular cartilage are bridged by a tough ligamentous structure called the transverse acetabular ligament. This ligament serves as a supportive anchor for the ligamentum teres and also blends imperceptibly at the periphery of the joint with the fibrocartilaginous labrum or limbus. This latter structure makes up the peripheral margin of the acetabulum and assists somewhat in deepening the concavity of the hip socket, thus lending some stability to the hip joint (Fig. 1-12). The labrum is also believed to contribute to the peripheral growth of the acetabulum during the development of the joint. The labrum lies inside the capsule, which renders it a potential source of obstruction to reduction of a dislocation (Fig. 1-13).

The fibrous capsule of the hip joint extends from the periosteum of the acetabular rim to the base of the neck. At the posterior superior attachment, the origin of the reflected head of the rectus femoris muscle blends with the capsule. The capsule is much more expansive an-

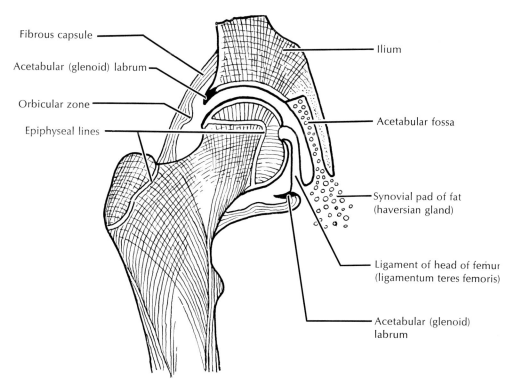

Fig. 1-13. Diagrammatic coronal section of the hip joint, showing clearly the relationships of the labrum to the capsule, to the transverse acetabular ligament, and to the ligamentum teres. The acetabular fossa containing the haversian fat pad (pulvinar) is also seen. (Reproduced by permission from J. C. B. Grant's An atlas of anatomy, ed. 7. Copyright © 1978, The Williams and Wilkins Co.)

16 *Congenital dysplasia and dislocation of the hip*

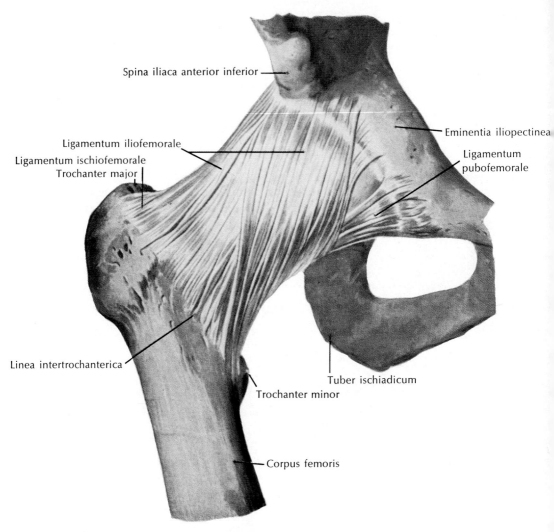

Fig. 1-14. The ligaments reinforcing the hip joint capsule follow a winding course about the neck of the femur. The large iliofemoral ligament appears to bifurcate as it passes from the ilium to its intertrochanteric attachment, thus giving rise to the name Y ligament (Bigelow). (From Spalteholz, W.: Hand-atlas of human anatomy, ed. 7, Philadelphia, 1933, J. B. Lippincott Co.)

teriorly than posteriorly. In front, the capsule extends as far distally as the intertrochanteric line (Fig. 1-14), but posteriorly it extends distally only as far as the middle of the neck (Fig. 1-15). These capsular structures become continuous with the periosteum of the femoral neck and are reflected backward and upward on the neck of the femur. At this point they are called retinacular fibers. The capsule is reinforced by three ligaments arising from the pelvis and inserting onto the femur. The ligaments are thickenings of the capsule and cannot be discretely dissected as separate entities. They arise from the ilium, pubis, and ischium and are respectively called the iliofemoral (Bigelow or Y) ligament, the pubofemoral

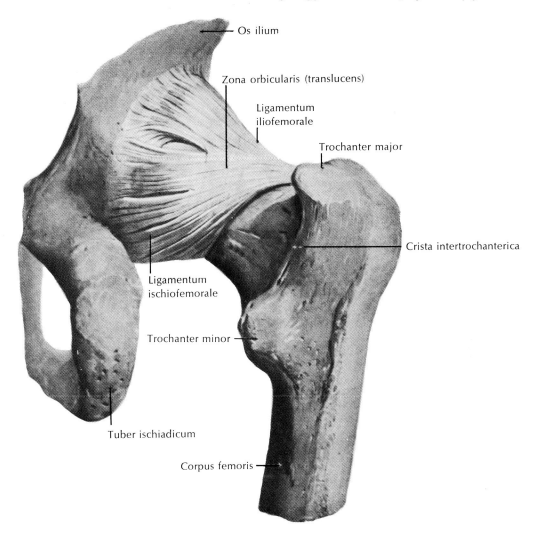

Fig. 1-15. The capsule does not extend as far distally over the posterior aspect of the femoral neck as it does anteriorly. The area of the zona orbicularis is indicated, but this ligamentous thickening is seen better in Fig. 1-16. (From Spalteholz, W.: Hand-atlas of human anatomy, ed. 7, Philadelphia, 1933, J. B. Lippincott Co.)

ligament, and ischiofemoral ligament (Fig. 1-14). In the anatomic (extended position of the hip, they take a winding course about the femoral neck so that further extension and inward rotation tend to tighten these ligaments. Conversely, flexion, abduction, and outward rotation relax them, thus explaining why an effusion or a painful intra-articular condition of the hip joint tends to produce a flexed, abducted, and outwardly rotated attitude of the thigh. In the deeper portions of the capsule posteriorly, the ligaments are arranged in a circular fashion, which is called the zona orbicularis (Fig. 1-16).

The ligamentum teres connects the bone of the ischium in the acetabular fos-

18 *Congenital dysplasia and dislocation of the hip*

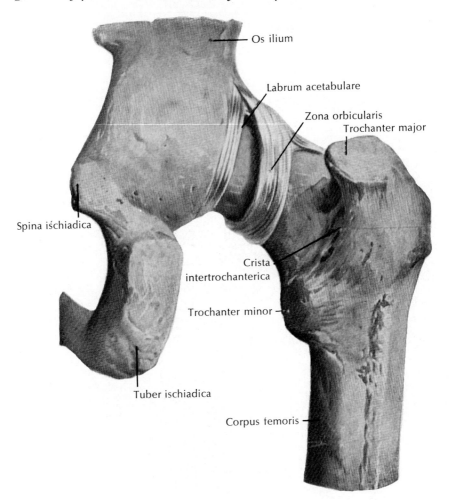

Fig. 1-16. In the posterior aspect of the femoral neck the thickened circular band of fibers is better seen. The zona orbicularis lies deep to the capsule and the ischiofemoral ligament. (From Spalteholz, W.: Hand-atlas of human anatomy, ed. 7, Philadelphia, 1933, J. B. Lippincott Co.)

sa with the femoral head. Its pelvic origin includes an attachment to the transverse acetabular ligament. On the femur the ligamentum teres inserts into the fovea capitus and subtly blends into the surrounding articular cartilage.

Joint cavity. The hip joint cavity is rather capacious and is lined by synovial membrane, which is attached to and blends with the glenoidal labrum and the transverse acetabular ligament. The synovial membrane lines the fibrous capsule as it extends down to its attachment on the neck of the femur; it then is reflected back up onto the femoral neck and stops at the osteochondral juncture of the femoral head. As with intra-articular fat pads and ligaments elsewhere, the ligamentum teres, the transverse acetabular ligament, and the haversian gland (pulvinar) are invested (as a visceral layer) by the synovial membrane, thus rendering these structures technically extrasynovial. Anteriorly there is an occasional

Embryology and anatomy of the hip joint 19

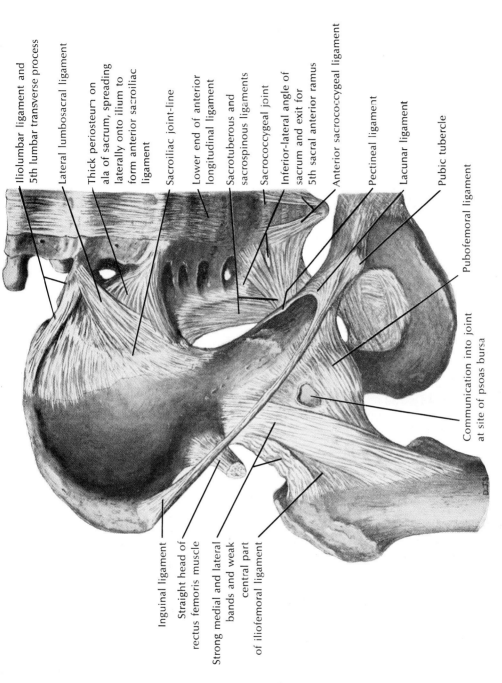

Fig. 1-17. Anteriorly there is a bursa that lies under the psoas muscle and tendon and on top of the capsule, as seen in this diagrammatic illustration of the anterior aspect of the hip. Occasionally there is a connection between this bursa and the hip joint (see text). (Reprinted by permission of Faber and Faber Ltd. from Anatomy of the human body by R. D. Lockhart, G. F. Hamilton, and F. W. Fyfe. Published in the United States by J. B. Lippincott Co., Philadelphia.)

20 *Congenital dysplasia and dislocation of the hip*

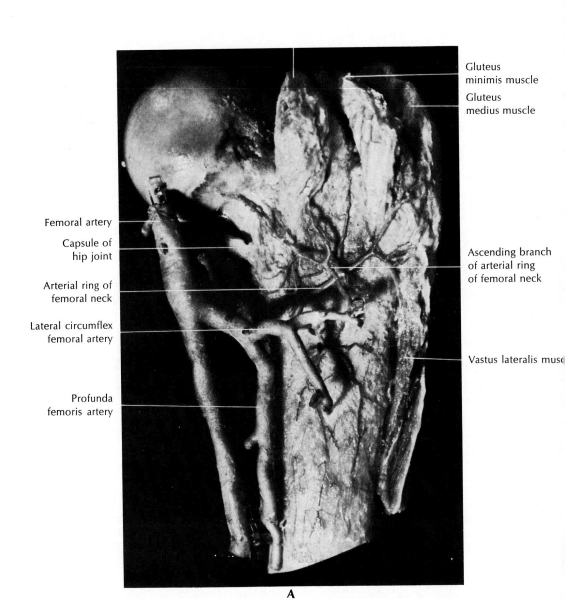

Fig. 1-18. Anatomic dissection of the proximal femur, showing the branches of the lateral circumflex femoral artery that contribute to the arterial ring of the femoral neck, **A.** The posterior dissection shows the contribution to the ring made by branches from the medial circumflex femoral artery, **B.** (From Crock, H. V., and Crock, C.: The blood supply of the lower limb bones in man (descriptive and applied), Edinburgh, 1967, E. & S. Livingstone.)

Embryology and anatomy of the hip joint 21

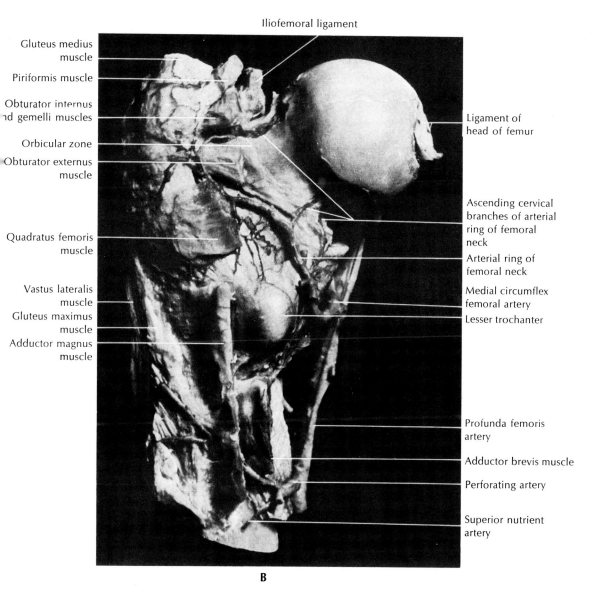

Fig. 1-18, cont'd. For legend see opposite page.

communication between the hip joint cavity and a bursa between the iliopsoas muscle and the capsule. This connection is extremely rare in children but is found in approximately 20% of adults (Fig. 1-17). In some instances, through this same synovial connection, an effusion originating in the hip joint can present itself as an inguinal swelling simulating hernia.

Blood supply of the hip. The vasculature of the hip joint is very rich, but because of the unique morphology of the femoral head and neck, the blood supply to the femoral head is somewhat precarious. Furthermore, the blood vessels supplying the femoral head assume differing degrees of importance at varying periods during postnatal development.*

The blood vessels principally involved in supplying the hip joint and femoral head are derived from the descending branch of the superior gluteal artery, the ascending branches of the lateral and medial circumflex vessels, and the inferior gluteal artery. In a variety of ways these vessels form a ring of arteries that surround the hip joint.[7] The posterior part of the ring is most often formed by a large branch of the medial circumflex femoral artery. Correspondingly, the anterior branch is formed by branches of the lateral circumflex femoral artery. Branches from this arterial ring ascend to the posterior capsule of the hip and infiltrate the capsule. They pass proximally under the synovial reflection to the osteochondral juncture of the femoral head. It is from these vessels that the epiphyseal and metaphyseal arteries of the upper femur are derived (Fig. 1-18). All of these vessels are firmly held against the femoral neck by the reflected portion (retinacular fibers) of the capsule and the periosteum. A modest arterial contribution is made by way of the round ligament. This artery is usually derived from a branch of the obturator artery and originates near the transverse acetabular ligament, where it enters the ligamentum teres. The artery supplies that ligament as well as a small but variable portion of the head about the attachment of the ligament into the fovea capitis.

The blood supply to the hip joint during its postnatal development deserves special mention because of its relationship to the behavior of the femoral head in certain hip disorders as well as its importance in the treatment of congenital dislocation of the hip. The medial circumflex femoral artery passes between the iliopsoas and adductor muscles, then wraps around the femoral neck posteriorly and enters the intraepiphyseal groove (Fig. 1-19). It passes forward in this groove and anastomoses with a comparable anterior vessel coming from a branch of the lateral circumflex artery (Fig. 1-20). It is these vessels, in the intraepiphyseal groove, that can become compressed between the femoral neck and the rim of the acetabulum when the hip is placed in the forced "frog-leg" position. Also, because of the unique relationship of these vessels to the surrounding muscles and soft tissues, forced inward rotation and extension of the thigh can "wring out" the capsular vessels, thus compromising the femoral head blood supply in still another way.[20] These observations are important because any extremes of position of the thigh following reduction of a congenitally dislocated hip may result in a serious compromise of the circulation, leading to partial or complete necrosis of the capital femoral epiphysis.

The artery to the ligamentum teres is virtually nonfunctional until the age of 8 years, when it assumes a relatively minor role in supplying the femoral head. Thus, when necessary, excision of the round ligament can be safely accomplished dur-

---

*See references 5, 6, 30, 31, and 33.

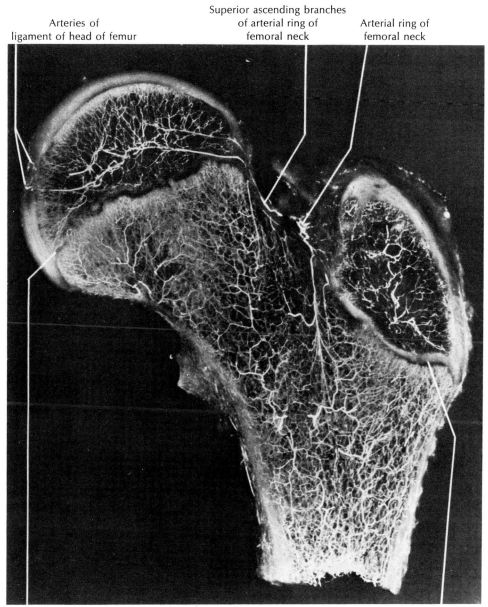

Fig. 1-19. Coronal section of proximal end of femur in a 13-year-old boy, showing the arterial ring of the femoral neck and its ascending branches that enter the epiphysis. (From Crock, H. V., and Crock, C.: The blood supply of the lower limb bones in man (descriptive and applied), Edinburgh, 1967, E. & S. Livingstone.)

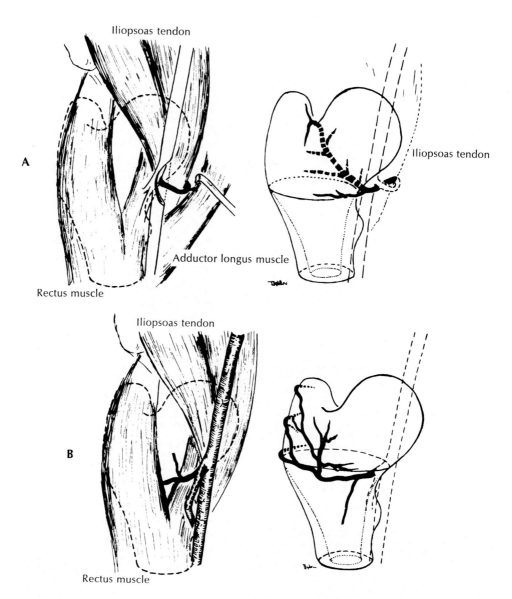

Fig. 1-20. Treatment of childhood disability. **A,** Medial circumflex arterial circulation. The artery usually stems from the profunda femoris. It crosses the iliopsoas tendon and then wraps around the iliopsoas tendon to reach the medial portion of the proximal femur. It then courses along the posterior intraepiphyseal groove, providing the major blood supply to the chondroepiphysis and central and medial portions of the growth plate. **B,** Lateral circumflex arterial circulation. The artery stems from the profunda femoris, crosses the iliopsoas tendon, and then goes between the two heads of the rectus femoris origin to reach the anterior proximal femur, where distribution is primarily to the trochanteric region. (From Ogden, J. [Ferguson, A. B., ed.]: Orthopedic surgery in infancy and childhood, ed. 4. Copyright © 1975, The Williams and Wilkins Co., Baltimore.)

ing open reduction of the hip in *young children* under age 8 years, without fear of significantly compromising the femoral head blood supply. Also, it is during this early period of childhood that the incidence of the Perthes disease (femoral head bone necrosis) is highest, and this observation has been indirectly associated with the fact that there is no arterial blood supply through the round ligament at this age.

Nerve supply. The nerve supply to the hip joint follows the same basic pattern found in joints elsewhere in the body; this means that the same nerves supply the joint as supply the pelvic girdle and lower limb. In the hip joint this includes the nerve to the rectus femoris muscle from the femoral nerve, the nerve to the quadratus femoris muscle from the sciatic nerve, and a branch from the anterior obturator nerve. The fact that these nerves innervate the muscles going down the thigh explains why lesions in the hip joint may produce painful referred pain into the lower thigh and knee. Thus it is not uncommon at all for a child with hip joint disease to complain of discomfort in his lower thigh or about his knee. This is extremely important from the standpoint of diagnosis, for knee and thigh pain must always suggest the possibility of ipsilateral hip joint disease.

Clinical correlations

From a diagnostic and therapeutic point of view, certain aspects of the gross anatomy of the hip joint are highly significant. The major considerations are those that relate to the characteristics of the capsule and ligaments and to the blood supply of the femoral head. For example, the capacity of the hip joint is greatest when the hip is flexed, abducted, and outwardly rotated. Thus, any irritating intra-articular lesion of the hip that produces a synovitis and effusion will cause the thigh to be held in some degree of flexion, abduction, and outward rotation. Conversely, efforts to extend and inwardly rotate the thigh will be resisted by any painful intra-articular lesion, such as that seen in bone or cartilage necrosis.

The blood supply to the femoral head and neck enters largely through the posterior capsule, especially in younger children. Thus incisions in the capsule are considered to be safer if they are made anteriorly, rather than posteriorly. Also, the fact that these capsular vessels are critical to the blood supply of the head renders these vessels susceptible to any extreme positions of the thigh that may "wring out" or compress the vessels. Furthermore, any fixed and extreme outward rotation and abduction of the hip in infants and young children can compress the posterolateral epiphyseal artery, which can severely compromise the circulation to the femoral head resulting in bone or cartilage necrosis. This observation is responsible for the development of the concept of the "human" position described by Salter and associates[23] and the employment of flexible abduction devices such as the Pavlik harness and the Frejka apron, which do not hold the thighs rigidly flexed and avoid any severely abducted or outwardly rotated position.

Other aspects of the gross and functional anatomy of the hip joint are very important from a surgical point of view, but these issues will be covered separately, in the specific sections that deal with the various operative procedures.

REFERENCES

1. Badgley, C. E.: Correlation of clinical and anatomical facts leading to a conception of the etiology of congenital hip dysplasias, J. Bone Joint Surg. **25:**503, 1943.
2. Bardeen, C. R.: Studies in the development of the human skeleton, Am. J. Anat. **4:**265, 1905.
3. Bardeen, C. R.: The development of the skeleton and the connective tissue. In Bardeen, C. R., Evans, H. M., and associates (Keibel, F., and

Mall, F. P., editors): Manual of human embryology, vol. 1, Philadelphia, 1910, J. B. Lippincott Co., p. 292, Chapter XI.
4. Bardeen, C. R., and Lewis, W. H.: Development of the limbs, body-wall and back in man, Am. J. Anat. 1:1, 1901.
5. Brodetti, A.: The blood supply of the femoral neck and head in relation to the damaging effects of nails and screws, J. Bone Joint Surg. 42B:794, 1960.
6. Chung, S. M.: The arterial supply of the developing proximal end of the human femur, J. Bone Joint Surg. 58A:961, 1976.
7. Crock, H. V., and Crock, C.: The blood supply of the lower limb bones in man (descriptive and applied), Edinburgh, 1967, E. & S. Livingstone.
8. DeSanto, D. A., and Colonna, P. C.: Embryology of the hip joint, Arch Surg. 39:448, 1939.
9. Dunn, P. M.: Congenital postural deformities, Br. Med. Bull. 32:71, 1976.
10. Ferguson, A. B.: Orthopedic surgery in infancy and childhood, ed. 4, Baltimore, 1975, The Williams & Wilkins Co., p. 57.
11. Gardner, E.: Prenatal development of the human hip joint, femur, and hip bone. In American Academy of Orthopaedic Surgeons: AAOS Instructional Course Lectures, vol. 21, St. Louis, 1972, The C. V. Mosby Co., p. 138.)
12. Gardner, E., and Gray, D. J.: Prenatal development of the human hip joint, Am. J. Anat. 87:163, 1950.
13. Grant, J. C. B.: An atlas of anatomy, ed. 6, Baltimore, 1972, The Williams & Wilkins Co.
14. Haines, R. W.: The development of joints, J. Anat. 81:33, 1947.
15. Keith, A.: Human embryology and morphology, ed. 5, Baltimore, 1933, William Wood and Co.
16. Last, R. J.: Anatomy, regional and applied, ed. 2, Boston, 1959, Little, Brown and Co., p. 192.
17. Laurenson, R. D.: Development of the acetabular roof in the fetal hip, J. Bone Joint Surg. 47A:975, 1965.
18. LeDamany, P.: Variation en potordeur du cotyle humain aux divers ages, Bull. Soc. Sci., et med de l'ouest, Rennes, 12:410, as cited by Gardner and Gray, D. J.: Prenatal development of the human hip joint, Am. J. Anat. 87:163, 1950.
19. Morville, P.: On the anatomy and pathology of the hip joint, Acta Orthop. Scand. 7:107, 1936.
20. Ogden, J. (Ferguson, A. B, ed.): Orthopedic surgery in infancy and childhood, ed. 4, Baltimore, 1975, The Williams & Wilkins Co., p. 59.
21. Ralis, Z., and McKibbin, B.: Changes in shape of the human hip joint during its development and their relation to stability, J. Bone Joint Surg. 55B:780, 1973.
22. Roberts, J.: Personal communication.
23. Salter, R. B., Kostuik, J., and Dallas, S.: Avascular necrosis of the femoral head as a complication of treatment for congenital dislocation of the hip in young children: a clinical and experimental investigation, Can. J. Surg. 12:44, 1969.
24. Siffert, R. S. (Rang, M., ed.): The growth plate and its disorders, Baltimore, 1969, The Williams & Wilkins Co.
25. Somerville, E. W.: Personal communication.
26. Spalteholz, W.: Hand-atlas of human anatomy, ed. 7, Philadelphia, 1933, J. B. Lippincott Co., p. 217.
27. Stanisavljevic, S., and Mitchell, C. L.: Congenital dysplasia, subluxation, and dislocation of the hip in stillborn and newborn infants, J. Bone Joint Surg. 45A:1147, 1963.
28. Strayer, L. M.: The embryology of the human hip joint, Yale J. Biol. Med. 16:13, 1943.
29. Strayer, L. M.: Embryology of the human hip joint, Clin. Orthop. 74:221, 1971.
30. Trueta, J.: The normal vascular anatomy of the human femoral head during growth, J. Bone Joint Surg. 39B:358, 1957.
31. Tucker, R. F.: Arterial supply to the femoral head and its clinical importance, J. Bone Joint Surg. 31B:82, 1949.
32. Watanabe, R. S.: Embryology of the human hip, Clin. Orthop. 98:8, 1974.
33. Wolcott, W. E.: The evolution of the circulation in the developing femoral head and neck, Surg. Gynecol. Obstet. 77:61, 1943.

CHAPTER 2

Etiology and pathogenesis

Incidence
Racial and ethnic influences
Sex and family influences
Birth factors
    Seasonal influence
    Associated congenital anomalies
Primary acetabular dysplasia and ligamentous laxity
    Primary acetabular dysplasia
    Ligamentous laxity
    Mechanical factors
Conclusions

INCIDENCE

Many extensive and detailed investigations have been made regarding the incidence of congenital dislocation of the hip. These studies, conducted in medical centers throughout the world, have included different racial and ethnic populations and have added considerably to our understanding of the pathogenesis of congenital dysplasia and congenital dislocation of the hip. Because of the wide variation in the incidence of congenital dislocation of the hip reported from different geographic areas and for different racial and ethnic groups, a review of some of the factors that seem to cause certain races or individuals to be more susceptible, or, conversely, more immune, to this condition will be presented in this chapter.

One of the principal problems encountered in any discussion about the incidence of congenital dislocation of the hip is the poorly standardized and often nebulous definitions of the different manifestations of congenital dislocation of the hip. Whether one is referring to dysplasia of the hip (that is, a dislocatable hip) in the newborn or the neonate or whether the condition under consideration is complete dislocation of the hip (that is, dislocated, not dislocatable), is an important distinction when incidence is being discussed. Another difficulty posed by these studies may be illustrated by the following example: In most studies performed on white neonates, the incidence of dysplastic hips is consistently reported at about one per 100 (1%); on the other hand, complete dislocation of the hip in the same ethnic population is usually reported at somewhere between eight and 10 per 10,000, or about 0.1%. This tenfold difference may well be explained by the commonly held concept that many dysplastic hips in the newborn must become stable spontaneously and that eventually they become normal, both clinically and roentgenographically. Correspondingly, about one in 10 of these dysplastic hips will become totally dislocated if untreated. It is important to emphasize that a certain number of the dysplastic hips that "do not heal" or that do not become dislocated will retain certain dysplastic features. The incidence of this particular manifestation, namely, residual dysplasia, has not been well established because of the difficulties encountered in making the diagnosis. These problems will be discussed in greater detail in Chapter 3.

In addition to the various manifestations of congenital dislocation of the hip, other variables must be considered in assessing its incidence. Much seems to depend on the thoroughness of the clinical examination, on the examiner's ability to detect abnormalities, and on the age at which the patient is examined.[23,74,77]

For example, Czeizel and associates[16] in 1974 found that the use of a routine newborn screening examination resulted in an increase in the reported incidence of dislocatable (dysplastic) hips from four to six times. In 1962 Barlow emphasized that not only was a competent examination important but that the age at which the examination was conducted had a great influence on the number of positive physical findings identified.[8] He found that at birth one infant in 60 demonstrated instability in one or both hips; these same infants were then reexamined at more than 3½ days of age, with the result that less than half the incidence of instability was encountered as in the earlier examination. He then suggested that his figures represented a spontaneous "cure" rate of 58% and proposed that antenatal asymmetric postural muscular tightness might be a significant factor in producing these unstable hips. However, he also believed that postnatal muscle action could be a significant factor leading to the spontaneous development of stability in many of these hips. Nelson[49] made similar observations.

The terms "newborn" and "neonate" have often been used interchangeably and synonymously. However, these two chronologic age groups should be defined. The newborn period is usually considered to encompass the first days after birth, whereas the neonatal age, by accepted definition, extends through the first 28 days of life. Because the clinical manifestations of congenital dysplasia and dislocation of the hip vary considerably during the first postnatal month, the temporal *distinction* between the newborn age and the neonatal age must be kept in mind. Thus the variations in the ways a congenital dislocation of the hip have been reported must be kept in mind during the discussion that follows; otherwise, the widely divergent statistical data that have been reported may be misleading and lead one to false conclusions.

RACIAL AND ETHNIC INFLUENCES

Early studies on the incidence of congenital dislocation of the hip report figures ranging between 0.7 and 2.2 patients per 1000 live births in western and northern Europe and vary only slightly for Canada and the United States.* More recent investigations, such as those from Hungary by Czeizel and associates,[16] report an incidence as high as 28.7 per 1000 live births. In sharp contrast, much lower incidences have been reported for blacks. Based on his evaluation of 16,678 black African neonates, Edelstein[21] was unable to find even one case of congenital dislocation of the hip. Van Meerdervoort,[65] who also had an extensive experience with black Africans, found a total of only three cases of congenital dislocation of the hip. These studies support the now well-established conclusion that blacks are essentially free from congenital dislocation of the hip.

Hodgson[34] reported a very low incidence of congenital dislocation of the hip in Koreans and Chinese. Yet, among the Lapps, the incidence of congenital dislocation of the hip is remarkably high, for Wessell[70] found from 20 to 50 dysplastic hips per 1000 live births.[16,26] For some North American Indian tribes, such as the Apaches, the Navajos, and some Cana-

---

*See references 27, 34, 46, 51, 57, and 67.

dian Indians, an incidence approximating 5% has been reported.[14,15,40,55]

Thus the data indicate that this condition, however the manifestation is defined, is rarely seen in some racial and ethnic groups, whereas other populations show a very high incidence. The careful reader is forced to conclude that a strong genetic or ethnic factor or both are involved. This is an issue that has been addressed by many and has led to the conclusion that the heritable factors that lead to congenital dislocation of the hip are probably transmitted as an autosomal dominant trait, having limited penetrance. The interrelationships displayed between certain obviously heritable factors and the many equally important environmental or mechanical factors contrive to make this a provocative subject for discussion.

Wynne-Davies[76,77] stressed the concept that the diagnosis of neonatal congenital dislocation of the hip is best made in the early days of life, before the infant has developed muscle tone. She believed that the improved muscle function tightened the hip and that this improved muscle tone might explain why the diagnostic "click" could not be elicited if the examination were made several days or weeks after birth. Wynne-Davies[77] also believed that a competent examination, if made at birth or in the newborn, would probably identify many of these very subtle findings; therefore, her observations supported those of Czeizel and associates[17] and explain the fourfold increase in the number of hip dysplasias reported in those studies where extensive routine newborn hip examinations are performed, as contrasted to those locations where such routine examination is not done.

SEX AND FAMILY INFLUENCES

Practically all clinical investigations on dysplasia and dislocation of the hip have consistently shown that girls are involved four to six times as frequently as boys, irrespective of the manifestation of the condition.* In an effort to explain these observations, Faber[22] and von Rosen[68] have considered the possible effects of the different hormones that circulate in the bloodstream as possible etiologic factors. The work of Thieme and associates,[64] however, argues against this theory. Despite efforts to uncover a plausible and defensible explanation for this difference in the boy-girl ratio, at present, agreement on a clearly defined answer has yet to be reached.

Most investigations have shown that there is a strong family influence in the occurrence of congenital dysplasia and dislocation of the hip. This increased in-incidence in family members is substantial when compared to the incidence for both in the general populace. Bjerkreim and Hagen[9] found that the overall occurrence of congenital dysplasia or dislocation of the hip in siblings of probands was 7.1%, which reflected approximately a sevenfold increase over the incidence of congenital dysplasia of the hip reported for the general population. He also demonstrated that the occurrence of dysplastic hip manifestations in the parents of all probands was 2.1%; this figure amounted to 10 times that for a control group. Wynne-Davies[76,77] found that the incidence of hip dysplasia in siblings of probands was between 12.1% and 13.5%, depending on whether they were diagnosed early or later in infancy.

These figures are in general agreement with those found in other similar studies.[9,18] Furthermore, familial influence was also reported by those who studied the occurrence of dysplasia in twin births, as illustrated by Idelberger,[38] who investigated 138 pairs of twins. He noted that in monozygous twins, if one child had

---

*See references 9, 14, 53, and 76.

congenital dislocation of the hip, there was a 42.7% likelihood of dislocation in the other twin. In the dizygous twins evaluated there was a 2.8% crossover rate.[9]

Such data leave little doubt that congenital dysplasia and dislocation of the hip in first-degree relatives and in twin siblings will significantly increase the probability that other relatives will show some manifestation of congenital dislocation of the hip.

BIRTH FACTORS

Most studies have shown that a child's order of birth is an important factor that is associated with an increased incidence of dysplasia and dislocation. Wynne-Davies,[77] Czeizel and associates,[16] and Carter and Wilkinson[10,11] have shown that there is an increased incidence of dislocation in the firstborn child. My own experience also supports this observation.[75] Wynne-Davies[76,77] also concluded that the incidence of congenital dislocation in firstborn infants was significantly increased, and she also demonstrated that it was not dependent on the mother's age.

Conversely, Barlow[8] in 1962 was unable to demonstrate any correlation between the order of birth and the incidence of congenital hip dislocation. Dunn[19] has postulated that the increased incidence of postural deformities, including a congenital dislocation of the hip, in firstborn children can possibly be explained by a variety of circumstances unique to the primigravida. These factors include an unstretched uterus and abdominal muscles, uteroplacental insufficiency, oligohydramnios, and the increased likelihood of breech presentations.

In the general population, breech deliveries comprise about 2% to 4% of all vaginal deliveries, although more infants may have maintained a breech posture in utero and then undergone spontaneous version just prior to birth. Bjerkreim and Hagen[9] demonstrated a 3.4% incidence of breech presentations in their studies. In the case of congenital dislocation of the hip, on the other hand, they found an 8.3% incidence of breech presentations in those patients who had been diagnosed after early infancy. They also found a 15.7% incidence in infants who were diagnosed during the neonatal period, thus representing a marked increase in incidence compared to the general populace.

In a similar observation, Carter and Wilkinson[11] found that 17.3% of the patients in their series with congenital dislocation of the hip were the product of a breech delivery. Ramsey and MacEwen,[56] in an unpublished study of 25,000 newborn infants, made the following statistical observations on breech births as they relate to congenital hip disease: one in 35 infants will have a completely dislocated hip; one in 25 will have a subluxatable hip; and one in 175 will have a dislocatable hip. They found the overall incidence of hip joint instability to be one in 15 for female infants who had a breech birth. From these data it would appear incontrovertible, therefore, that breech presentation and delivery definitely increase the likelihood of a congenital dislocation of the hip in one of its various manifestations.

The explanation for this increased incidence in infants who have had breech births probably lies in the observation that intrauterine pressure and position can have a profound effect on the development of the thigh and hip joint. It is now generally agreed that such antenatal environmental (mechanical) factors may exert a causal relationship on the development of a congenital dislocation of the hip. This concept has been further reinforced by the investigative conclusions of Salter and associates[60,61] and Smith and associates,[62,63] who demonstrated that dysplastic hips can be produced by the prolonged maintenance of an abnormal position of the thighs in growing animals. Further circumstantial evidence to support this impression is found in the observation that dislocation of the hip is rarely found in any fetus aborted during the first 20 weeks of pregnancy, for at 20 weeks the fetus is still very small and probably not subject to intrauterine pressures sufficient to produce a mechanical effect on the developing hip.[24,25,50]

In view of the theoretic and circumstantial considerations outlined above, it would appear that intrauterine postural influences must play an important but poorly quantitated role in the pathogenesis of congenital dislocation of the hip. That such factors are not the prime or the exclusive etiologic factors involved, however, has already been demonstrated by the importance of the heritable influences discussed earlier.

It has been demonstrated by Bjerkreim and Hagen[9] that there is an increased birthweight in neonatal females with congenital dislocation of the hip as compared to a control series. But, conversely, Bjerkreim and Hagen[9] also found that there was no difference in neonatal males with congenital dislocation of the hip. At the present time it appears that no clearly defined agreement has been reached on this issue.

Seasonal influence

The unusual observation that there is a seasonal element in the incidence of congenital dislocation of the hip has been explored by several authors. Bjerkreim and other authors* have shown that the incidence of congenital dislocation of the hip is increased for those children born in the fall and winter months in temperate climates. This ostensibly unique observation has been explained in a variety of ways, including such factors as seasonal

---

*See references 5, 9, 16, and 77.

hormonal changes[5] and the heavy clothing on the infant that holds the lower limbs in an adducted and extended position. This custom has been well documented among the Japanese, the northern Italians, and the Czechs, where the children are often swaddled during the cold months. The swaddled position holds the limbs in adduction and extension and could contribute to an unstable position of the hip joint.

Other authors have been unable to show a substantial variation in the incidence of congenital dislocation of the hip as being convincingly related to the season of birth. Barlow[8] and Coleman[14] have emphasized that, in their evaluation, the seasonal considerations have very little if any bearing on the manner in which the infant is clothed in the early months. Wilkinson's[72] theories even suggest that in England a higher incidence of hip dislocation occurs in those children who are born during the summer months, but he offered no explanation for this apparent discrepancy.

Associated congenital anomalies

It is generally accepted that concomitant congenital anomalies occur with a greater frequency in those children with congenital dislocation of the hip than is found in the general population. Muller and Seddon[48] found an important increase in the incidence of talipes equinovarus and other congenital deformities in infants who also had congenital dislocation of the hip. Bjerkreim and Hagen[9] demonstrated a 9% incidence of other congenital anomalies in infants with a neonatal congenital dislocation of the hip and a 14% incidence in infants who were diagnosed as having a congenital dislocation of the hip after 4 weeks of age. Hummer and MacEwen[37] observed a very substantially increased incidence of congenital dislocation of the hip in children with torticollis; Jacobs[39] demonstrated that there is a much higher probability of hip dysplasia in infants with metatarsus varus than in the normal infant population. Even more recently, an association has been demonstrated between the incidence of calcaneovalgus (pes planus) and dysplasia of the hip.[52]

Many of these conditions seem to have strong environmental influences in their causation (that is, the intrauterine position), and it is attractive to propose that some sort of postural cause-and-effect relationship exists. The most important element to weigh in this consideration, however, is to emphasize that an infant having any anomaly, either skeletal or visceral, should be seriously suspected of having an associated congenital dysplasia or dislocation of the hip.

PRIMARY ACETABULAR DYSPLASIA AND LIGAMENTOUS LAXITY

Much controversy has centered on the arguments regarding the relative importance of a *primary* defect in the acetabulum, as opposed to excessive ligamentous laxity, as the cause of congenital dislocation of the hip. To what extent each of these conditions plays a role in the pathogenesis of hip dysplasia and dislocation remains somewhat clouded, even today. However, in recent years considerable evidence has been presented to support *both* concepts, indicating that each may have a role, varying in relative importance according to the nature of the problem presented by the individual patient.

Primary acetabular dysplasia

The concept that congenital dislocation of the hip is the result of developmental abnormalities that occurred during prenatal growth was advanced as early as 1842 when VonAmmon[66] suggested that the process was an ectopia of the femoral head, wherein the proximal femur actually developed outside the acetabulum. This theory argued that a dislocation actually did not occur, because the hip was never truly located. This concept was later disproved by the early embryologic studies discussed in Chapter 1. It is now proved that the femoral head and acetabulum are derived from the same cell mass and develop as a unit. However, the belief that in the pathogenesis of hip dysplasia and dislocation some form of primary developmental abnormality in the hip joint is involved has continued to be a source of controversy.

In 1937 Faber[22] performed studies that were based on the concept that the dislocation itself is not inherited, but rather that a deformation of the acetabular socket was most likely the inherited characteristic. He concluded that it was this deformity, which consisted of a flattening of the socket, that permitted the hip to dislocate. His investigations supported the conclusions that there was no genetic factor per se that produced dislocation, but rather he believed that there was an inherited "hip dysplasia" factor. He also showed in his data that dysplasia of the hip, without dislocation, was three times as frequent as complete dislocation.

In 1942 Hart[28] further advanced the primary dysplasia theory; he stated that a condition known as primary acetabular dysplasia did indeed exist and was genetically determined by a dominant autosomal gene. He believed, however, that primary dysplasia was substantially affected by environmental and biomechanical factors; he also believed that different genotypes would vary in their clinical presentations. He appropriately pointed out that hip dysplasia not only involves the acetabulum but also involves the other "joint-forming" parts of the hip joint. He agreed with Putti[53,54] and Faber[22] that dysplasia of the hip without dislocation was substantially more common than complete dislocation. Later in 1949 Hart[29] described the various stages of hip dysplasia, beginning with the hip that spontaneously becomes normal, both clinically and radiologically, and ending with the hip that eventually becomes completely dislocated.[28,29,30] Hass[31] also believed that actual dislocation of the hip was not primarily a true congenital condition but rather that only the *predisposition* to luxation was congenital and was seen as some form of acetabular dysplasia. Hass concluded that a demonstrable retardation of growth in the triradiate cartilage could be identified, but he could not determine whether it was primary or secondary. He agreed with Faber[22] that a flattening of the acetabular roof was the principal pathologic feature, but he also believed that there was an "unknown hereditary factor" that was largely responsible for the growth disturbances involving the upper end of the femur and the soft tissues about the hip joint. Hass[31] further concluded that if the hip could be maintained in a normal relationship to the acetabulum, normal hip joint development would take place.

In the effort to establish the validity of the primary acetabular dysplasia concept, Wynne-Davies,[76,77] Bjerkreim and Hagen,[9] and Czeizel and associates[16,17,18] have recently been the most productive. Wynne-Davies[76,77] studied 589 patients with congenital dislocation of the hip, along with many of their first-degree relatives, from the standpoint of acetabular configuration and ligamentous integrity. She found it convenient to separate these patients into two large groups. The first she called the "neonatal dislocation" or early-diagnosis group; these included patients whose diagnosis was made during the first 4 weeks of life on the basis of having a subluxatable hip. The second was the "late diagnosis" group, that is, those whose diagnosis was determined *after* 4 weeks of age and in many cases months or even several years after birth. Recognizing the technical difficulties involved in evaluating the unossified acetabulum in neonates and young infants, she elected to employ the pelvic x-ray films of the parents of 162 index patients who had been diagnosed as having congenital dislocation of the hip. She concluded that the parents of children who were diagnosed after 4 weeks of age showed a much shallower acetabulum than did the parents of a control group. Furthermore, the parents of the patients in the neonatal group showed similar manifestations, but to a lesser degree. Moreover, Wynne-Davies[76,77] was able to demonstrate that the parents whose pelvic films revealed a more severe acetabular dysplasia also had more relatives who were affected with congenital dislocation of the hip than did a control group. She believed that these findings offered rather convincing evidence in support of acetabular dysplasia being a "primary genetic disorder with polygenic inheritance."

More recent studies by Czeizel and associates[18] and Bjerkreim and Hagen[9] have supported the conclusions of Wynne-Davies and have added greater credence to the concept that acetabular dysplasia is a primary etiologic factor in the development of congenital dislocation of the hip.

Ligamentous laxity

As early as 1902, in a study of stillborn infants, Heusner[32] observed that ligamentous laxity was much greater in female infants than in male infants. However, he apparently did not conclude that there was any association between this observation and the already known and accepted increased incidence of congenital dislocation of the hip in female infants. In 1920 Lorenz[43] observed evidence of a generalized joint laxity in some patients with congenital dislocation of the hip, but he believed that it was an infrequent association.

In 1947 Howorth[35] reported his observations on the pathology of congenital hip dislocation as a consequence of his experiences in open surgery on the hip. He concluded that the capsule was always elongated in these instances and reasoned that capsular laxity was probably the prime factor in the development of congenital dislocation of the hip. At the same time Howorth[35] recognized that excessive femoral anteversion and intrauterine posture were probably contributing factors. He also postulated that the commonly encountered posterior dislocation develops originally as an anterior dislocation and that the femoral head then moves upward and posteriorly as a result of the capsular elongation.

In 1951 Massie and Howorth[45] disputed the concept of primary acetabular dysplasia because they believed that it could not explain their observations that completely dislocated hips in young infants often had normal acetabula. They also observed that most dislocated hips that were treated early in infancy usually became normal, and they reasoned that this observation could not be explained by a primary acetabular defect nearly so well as by a defect in capsular integrity. The precise reason for the apparent relaxation of the capsule eluded these authors, but they believed that it was caused by a possible combination of genetic, mechanical, hormonal, and possibly even nutritional factors. These and subsequent studies led Howorth[36] to the rather sweeping and provocative conclusion that he voiced in 1963 that "all the facts of dysplasia of the fetal and infant hip are explained by the concept of primary elongation of the capsule and action of purely mechanical forces. No other theory is necessary to explain the facts and no other theory is consistent with the facts."

In 1958[63] and later in 1963,[62] Smith and his colleagues were able to produce acetabular dysplasia by surgically dislocating the hip in dogs. On the strength of their observations, they believed that acetabular dysplasia was most likely the result, rather than the cause, of dislocation. As a consequence of a series of well-controlled animal studies, they therefore added credence to the ligamentous laxity theory of dislocation. Similar investigations by Langenskiöld and associates[41] in 1962 supported the observations of Smith.

Andrén[2,3,4] noted the consistent coexistent instability of the pelvic symphysis in three children with a congenital dislocation of the hip, and he related the instability to the possible presence of the hormone known as "relaxin." The possible relationship of relaxin to ligamentous laxity had been earlier demonstrated in parturient women by Hisaw and associates.[33]

Subsequently evidence to support the causal relationship of the gonadal hormones to an increase in the laxity of the pelvic ligaments was produced by many observers, and all proposed that the laxity may be one of the explanations for the greater incidence of dysplasia and dislocation of the hip in females. The experimental work of Wilkinson[73] in this area is especially impressive. He gave rabbits esterone and progesterone and splinted one hind limb in the breech position. The female rabbits developed hip joints similar to those found in patients with congenital dislocation of the hip, whereas the male rabbits showed only a torsional deformity of the femur. None of the unsplinted control limbs showed any abnormalities. Wilkinson thus concluded that congenital dislocation of the hip was probably the result of a combination of hormonally induced ligamentous laxity and intrauterine mechanical factors, with particular emphasis on the breech position. He further emphasized the long accepted concept that forcible extension of the hips during delivery and immediately after birth may contribute to hip joint instability and, ultimately, to dislocation.

However, not all studies support the cause-and-effect concept of gonadal hormones and relaxin in dislocated hips. Aarskog and associates[1] in 1966 and Thieme and associates[64] in 1968 were unable to demonstrate any increased estrogen secretion in patients having congenital dislocation of the hip as compared to a control group. Each inferred, therefore, that there was no conclusive evidence to support the hormonal theory of ligamentous laxity and its etiologic relationship to congenital dislocation of the hip.

These investigators believed that there are two forms of ligamentous laxity: (1) a temporary type of laxity, which disappears during the neonatal period, and (2) a persisting form, which extends into adult life. Patients with this latter condition showed excessive ranges of motion of many of the peripheral joints; also the incidence of hip disorders was significantly higher in this group of patients as compared to a control group. These authors reasoned that a generalized pattern of joint laxity was often familial and that it predisposed these individuals to congenital dislocation of the hip. They also supported an earlier conclusion of Wilkinson's[73] that argued that intrauterine mechanical factors played a large role in the causation of hip dislocation.

In 1968 Salter[59] designed a provocative flow sheet in an effort to explain the pathogenesis of congenital dislocation of the hip. It represented an editorialization of the many concepts and theories proposed earlier and generally supported the principle of ligamentous laxity as the primary cause of congenital dislocation of the hip. Somewhat later in 1970, McKibbin[47] found evidence to support the ligamentous laxity concept in his study of a newborn with congenital dislocation of the hips.

In 1970 Wynne-Davies[77] also explored the issue of ligamentous laxity with respect to its etiologic relationship to congenital hip dislocation. She found that there was a higher proportion of children with dislocation who also had ligamentous laxity than was seen in a control population. Furthermore, first-degree relatives of these patients demonstrated an increased incidence of joint laxity along with other developmental abnormalities such as hernia, plagiocephaly, talipes equinovarus, and idiopathic scoliosis. She therefore postulated a possible disorder in collagen as a factor in the etiology of these various conditions.

She concluded that ligamentous laxity is causally related to congenital dislocation of the hip and that it is probably a dominant trait. In addition, she believed that either the dysplasia trait or the ligamentous laxity trait may be present separately or in combination. However, she did find a preponderance of ligamentous laxity in those patients who were diagnosed as having dislocation of the hip in the neonatal period, whereas primary acetabular dysplasia predominated in the late diagnosis group. Others have drawn similar conclusions.

Czeizel and associates[18] in 1975 found a higher incidence of joint laxity in male infants with congenital dislocation of the hip; they also found an increase in joint laxity in the first-degree relatives of these patients. He endorsed the proposed concept of a dominant mode of inheritance proposed by Wynne-Davies.

Mechanical factors

The concept of mechanical forces serving as factors in the causation of congenital dislocation of the hip is based on the belief that external forces and abnormal positions, both antenatal and postnatal, may play a major role in the development of the hip joints. As noted in the section on embryology in Chapter 1, the hip joint develops from a single mass of mesoderm, and the joint itself does not really begin to differentiate until the end of the third month. Watanabe[69] has also demonstrated that the hip joint cannot be physically dislocated until this fetal age. Therefore, if one is to evaluate the effects that mechanical forces have on dislocation of the hip joint, it is essential to keep these embryologic facts in mind.

Normally, by the last month of gestation, the thighs of the fetus assume a position of flexion and slight abduction; the hip joint is stable in this position. However, the frank breech attitude, with the thighs and knees fully extended, has been shown to be a position of increased risk for the development of hip dislocation. Experimentally in lower animals the frank breech position predictably produces hip dislocation, and, as discussed earlier in this chapter, many clinical studies support a greatly increased incidence of congenital dislocation of the hip as a consequence of any breech presentation at birth.

Badgley[6,7] demonstrated that in order for normal development of the hip joint to occur, normal relationships of the femoral head and acetabulum must exist. Thus any external force or position that alters these normal relationships can exert an important influence on the development of hip disorders, especially dysplasia and dislocation. As early as 1800, Dupuytren[20] considered the intrauterine factors of fetal position and oligohydramnios as causal agents in the development of congenital dislocation of the hip. Roser[58] and Ludloff[44] held similar views, and they also incriminated any sudden extension of the thigh that might occur at birth or immediately after birth as additional contributing factors. Chuinard and Logan[12] and Salter[59] agree with this concept. von Friedlander,[67] Lorenz,[43] Codivilla,[13] and Hass[31] have also expressed the view that intrauterine factors are significant in the etiology of dislocation of the hip.

LeDamany[42] proposed an interesting but poorly accepted anthropological theory to explain the development of hip dislocation. He believed that the relative size of man's pelvis and femur, along with the upright posture, were among the cogent etiologic factors.

Recently the mechanical concept has been put into a more logical perspective by Howorth,[36] Wynne-Davies,[77] Carter and Wilkinson,[11] Czeizel and associates,[16] and Wilkinson.[71,72] They have shown that congenital dislocation of the hip is the ultimate result of multiple factors, of which abnormal external forces and positions of the thigh are only two. Few can now discount the well-known observations that support the increased incidence of dislocation of the hip in breech births and in populations in which infants are swaddled with the thighs in extension. The fact that correcting these factors by splinting results in a reversal of the hip abnormalities in a high percentage of the cases adds further support to the proposals on the importance of mechanical factors.

CONCLUSIONS

In analyzing and evaluating the many determinants that have been found causally related to congenital dislocation of the hip, several general conclusions seem justified. That racial and genetic factors are important seems incontrovertible. These factors appear to operate as an autosomal dominant, producing either ligamentous laxity, acetabular dysplasia, or both. To what extent they operate together, or each to the exclusion of the other, will vary considerably, depending on many other factors. Clearly, much scientific support seems to favor the concept of genetically determined ligamentous laxity as the single most important factor.

Environmental and mechanical factors also seem to play a substantial role in the etiology and pathogenesis of congenital dislocation of the hip, as evidenced by the increased incidence of dislocated hips as a consequence of breech births and the practice of swaddling infants. There is also evidence of an increased incidence of congenital dislocation of the hip found in other posturally related conditions.

Therefore, the condition known generally as congenital dislocation of the hip, whether the hip is dysplastic, subluxated, or dislocated, is the product of a complex series of factors and circumstances. An understanding of these issues and of their interrelationship is extremely important when it comes to the diagnosis and treatment of this highly capricious and potentially crippling condition.

REFERENCES

1. Aarskog, D., Støa, K. F., and Thorsen, T.: Urinary oestrogen excretion in newborn infants with congenital dysplasia of the hip joint, Acta Paediatrica Scand. **55**:394, 1966.
2. Andrén, L.: Instability of the pubic symphysis and congenital dislocation of the hip in newborns, Acta Radiol. (Stockh.) **54**:123, 1960.
3. Andrén, L.: Pelvic instability in newborns with special reference to congenital dislocation of the hip and hormonal factors: a roentgenologic study, Acta Radiol. Scand. [Suppl.] 212, 1962.
4. Andrén L., and Borglin, N. E.: Disturbed urinary excretion pattern of oestrogens in newborns with congenital dislocation of the hip. II. The excretion of exogenous oestradiol-17β, Acta Endocrinol. **37**:427, 1961.
5. Andrén, L., and Palmén, K.: Seasonal variation of birth dates of infants with congenital dislocation of the hip, Acta Orthop. Scand. **33**:127, 1963.
6. Badgley, C. E.: Correlation of clinical and anatomical facts leading to a conception of the etiology of congenital hip dysplasia, J. Bone Joint Surg. **25**:503, 1943.
7. Badgley, C. E.: Etiology of congenital dislocation of the hip, J. Bone Joint Surg. **31A**:341, 1949.
8. Barlow, T. G.: Early diagnosis and treatment of congenital dislocation of the hip, J. Bone Joint Surg. **44B**:292, 1962.
9. Bjerkreim, I., and Hagen, C. B. van der: Congenital dislocation of the hip joint in Norway, Clin. Genet. **5**:433, 1974.
10. Carter, C. O., and Wilkinson, J.: Congenital dislocation of the hip, J. Bone Joint Surg. **42B**:669, 1960.
11. Carter, C. O., and Wilkinson, J. A.: Genetic and environmental factors in the etiology of congenital dislocation of the hip, Clin. Orthop. **33**:119, 1964.
12. Chuinard, E. G., and Logan, N. D.: Varus-producing and derotational subtrochanteric osteotomy in the treatment of congenital dislocation of the hip, J. Bone Joint Surg. **45A**:1397, 1963.
13. Codivilla, A., as cited by Hass, J.: Congenital dislocation of the hip, Springfield, Ill., 1951, Charles C Thomas, Publisher.
14. Coleman, S. S.: Congenital dysplasia of the hip in the Navajo infant, Clin. Orthop. **56**:179, 1968.
15. Corrigan, C., and Segal, S.: The incidence of congenital dislocation of the hip at Island Lake, Manitoba, Can. Med. Assoc. J. **62**:535, 1950.
16. Czeizel, A., Szentpétery, J., and Kellermann, M.: Incidence of congenital dislocation of the hip in Hungary, Br. J. Prev. Soc. Med. **28**:265, 1974.
17. Czeizel, A., Szentpétery, J., Tusnády, G., and Vizkelety, T.: Two family studies on congenital dislocation of the hip after early orthopaedic screening in Hungary, J. Med. Genet. **12**:125, 1975.
18. Czeizel, A., Tusnády, G., Vaczó, G., and Vizkelety, T.: The mechanism of genetic predisposition in congenital dislocation of the hip, J. Med. Genet. **12**:121, 1975.
19. Dunn, P. M.: Congenital dislocation of the hip (CDH): necropsy studies at birth, Proc. R. Soc. Med. **62**:1035, 1969.
20. Dupuytren, J.: Mémoire sur un déplacement original de la tête des fémurs, Repertoire Gén. d'Anat. et de Phys. **2**:151, 1826; Leçons Orales de Clinique Chir. Paris **1**:3, 1833, as cited by Hass, J.: Congenital dislocation of the hip, Springfield, Ill., 1951, Charles C Thomas, Publisher.
21. Edelstein, J.: Congenital dislocation of the hip in the Bantu, J. Bone Joint Sur. **48B**:397, 1964.
22. Faber, A.: Erbbiologische Untersuchungen über die Anlage zur "angeborenen" Hüftverrenkung, Z. Orthop. **66**:140, 1937.
23. Finlay, H. V. L., Maudsley, A. H., and Busfield, P. I.: Dislocatable hip and dislocated hip in the newborn infant, Br. Med. J. **4**:377, 1967.
24. Gardner, E.: Personal communication.
25. Gardner, E., and Gray, D. J.: Prenatal devel-

opment of the hip joint, Am. J. Anat. **87:**163, 1950.
26. Getz, B.: The hip in Lapps and its bearing on the problem of congenital dislocation, Acta Orthop. Scand. [Suppl.] **22:**1955.
27. Harris, L. E., Lipscombe, P. R., and Hodgson, J. R.: Early diagnosis of congenital dysplasia and congenital dislocation of the hip: value of the abduction test, J.A.M.A. **173:**229, 1960.
28. Hart, V. L.: Primary genetic dysplasia of the hip with and without classical dislocation, J. Bone Joint Surg. **24:**753, 1942.
29. Hart, V. L.: Congenital dislocation of the hip joint: relationship between subluxation and congenital dislocation, J. Bone Joint Surg. **31A:**357, 1949.
30. Hart, V. L.: Congenital dysplasia of the hip joint and sequelae in the newborn and early postnatal life, Springfield, Ill., 1952, Charles C Thomas, Publisher.
31. Hass, J.: Congenital dislocation of the hip, Springfield, Ill., 1951, Charles C Thomas, Publisher.
32. Heusner, L.: Über die angeborene Huftluxation, Z. Orthop. Chir. **10:**571, 1902.
33. Hisaw, F. L., Zarrow, M. X., Money, W. L., Taluage, R. V. N., and Abramowitz, A. A.: Importance of the female reproductive tract in the formation of relaxin, Endocrinology **34:**122, 1944.
34. Hodgson, A. R.: Congenital dislocation of the hip, Br. Med. J. **2:**647, 1961.
35. Howorth, M. B.: Congenital dislocation of the hip, Ann. Surg. **125:**216, 1947.
36. Howorth, M. B.: The etiology of congenital dislocation of the hip, Clin. Orthop. **29:**164, 1963.
37. Hummer, C. D., and MacEwen, G. D.: The coexistence of torticollis and congenital dysplasia of the hip, J. Bone Joint Surg. **54A:**1255, 1972.
38. Idelberger, K.: Die Erbpathologie der sogennanten angeborenen Hüftverrenkung, Munich, 1951, Verlag Urban & Schwarzenberg.
39. Jacobs, J. E.: Metatarsus varus and hip dysplasia, Clin. Orthop. **16:**203, 1960.
40. Kraus, B. S., and Schwartzman, J. R.: Congenital dislocation of the hip among the Fort Apache Indians, J. Bone Joint Surg. **39A:**448, 1957.
41. Langenskiöld, A., Sarpio, O., and Michelsson, J. E.: Experimental dislocation of the hip in the rabbit, J. Bone Joint Surg. **44B:**209, 1962.
42. LeDamany, P.: Congenital luxation of the hip, Am. J. Orthop. Surg. **11:**541, 1914.
43. Lorenz, A.: Die sogenannte angeborene Hüftverrenkung. Ihre Pathologie und Therapie, Stuttgart, 1920, Ferdinand Enke Verlag.
44. Ludloff, L., as cited by Hass, J.: Congenital dislocation of the hip, Springfield, Ill., 1951, Charles C Thomas, Publisher.
45. Massie, W. K., and Howorth, M. B.: Congenital dislocation of the hip. Part III. Pathogenesis, J. Bone Joint Surg. **33A:**190, 1951.
46. McIntosh, R., Merritt, K. K., Richards, M. R., Samuels, M. H., and Bellows, M. T.: The incidence of congenital malformations: a study of 5,964 pregnancies, Pediatrics **14:**505, 1954.
47. McKibbin, B.: Anatomical factors in the stability of the hip joint in the newborn, J. Bone Joint Surg. **52B:**148, 1970.
48. Muller, G. M., and Seddon, H. J.: Late results of treatment of congenital dislocation of the hip, J. Bone Joint Surg. **35B:**342, 1953.
49. Nelson, M. A.: Early diagnosis of congenital dislocation of the hip, J. Bone Joint Surg. **48B:**388, 1966.
50. Nishimura, H.: Incidence of congenital malformations in abortions. In Fraser, C., and McKusick, V. A., editors: Congenital malformations, Amsterdam, 1970, Excerpta Medica, p. 275.
51. Palmén, K.: Preluxation of the hip joint: diagnosis and treatment in the newborn and the diagnosis of the hip joint in Sweden during the years 1948-1960, Acta Paediatr. [Suppl.] (Uppsala) **50**(129):1, 1961.
52. Paterson, D.: Presented at 5th International Pediatric Orthopedic Seminar, Chicago, June 1977.
53. Putti, V.: Congenital dislocation of the hip, Surg. Gynecol. Obstet. **42:**449, 1926.
54. Putti, V.: Early treatment of congenital dislocation of the hip, J. Bone Joint Surg. **11:**798, 1929.
55. Rabin, D. L., Barnett, C. R., Arnold, W. D., Freiberger, R. H., and Brooks, G.: Untreated congenital hip disease: a study of the epidemiology, natural history and social aspect of the disease in a Navajo population, Am. J. Public Health **55**(2):1, 1965.
56. Ramsey, P. L., and MacEwen, G. D.: Personal communication.
57. Record, R. G., and Edwards, J. H.: Environmental influences related to the etiology of congenital dislocation of the hip, Br. J. Prev. Soc, Med. **12:**8, 1958.
58. Roser, K., as cited by Hass, J.: Congenital dislocation of the hip, Springfield, Ill., 1951, Charles C Thomas, Publisher.
59. Salter, R. B.: Etiology, pathogenesis and possible prevention of congenital dislocation of the hip, Can. Med. Assoc. J. **98:**933, 1968.
60. Salter, R. B.: Congenital dislocation of the hip. In Graham, W. D., editor: Modern trends In orthopedics, No. 5, New York, 1967, Appleton-Century-Crofts.
61. Salter, R. B., Kostuik, J., and Schatzker, J.: Ex-

perimental dysplasia of the hip and its reversibility in newborn pigs, J. Bone Joint Surg. **45A:**1781, 1963.
62. Smith, W. S., Coleman, C. R., Olix, M. L., and Slager, R. F.: Etiology of congenital dislocation of the hip, J. Bone Joint Surg. **45A:**491, 1963.
63. Smith, W. S., Ireton, R. J., and Coleman, C. R.: Sequelae of experimental dislocation of a weight-bearing ball-and-socket joint in a young growing animal, J. Bone Joint Surg. **40A:**1121, 1058.
64. Thieme, W. T., Wynne-Davies, R., Blair, H. A. F., Bell, E. T., and Lorraine, J. A.: Clinical examination and urinary oestrogen assays in newborn children with congenital dislocation of the hip, J. Bone Joint Surg. **50B:**546, 1968.
65. Van Meerdervoort, H. F.: Congenital dislocation of the hip in black patients, South African Med. J. **48:**2436, 1974.
66. VonAmmon: Die angeborenen chirurgischen Kranxheiten des Menschen, Berlin, 1842, as cited by Hass, J.: Congenital dislocation of the hip, Springfield, Ill., 1951, Charles C Thomas, Publisher.
67. von Friedlander, F., as cited by Hass, J.: Congenital dislocation of the hip, Springfield, Ill., 1951, Charles C Thomas, Publisher.
68. von Rosen, S.: Diagnosis and treatment of congenital dislocation of the hip joint in newborns, J. Bone Joint Surg. **44B:**284, 1962.
69. Watanabe, R. S.: Embryology of the human hip, Clin. Orthop. **98:**8, 1974.
70. Wessell, A. B.: Laughatte Slegter: Finnmarken, T. Nor. Laegeforen **38:**337, 1918, as cited by Getz, B.: The hip in Lapps and its bearing on the problem of congenital dislocation, Acta Orthop. Scand. [Suppl.] **22:**186, 1955.
71. Wilkinson, J. A.: Breech malposition and intrauterine dislocations, Proc. R. Soc. Med. **59:**1106, 1966.
72. Wilkinson, J. A.: A post-natal survey for congenital displacement of the hip, J. Bone Joint Surg. **54B:**40, 1972.
73. Wilkinson, J. S.: Prime factors in the etiology of congenital dislocation of the hip, J. Bone Joint Surg. **45B:**268, 1963.
74. Wilson, D. W.: Congenital dislocation of the hip, J. Bone Joint Surg. **46B:**163, 1964.
75. Woolf, C. M., Koehn, J. H., and Coleman, S. S.: Congenital hip disease in Utah: the influence of genetic and nongenetic factors, Am. J. Hum. Genet. **20:**430, 1968.
76. Wynne-Davies, R.: A family study of neonatal and late-diagnosis of congenital dislocation of the hip, J. Med. Genet. **7:**315, 1970.
77. Wynne-Davies, R.: Acetabular dysplasia and familial joint laxity: two etiologic factors in congenital dislocation of the hip, J. Bone Joint Surg. **52B:**704, 1970.

CHAPTER 3

Diagnosis and treatment in the newborn, neonate, and young infant

Definition of terms
History and physical examination
Congenital hip dysplasia
    Pathology
    Diagnosis in the newborn and neonate
    Diagnostic physical features
    High-risk infants
    Roentgenography
    Treatment
Subluxation of the hip in early infancy
    Pathology
    Physical findings
    Roentgenographic changes
    Treatment
Neonatal dislocation of the hip
    Pathology
    Physical findings
    Roentgenographic findings
    Treatment
"Irreducible" neonatal dislocation

The problems encountered in the newborn and the neonate represent some of the most difficult problems to define. However, once defined, they are fortunately the easiest to treat and produce the most predictable and satisfactory results. The newborn period includes the first few days of life, whereas the neonatal period has been arbitrarily defined by the neonatologists as the first 28 days of life. During these early days and weeks of life the clinical findings and manifestations are extremely variable as one proceeds from birth through the early weeks of infancy. Instability of the hip, for example, is largely a manifestation of the newborn, whereas adduction contractures, apparent shortening, and significant asymmetry of the skin folds are later expressions of hip abnormality.

In order to make the earliest diagnosis possible, it is extremely important for the physician to learn the great variability in the ways the physical findings can present themselves at different times during the first few months of infancy. The earlier the diagnosis, the more effective the treatment will be. During the first year of life, the pelvis develops more rapidly than during any single subsequent year; because skeletal growth is the single most important factor necessary for the correction of congenital abnormalities, early detection and treatment become critical.

One of the greatest sources of confusion associated with this condition is the poorly documented and often controversial relationship between dysplasia and dislocation. Gradually over the years the concept has evolved that the condition known as congenital dislocation of the hip is a clinical complex involving antenatal factors, which may be both genetic and environmental (mechanical), and postnatal factors, which by definition must be exclusively environmental. It has been difficult to prove or substantiate the cause-and-effect relationship that operates between dysplasia and dislocation, even though intuitively the relationship appears clear and undeniable. These uncertainties are primarily the result of a lack of convincing and well-documented studies of both the clinical and radiologic pathology of children who have either dysplasia or dislocation of the hip. This is largely because the hip of the newborn lends itself poorly to accurate radiographic examination and because some of the diagnostic clinical criteria are still controversial. Nevertheless, the recent experiences of several observers* have provided a considerably greater understanding of the interrelationships between dysplasia and dislocation, and it now appears that most hip abnormalities that can be demonstrated at birth (usually hip dysplasia) are simply a part of a broad spectrum of a condition popularly described as congenital dislocation of the hip.

DEFINITION OF TERMS

The semantics of this clinical problem have been abused in the literature as well as by our daily usage. In order to establish a sound basis for discussion, it is necessary that we define and hopefully agree on the terms used to categorize the various manifestations. The entities that need definition are dysplasia, subluxation, dislocation, and the residuals or sequelae of either dysplasia or dislocation.

According to Hart,[15,16] *congenital dysplasia* of the hip may be defined as an interruption in the growth forces of the elements that form the anatomic structures of the hip joint as a whole; these should include the innominate bone, the femur, the capsule, the ligamentum teres,

---

*See references 2, 5, 9, 25, 31, 42, and 43.

and the musculotendinous structures. He emphasized that the term *hip dysplasia* refers not only to the acetabulum, but also to the other parts of the hip joint. In concept I agree with this definition because it takes into account not only acetabular deficiencies and the deformities of the proximal femur, but also capsular and soft tissue abnormalities that may contribute to instability of the hip joint.

Subluxation of the hip simply states that there is contact between the articular surfaces of the femoral head and acetabulum, although the head is not concentrically reduced, and there is, therefore, an abnormal relationship between the head and acetabulum.

Dislocation means that there is no contact between the femoral head and acetabulum; as a result, the head lies completely outside the socket.

As a result of common clinical usage, the term *hip dysplasia* embraces two entirely separate conditions: On the one hand, the term *dysplasia* has been applied to the newborn and neonatal hip in which some degree of clinical instability or abnormality can be demonstrated by physical examination or roentgenographic study. The cause of this instability and its significance have been the source of a great deal of speculation, and not all clinicians agree about the many nebulous and poorly documented manifestations of the condition. On the other hand, the word *dysplasia* has also been identified with other conditions seen in later infancy, childhood, adolescence, and even through adult life. These later hip problems are characterized by either an inadequate acetabulum or a significant deformity of the upper femur, or both. Such abnormalities are easier to identify and to recognize roentgenographically, and they lend themselves to more accurate documentation by x-ray examination (Fig. 3-1). Furthermore, their clinical importance has been well accepted and the

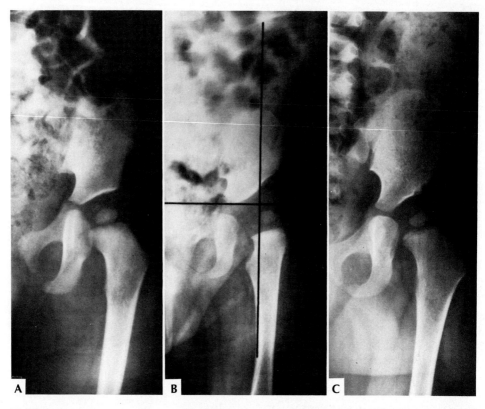

Fig. 3-1. Hip roentgenograms illustrating the difference between dysplasia and subluxation in an infant about 12 months of age. **A,** The hip is normal. **B,** The acetabular roof is slightly convex, the femur is displaced upward slightly, and the femoral head is located in the lower outer quadrant of the hip. This is considered subluxated. **C,** The femoral head seems concentrically located within the acetabulum, but the acetabular roof does not cover the head well, the roof is abnormally high, and the articular cortex is developed only over the lateral portion of the socket. This is a dysplastic hip. (From Coleman, S. S.: N. W. Q. Bull. **36:**222, 1962.)

need for treatment well established. Paradoxically, however, they are extremely difficult to diagnose by means of the physical examination. Hip dysplasia in these older patients almost always exhibits an abnormal acetabulofemoral head relationship by roentgenographic examination, and the subsequent development of some degree of secondary degenerative arthritis in adult life becomes almost inevitable. This eventuality has been emphasized by Putti,[33] who estimated that 40% of all osteoarthritis of the hip in Italy is the result of the sequelae of dysplasia or dislocation of the hip; Salter[38] states that this same causal relationship can be seen in at least one third of all instances of osteoarthritis of the hip in adult life. Recent studies by Harris[12] may show that the incidence is even higher.

Obviously, the differences between these two hip dysplasias are great. On the one hand, in the newborn and neonate infant the validity of the diagnostic disciplines has not been unequivocally proved, and the requirement that all cases receive routine treatment could be contested. In the second instance, in those instances dealing with older infants, children, and adults, any grossly deficient or biomechanically abnormal hip mandates the correction, wherever possible, of an established, proved deformity that, if untreated, has reasonably predictable and significant adverse sequelae. Because of these distinctions, the two conditions will be discussed separately.

HISTORY AND PHYSICAL EXAMINATION

Although perhaps self-evident, it is important to emphasize the value of recording the history of the patient; one should determine first whether the infant was full term or not; whether the gestation was uneventful; whether the birth was normal; and whether the infant was delivered by breech or cephalic presentation. The physician should know whether there was anything unusual about the birth and neonatal history, whether the dislocation existed at birth (antenatal), and whether there is, or was, a family history of congenital hip disease. These types of historical data should help to identify whether one patient is a member of the high-risk group discussed later in this chapter. In older infants and children it is obviously important to know whether any treatment has been given as well as the results of that treatment, including any special problems that might have been encountered.

As a part of the physical examination, a complete orthopedic evaluation must be made, including the neck, spine, upper limbs, and lower limbs, as well as an appropriate neurologic examination. During these examinations any associated abnormalities in the musculoskeletal system should be carefully considered, with specific attention directed to the length and girth of the lower limbs and to any palpable abnormalities about the hip joint area. This must be done in order to determine the possible presence of a neuromuscular disorder or other more complex problems, such as proximal femoral deficiencies and other limb deficiencies. The range of motion and flexibility (or rigidity) of the hip should be assessed, and the overall muscle tone and general appearance of the lower limbs must be evaluated. At the conclusion of such an examination it should be possible in nearly all instances to establish whether this is a hip disorder in an otherwise normal infant or whether there are complicating circumstances that will require further clinical and specialized investigation.

In the case of otherwise normal infants who are suspected of having a congenital hip abnormality, a pelvic x-ray examination is mandatory. In the newborn there is some controversy about the validity and diagnostic value of pelvic radiography. Nevertheless, I believe that it is appropriate to have a pelvic film made at this time *if* it can be done accurately, can be interpreted properly, and is placed into proper perspective with the clinical examination. With it, such disorders as coxa vara and other skeletal abnormalities can be ruled out. In older infants the x-ray examination assumes much greater validity and, by the time the infant is 6 months of age, a very reliable evaluation of the infant's hips is possible. In still older infants and young children more extensive radiography is usually necessary; the minimum acceptable radiographic examination requires an anteroposterior view of the pelvis with the femora in neutral rotation, an anteroposterior view of the pelvis with the thighs in abduction and internal rotation, and a cross-table (groin) lateral view of the hip (the so-called Laage view).

In some instances arthrography will be necessary. This examination, however, requires the presence of certain specific indications to justify its accomplishment. Although some believe that routine arthrography is indicated whenever a dislocated hip is treated, as will be discussed later, I have found that it is rarely necessary to perform arthrography on infants and young children unless there is some strong doubt about the concentricity of reduction after a review of the *plain roentgenograms*. At the conclusion of the x-ray evaluation, including arthrography when necessary, and when accompanied by the history and physical examination mentioned earlier, a reasonably accurate definition of the problem is usually possible.

CONGENITAL HIP DYSPLASIA

Congenital dysplasia in the newborn and neonate consists of one or a combination of two or three possible abnormalities in the hip. These are: (1) a shallow, deficient acetabulum, (2) excessive capsular laxity, and (3) a deformity of the proximal femur.

Pathology

Several studies on premature and full-term stillborn infants have been made that have established to some extent the pathology involved in neonatal dysplasia. In newborn and neonatal hip dysplasia, the acetabulum may be slightly reduced in circumference but is of a normal shape and depth. There may be some deficiency of the posterior rim of the socket, as demonstrated by Stanisavljevic[41] and Ortolani.[30] The femoral head may be slightly smaller than normal, but it may have a normal configuration. Anteversion of the femoral head and neck may be slightly increased, and usually there is some degree of capsular laxity present.[21,37]

Hass[17] believed that a dysplastic hip varies anatomically only slightly from the normal hip; he further proposed that there was some degree of hypoplasia of the acetabulum, which made the hip more susceptible to dislocation. This "predislocation" concept is one that I fully support.

However, despite these very sophisticated studies of shallow, deficient acetabula, excessive capsular laxity, and deformities of the proximal femur, it has still not been definitely proved whether the existence of one or the other, or all three, is essential to produce an unstable hip. It is also controversial as to which of the three is the primary problem. This controversy, in addition to the incidence, etiology, and pathogenesis of the whole problem, has been thoroughly reviewed in Chapter 2. At this point the major challenge to the physician is to identify an unstable hip, or the sequelae of an unstable hip, so that appropriate treatment can be administered.

Diagnosis in the newborn and neonate

Ever since Ortolani[30] introduced and popularized the "jerks" of entry and exit and established their diagnostic significance in the infant hip, there has been an increased enthusiasm for developing examination programs whose aim is the early diagnosis of an unstable hip in the newborn and neonatal period. Several clinical studies have been made in different countries that have attempted to identify the salient physical and roentgenographic manifestations of newborn and neonatal hip dysplasia; correspondingly, treatment programs have been carried out that have indirectly attached some degree of validity to these diagnostic criteria.

My own studies on congenital dysplasia of the hip have been largely substantiated by several other investigators. In a study of newborn and neonatal Navajo infants,[6] it was possible for me to assess the clinical consequences of untreated hip dysplasia, because many of the parents of infants with dysplastic hips had refused any form of therapy. It was thus possible to follow these cases and observe the results of the lack of treatment. Such observations lend additional support to the conclusions that have been derived from the data published by others. These observations are as follows: if untreated, the dysplastic hip can follow any one of four courses: (1) it may become normal; (2) it may become subluxated; (3) it may proceed to dislocation; or (4) it may retain certain dysplastic features that persist throughout adult life.

It has been shown* that the great majority of unstable hips identified by physical examination during the newborn and neonatal period become stable during the first few days or weeks of life. Also, many of those that eventually become stable become completely normal, both clinically and roentgenographically, whether they are treated or not. This observation is supported by several statistical data. For example, the incidence of a dislocatable hip in newborn white infants is about one in 100, yet the overall incidence of a true dislocation of the hip in similar racial and ethnic groups has been established as approximately one in 800 or one in 1000. Because many newborn infants with unstable hips are not identified and, therefore, are not treated, it must be assumed that spontaneous correction must take place in a significant number of cases. Although the percentage must be high, the exact figure is unknown. The answers to two other very important related questions are also as yet unknown, namely; (1) how many of these dysplastic, or initially unstable, hips that never proceed to dislocation will retain certain stigmata of dysplasia, and (2) how does the physician determine at the time of the newborn examination which ones will proceed to a frank dislocation and which ones will develop normally? In my opinion it is the lack of answers to these two questions that mandates the treatment and appropriate follow-up of all infants who show demonstrably unstable hips at birth or in early infancy.

Diagnostic physical features

My own personal experience with hip dysplasia in the newborn and neonate supports the conclusion that the most valuable diagnostic physical finding is the ability of the examiner to displace, or subluxate, the femoral head from the socket. This particular physical feature can be elicited in about 1% of newborn white infants during the first or second day after birth. The maneuver required to elicit this finding is illustrated in Fig. 3-2. The infant's hips and knees are flexed to 90 degrees and the examiner grasps both knees and thighs. The pelvis is stabilized on one side by firmly holding the lower limb with one hand, and the thigh on the opposite (tested) side is *gently* manipulated downward and outward (posterolaterally) so that the femoral head may, if unstable, be displaced partially or completely from the acetabulum. When positive, the examiner will feel the femoral head ride posteriorly over the acetabular rim. As the gentle pressure is released, the femoral head will immediately slip back into the acetabulum with an impressive "jerk."

It should be emphasized that this maneuver must be done gently and without force. To acquire the technical skill necessary to elicit a positive result requires not only patience, but also experience. Generally speaking, until one has experienced a true "subluxation provocation" as described above, it is difficult to feel confident about whether the maneuver has been appropriately or effectively accomplished. Furthermore, even the most experienced examiner may fail to elicit

---

*See references 6, 10, 14, 15, and 31.

46 Congenital dysplasia and dislocation of the hip

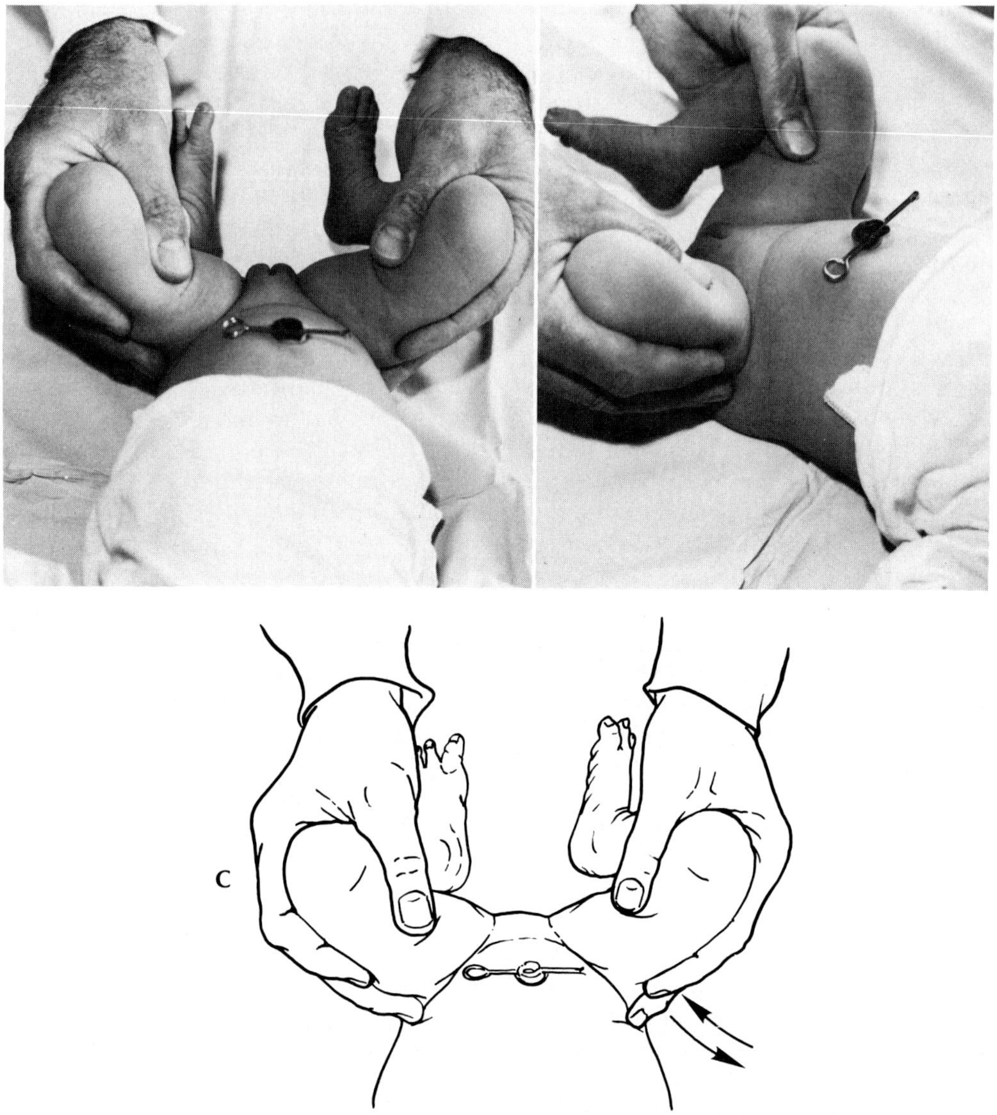

Fig. 3-2. Photographs and diagrammatic illustration of method by which the newborn hip is examined for instability. The surgeon faces the infant and grasps both thighs firmly, **A.** The examiner's thumbs are placed over the medial aspect of the upper thigh and the fingers are placed over the greater trochanters. With the pelvis being stabilized with one hand, the opposite hip and thigh are gently forced posteriorly and laterally in an effort to displace the femoral head from the socket, **B.** The maneuver is illustrated diagrammatically in **C.**

this finding during the newborn period and yet find several weeks or even months later that the hip is abnormal by some other criteria. This distressing but realistic frailty of the ability to accomplish this maneuver emphasizes and underscores the need for repeated periodic examinations of all infants' hips during the first year of life.

Although the identification of this abnormality is best accomplished during the newborn period, it is more important to recognize that such a finding can be missed during this early period even with conscientious examination. Realizing this, the clinician should carefully and faithfully carry out periodic examinations of the infant's hips. However, one should reemphasize that the physical findings in congenital hip disease are manifested decidedly differently when the infant is examined in later weeks and months than they are in hip dysplasia encountered during the newborn period. An example of this variation in physical findings at different infant age groups is shown by Ramsey and MacEwen.[36] In 25,000 infant examinations they encountered the following:

	Birth to 1 month	1 to 3 months	3 to 6 months
Instability	100%	29%	15%
Limited abduction	7%	67%	86%

Thus, as noted above, the physical findings often associated with true, complete dislocation of the hip are usually conspicuously absent in the newborn infant. For example, a true or apparent shortening of the limb is extremely difficult to identify in the newborn who has hip dysplasia. Asymmetric skin creases are virtually meaningless diagnostically, since approximately 50% of all newborns will have some asymmetry of the thigh and inguinal skin creases, presumably as a result of the intrauterine position and temporary congenital asymmetric hip flexion contractures. A significant restriction of hip abduction is rarely found in newborn infants, even when the hip is grossly unstable. However, I believe that some degree of diagnostic importance can be assigned to *persistent* and especially asymmetric restriction of abduction of the flexed thigh.

Therefore, from the standpoint of the newborn examination, I believe that the most reliable physical sign of dysplasia is the ability to subluxate or dislocate the femoral head from the socket by the maneuver described on p. 45. The second most reliable physical finding is a *persistent* limitation of abduction of the flexed thigh. This sign is especially helpful if it is unilateral. Other physical manifestations, unless an obvious complete and irreducible dislocation exists, can largely be ignored because they rarely have diagnostic significance for this particular age group.

Utilizing these evaluation criteria, I have found that it is very uncommon to encounter a true dislocation of the hip in the *newborn* infant *who is otherwise normal*. Most antenatal dislocations have been found to be associated with additional abnormalities, such as paralysis caused by meningomyelocele, arthrogryposis, and other significant congenital deformities. This does not mean that in the absence of other abnormalities dislocation of the hip cannot be present at birth, but in my experience it is rare. Thus the physical abnormalities found in dislocation (p. 67) will uncommonly be encountered in hip dysplasia of the newborn.

High-risk infants

Although all newborn children should be given the dignity of a thorough orthopedic examination and each child should be studied with a high index of suspicion for possible signs of hip dysplasia, there are certain infants whose unique genetic and/or environmental characteristics make them more susceptible to this particular problem than the average infant. These are members of the high-risk group, which includes infants with one or more of the following characteristics: a breech birth (or breech presentation in the case of a cesarean section), an infant with a family history of congenital hip disease (Fig. 3-3), a female infant with a deformity of the lower limbs (metatarsus varus, talipes equinovarus, congenital vertical talus, etc.), an infant with *significant* and persistent asymmetry of the thigh folds, an infant with excessive laxity of the joint ligaments, an infant with torticollis or any other significant musculoskeletal abnormality, and any child whose heritable or genetic background is associated with an increased incidence of congenital hip dislocation, such as the American Indian, Japanese, and northern Italians.

These children should probably be followed more closely, both clinically and

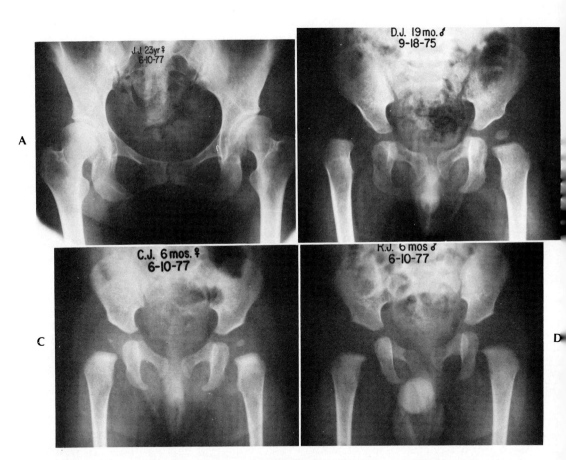

Fig. 3-3. An example of subluxation in the high-risk group. **A,** This 23-year-old mother had undergone treatment for bilateral CDH as an infant. The pelvic film shows bilateral dysplastic hips. **B,** Her 19-month-old son with CDH was not diagnosed as having hip disease until age 19 months. **C,** Specific efforts were made at early diagnosis in fraternal twins; physical examination was totally normal. At 6 months of age a clearly dysplastic right hip is seen in the female, **C,** and the same problem is definite but less clearly seen in the right hip of the male, **D.** This demonstrates the frailty of the physical examination in this high-risk group.

Diagnosis and treatment in the newborn, neonate, and young infant   49

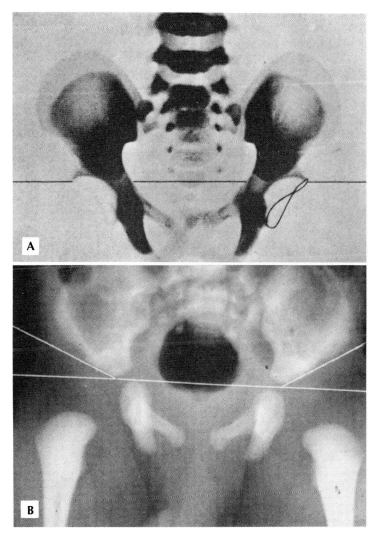

Fig. 3-4. A, Roentgenographic study of newborn. The left acetabular edge has been painted with aluminum bronze. The cartilaginous acetabulum is of the same extent, relatively, as in the adult. **B,** Roentgenographic study of a normal newborn (age 1 day). Note the acetabular index. (**A** from Severin, E.: Arthrography in congenital dislocation of the hip, J. Bone Joint Surg. **21:**304, 1939; **B** from Hart, V. L.: Congenital dysplasia of the hip joint and sequelae (in the newborn and early postnatal life), Springfield, Ill., 1952. Courtesy of Charles C Thomas, Publisher.)

radiographically, during early infancy and childhood than infants who do not have any of these characteristics. Routine pelvic films on the newborn are not necessarily indicated, however. In fact, if the films are normal, they may even contribute to a false sense of security in the absence of clinical abnormalities. A film taken when the child is between 3 and 6 months of age will have a high degree of validity, particularly when combined with clinical findings that support the diagnosis of dysplasia and potential dislocation.

Roentgenography

Roentgenographic findings. The significance of the roentgenographic features of the newborn hip have long been a source of considerable controversy and misunderstanding. The reasons for this skepticism and confusion are understandable: the bony structures seen roentgenographically represent only the ossification centers about the hip and cannot accurately reflect the true configuration or the size of the cartilaginous anlage. These bony centers are also widely spaced and develop at variable rates in different individuals. Severin[39] has shown that the normal newborn cartilaginous acetabulum has the same general configuration as the fully ossified adult acetabulum (Fig. 3-4). The ossified portion of the acetabulum in the newborn, however, usually bears very little resemblance to its mature counterpart. Thus one must be very cautious about attaching too much importance to the roentgenographic observations discussed below. Furthermore, the potential for a misinterpretation of the results that can be obtained from a newborn pelvic x-ray film has led some observers to discount the value of the film completely. I believe that there are certain determinations that can be made from such examinations that, when placed into proper perspective, can be helpful in establishing the presence or absence of hip dysplasia. However, under no circumstances should the clinician rely heavily on the interpretation of a *newborn's* pelvic x-ray film *unless it is unequivocally abnormal*. Correspondingly, and even more importantly, a "negative" roentgenogram has no meaning in the presence of other convincing diagnostic physical findings.

Radiographic techniques for the newborn pelvis. Several radiographic techniques have been employed to evaluate the pelvis and hip joints of the newborn and neonate most accurately. One commonly used is that described by Andrén and von Rosen,[1] which attempts to identify an unstable hip by the special positioning of the thighs in abduction (Fig. 3-5). I prefer to employ a simple anteroposterior view of the pelvis with the thighs held in neutral rotation and parallel to each other, in about 30 degrees of flexion (Fig. 3-6). In this way the hips and pelvis are uniformly positioned on the x-ray film, and any asymmetric hip flexion contracture, often present normally in newborns, is neutralized. With this position there is greater assurance that a true anteroposterior view of the pelvis will be taken. If the film is taken with the pelvis having any significant rotation, obliquity, or tilt, then nearly all of the determinants discussed below are invalidated. It is, therefore, important to emphasize that the technique of radiography is critical if it is to be diagnostically helpful and that the film *must* be a true anteroposterior view of the pelvis.

Roentgenographic determinants. The well-established x-ray determinants that can be made on the newborn pelvis include the acetabular index, the relationships of the proximal femoral metaphysis to the vertical line of Perkins,[32] and the "H" and "D" lines of Hilgenreiner.[20] Under differing circumstances each of these has special, although limited, diagnostic significance. A diagram of a roent-

Diagnosis and treatment in the newborn, neonate, and young infant 51

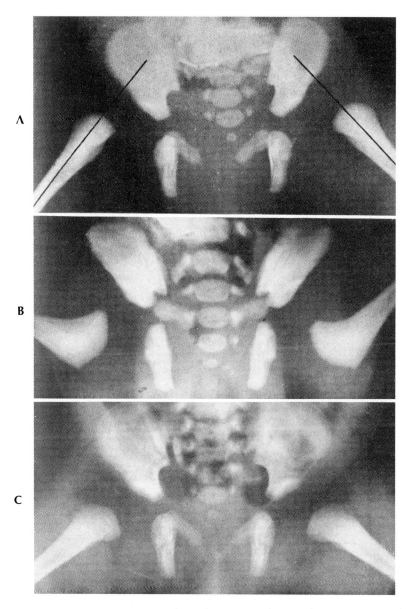

Fig. 3-5. Bilateral dislocations. **A,** Shafts directed approximately toward superior-anterior iliac spines despite limited rotation of femora. **B,** Roentgenogram of hips in reduced positions on same occasion. **C,** Same case after 16 days' treatment. Dislocation no longer possible. (From Andrén, L., and von Rosen, S.: The diagnosis of dislocation of the hip in newborns and the primary results of immediate treatment, Acta Radiol. **49:**89, 1958.)

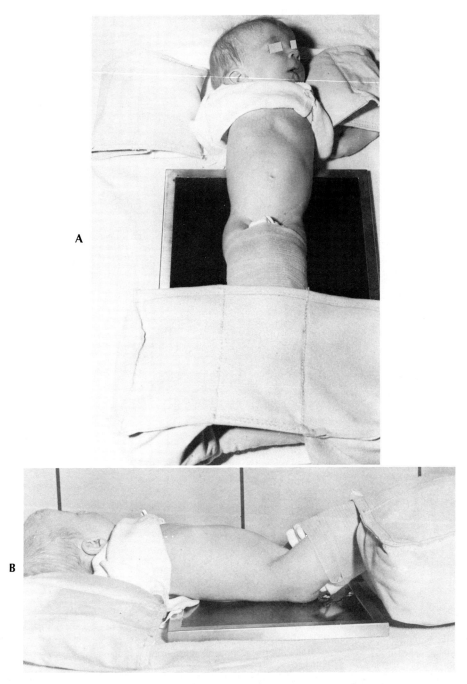

Fig. 3-6. An illustration of the technique for taking a pelvic x-ray film in a neonate. The lower limbs are lightly bound or held together parallel with the thighs extended, **A.** The hips should be flexed about 30 degrees in order that the pelvis can be positioned flat against the x-ray cassette, **B.**

genogram of the pelvis of a newborn is seen in Fig. 3-7.

Many observers have studied roentgenograms of the pelvis in the newborn, the neonate, and young infants and children in an effort either to make an early diagnosis or to make some prediction as to which children had dysplasia of the hip with the potential for dislocation. Soutter and Lovett[40] in 1924 were among the first to show an interest in the acetabular slope in young children as a diagnostic aid. They classified the "acetabular shelf" as being normal when horizontal; good when 30 degrees or less; fair when between 30 and 60 degrees; and poor when over 60 degrees. Most of their observations were made on older infants and children and therefore could not be applied to newborns. They were also responsible for establishing that x-ray examination in young infants and children did not reveal the true configuration of the acetabulum, because the cartilage could not be visualized on the routine roentgenogram.

Hilgenreiner[20] in 1925 studied the angle of inclination of the acetabulum and concluded that normally it should not exceed 20 degrees. He believed that any upward deviation from this value indicated dysplasia. His observations were not confined to neonates. In 1933 Putti[35] stressed the value and validity of the pelvic x-ray examination and suggested that *every* newborn child should have an x-ray

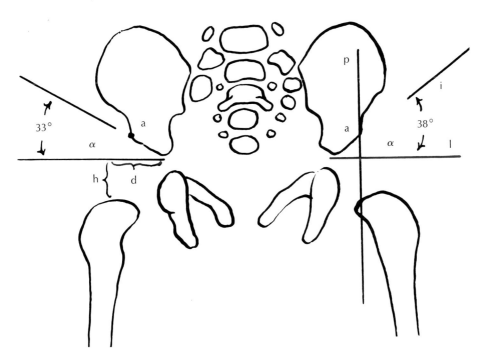

Fig. 3-7. A, Drawing from roentgenogram of the pelvis of a newborn infant. (This infant's hips were normal on physical examination.) *a,* Anterior inferior iliac spine; *l,* horizontal line of Hilgenreiner, drawn through comparable points on the triradiate cartilage; *i,* line drawn parallel to acetabular roof—angle formed between *i* and *l* is acetabular index (α); *p,* Perkins line, a perpendicular dropped through the anterior inferior iliac spine at right angles to *l;* *h,* distance between *l* and the highest point on the femoral neck; *d,* distance between the triradiate cartilage and the intersection of *h* and *l.* (From Coleman, S. S.: Diagnosis of congenital dysplasia of the hip in the newborn infant, J.A.M.A. **162:**548, 1956. Copyright 1956, American Medical Association.)

film routinely made of the pelvis. He considered radiographic evaluation a very good diagnostic aid in determining predislocation and believed that children with abnormal roentgenographic findings should be treated. He stated that he had seen "a state of predislocation, evidenced merely by an increased tilt of the roof of the acetabulum and a few clinical signs develop into a complete dislocation."

Kleinberg and Lieberman[23] introduced the term "acetabular index" in 1936. These authors studied twenty-three normal infants from 1 to 7 days old and concluded that the normal acetabular index averaged 27.5 degrees. In twenty normal children between the ages of 1½ and 2 years they found that 20 degrees was a normal value. In twenty-five patients with a congenital hip dislocation, they noted that the values for the abnormal hip were greater than those for the "normal" hip. They also concluded that "an acetabular index of above 30 degrees foreshadows a *possible* dislocation of the hip." However, these authors did not believe that such a determination was diagnostic. Even as recently as 1958, Hass[18] agreed with Kleinberg and Lieberman that 30 degrees was a reasonable upper limit of normal for the acetabular index; he further recommended routine pelvic roentgenograms on newborns and neonates. Ostensibly the importance of properly positioning the patient during the roentgenographic examination was not recognized or appreciated until 1940. At that time Burman and Clark[3] measured thirty-eight acetabular roof angles and concluded that the positioning of the patient could effect a significant change in the acetabular index. They therefore suggested that radiographic findings should be interpreted according to the clinical findings, and they further believed that the acetabular index warranted little emphasis.

In 1948 Heublein and associates[19] reported their observations on evaluations they had made on 300 normal hips. They concluded that the acetabular index was fairly constant and that it could be used as a helpful aid in evaluating the acetabulum. As with Kleinberg and Lieberman, they emphasized that an elevated acetabular index could be employed as a "*possible* indicator of an abnormal hip." Others supported this thesis.[8,18]

In the 1950s several large studies were reported that largely refuted the previously established upper range for a normal acetabular index value of 30 degrees, as suggested by Kleinberg and Lieberman. These authors believed that if the predislocation theory was valid then routine roentgenograms of newborn infants would permit the identification of those children with excessive acetabular indices to be selected for prophylactic treatment. Because of this confusion regarding normal values for the acetabular index, Caffey and associates[4] studied 627 normal children at birth and then at ages 6 months and 1 year. They found that the mean acetabular values varied between 25 and 29 degrees for all groups. They also established that the *mean value* for female infants was 30 degrees, a figure identical to that used as the upper limit of normal prior to their study. As a result of this well-done radiographic study, they concluded that radiographic evidence of an elevated acetabular index, in and of itself, was not sufficient basis on which to make a diagnosis of dysplasia or to start prophylactic treatment.

In 1956 I reported my evaluation of 3500 newborn infants.[5] In an effort to establish a baseline value for the acetabular index, 150 newborn infants were subjected to combined physical and roentgenographic examination. A wide range in the value of the acetabular indices was found, varying from 20 to 42 degrees, with the mean being 30.86 degrees. Utilizing a standard deviation of 3.8

degrees, the lower and upper limits of normal ranged from 23.3 to 38.5 degrees. I therefore concluded that the value of 30 degrees was actually an average value rather than the upper limit of normal; this conclusion supports the observations of Caffey and associates.[4]

Laurenson[21] reported in 1959 a very thorough and critical analysis of the significance and value of the acetabular index. He also concluded that 30 degrees was probably the upper limit of normal. However, he believed that routine films of the pelvis were not indicated until radiographic techniques could be better standardized.

In 1968 I again reported my findings from 1956 x-ray examinations of the pelvis in *randomly* selected Navajo neonates.[6] In 1155 cases both roentgenographic and physical examinations were accomplished: 1078 were clinically normal and seventy-seven were clinically abnormal, according to the criteria outlined earlier. It was my conclusion that during the first 3 months of life the acetabular index averages 28.6 degrees in normal infants. On the other hand, the infants showing abnormal physical findings had an average acetabular index of 34.8 degrees. I concluded that a *single* determination of the acetabular index was of little value unless it was in excess of 40 degrees. Even in these cases, in the absence of abnormal physical findings, the diagnosis of dysplasia was purely presumptive. Thus *in and of itself* the acetabular index has little diagnostic value.

In 1925 Hilgenreiner[20] described determinations that could be made by a

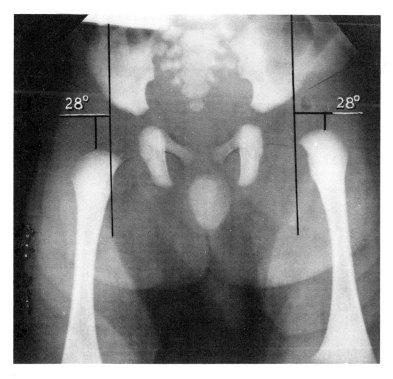

Fig. 3-8. The value of the foreshortened H distance is seen in this roentgenogram. The left hip was easily displaceable and very unstable. The hip is also laterally displaced, showing the value of the increased D distance. Note almost true anteroposterior view of the pelvis.

roentgenographic examination of hips in neonates (Fig. 3-7). He drew a horizontal line between the companion triradiate cartilages and concluded that the distance from the upper metaphyseal tip of the femur to this horizontal connecting line is normally 1 cm (the H distance) and that the distance from the same upward tip to the acetabular floor is 1.2 cm (the D distance). These absolute metric determinations were ultimately shown to be invalid because they were subject to variations depending on the size of the infant and could be greatly influenced by slight degrees of rotation of the pelvis at the time the roentgenograph was taken. However, when the H distance is unilaterally foreshortened or is compared to a similarly computed distance on its companion hip, abnormal upward displacement of the femur must be viewed as strongly suspicious of a dysplastic hip (Fig. 3-8). When the D distance is found to be greater than that on its companion hip, then abnormal lateral displacement of the femur should be suspected (Fig. 3-8). It can be seen that these evaluations are valid only when the comparison is made between measurements of the supposed abnormal hip and the normal hip. By the same token, in instances of bilateral dysplasia, the significance of these determinations is essentially invalidated (Fig. 3-9).

In 1928 Perkins[32] showed that the relationship of the proximal femoral metaphysis to the acetabulum could be established by means of a vertical line drawn through the superolateral rim of the ossified portion of the acetabulum. In

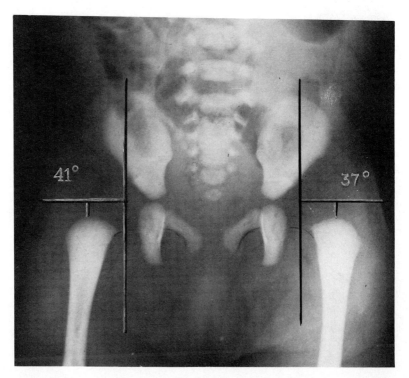

Fig. 3-9. This pelvic film shows why the H and D distances are invalid in bilateral dysplasias or dislocations. Both of these hips were easily subluxable, and the femoral metaphyses are well lateral to the vertical line of Perkins. However, the H and D Hilgenreiner distances are the same on both sides.

a normal pelvis the proximal femoral metaphysis ("beak") should lie well inside (that is, medial to) the line. Conversely, when the metaphysis lies lateral to the line, the hip is considered abnormal (Fig. 3-10). I believe that this particular determination provides the greatest value to be derived from all roentgenographic evaluations of the pelvis, *provided* that the film is an accurate anteroposterior view. This determination does not rely on a specific distance or number of degrees, and it is equally valid whether the condition is unilateral or bilateral. Furthermore, there is a high correlation in my experience between this factor and the demonstration of hip instability by the subluxation-provocation test (as described on p. 45). In my experience instability can be demonstrated in nearly 100% of the hips of *newborn infants* wherein the proximal femoral metaphysis lies lateral to the Perkins line, in an appropriately conducted x-ray examination (as described on p. 50).

Some observations of a temporal nature can be made that may also have diagnostic value during the first few weeks or months of infancy on the basis of an x-ray film. Unfavorable roentgenographic find-

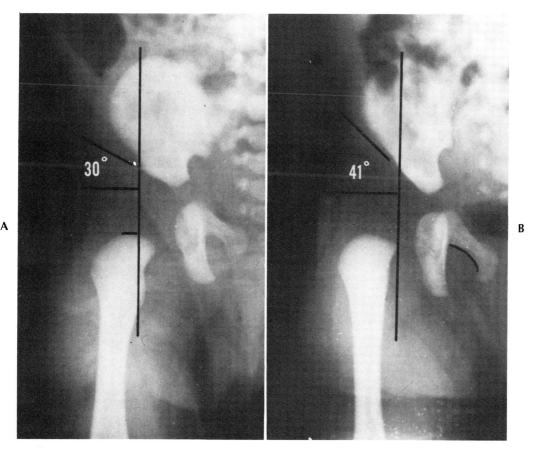

Fig. 3-10. The Perkins line is an absolute measurement because it shows the relationship of the proximal femur to the acetabulum. Normal acetabular femoral relationships are seen in **A,** and the laterally disposed femoral metaphysis ("beak") is well seen in the dysplastic (displaceable) hip in **B.**

58 Congenital dysplasia and dislocation of the hip

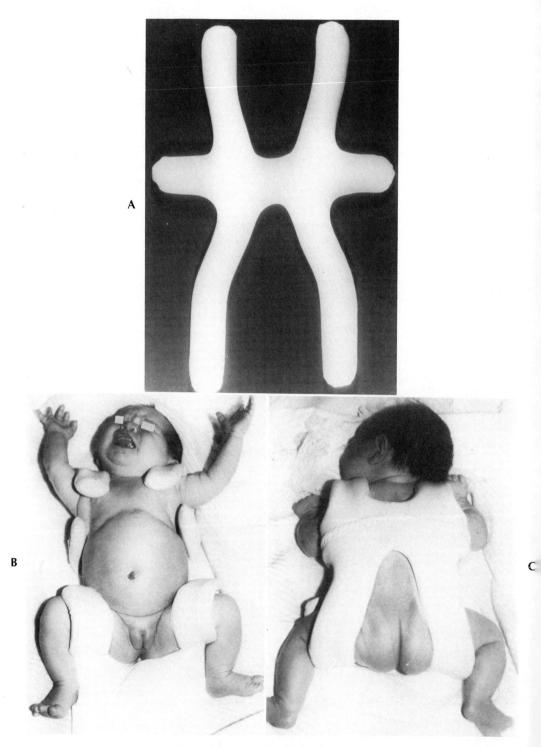

Fig. 3-11. For legend see opposite page.

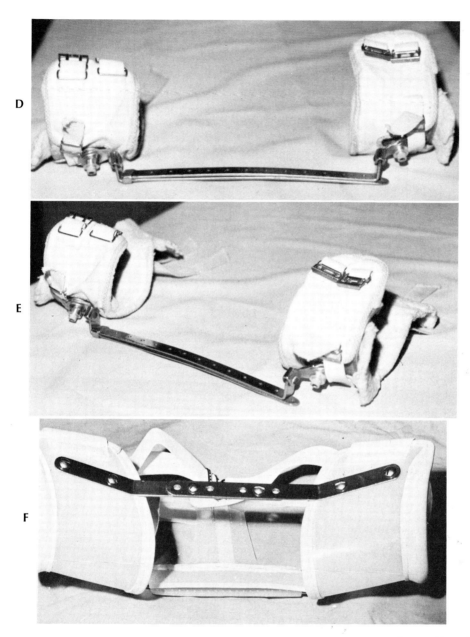

Fig. 3-11. The von Rosen splint is a rigid but malleable device made of flexible metal and covered by soft padding, **A.** When it is applied to the infant, the child's lower limbs can be placed into variable positions of flexion and abduction as needed, **B** and **C**. The Ilfeld splint is rigid, consisting of a transverse adjustable metal bar attached on two universal joints that can be adjusted and locked, **D.** These are, in turn, attached to two padded, trough-shaped devices designed to encircle the thighs, **E.** The major disadvantage of the Ilfeld splint is the difficulty in controlling abduction. The modified Craig splint, **F,** is semi-rigid and easy to clean. It is my preference for older infants. (**A** through **C** courtesy Dr. David Levine.)

ings that strongly suggest dysplasia include the following: a significant delay in the appearance of the femoral head ossification center; failure of the ossified acetabular index to reduce its angle with growth of the pelvis; failure of the ossified articular surface of the acetabulum to develop a concavity; and the delayed ossification of the ischiopubic synchondrosis. Most of these are findings that are related to either an opposite normal hip or to comparable findings in normal children of the same general age. Though not critically reliable, they can be valuable diagnostic adjuncts when properly interpreted.

Treatment

The beneficial results of appropriately instituted conservative therapy in newborn and neonatal dysplasia have been proved in numerous published studies. If the following principles of treatment are carefully observed, the incidence of complete congenital hip dislocation and residual dysplasia will be greatly reduced. Furthermore, the treatment, *appropriately administered,* is so innocuous that no infant with signs of dysplasia should ever be denied such therapy once the diagnosis has been established.

The indications for treatment of newborn and neonatal hip dysplasia are very simple if one accepts the foregoing conclusions. Thus any infant manifesting physical and/or roentgenographic signs of hip dysplasia should be treated with some type of abduction device. The nature of the device is not so important as the goal that it intends to accomplish and the technique with which it is used. Conceptually, the hips should be kept gently

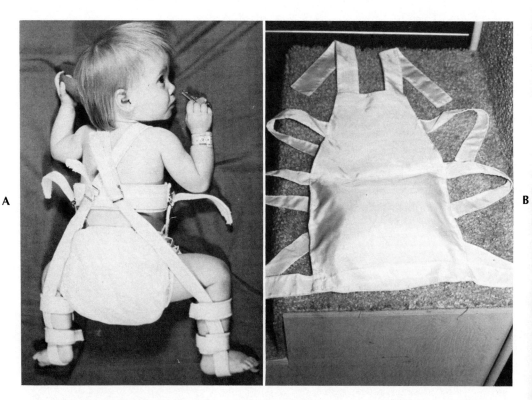

Fig. 3-12. Some flexible abduction devices include the Pavlik harness, **A,** and the Frejka apron, **B.** (From Coleman, S. S., and MacEwen, G. D.: Congenital dislocation of the hip in infancy. In American Academy of Orthopaedic Surgeons: AAOS instructional course lectures, vol. 21, St. Louis, 1972, p. 159.)

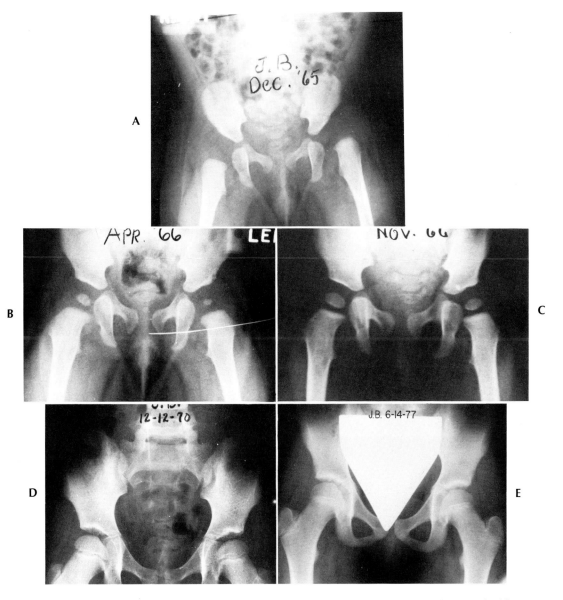

Fig. 3-13. Severe restriction of abduction and instability of the left hip seen in x-ray films of a 5-month-old girl. Prior examinations at birth and at age 3 months were considered normal. Pelvic roentgenogram shows a definite dysplasia (or subluxation?) of the left hip, **A.** After 4 months of treatment in a flexible abduction device the hip was better centered and the femoral head ossification center has appeared, **B.** Six months later, **C,** and 4 and 10½ years later, **D** and **E,** the hip has become progressively normal.

flexed and abducted, preferably in a nonrigid apparatus that does not exert any significant abduction force on the thighs. There are many of these devices available, and they can be arbitrarily placed into two groups: the rigid and the flexible. Although rigid devices may occasionally be necessary, when one is faced with an unusually unstable hip, I believe that a flexible apparatus offers greater safety and provides an opportunity for more normal physiologic functioning of the developing hip joint. Some rigid abduction devices are illustrated in Fig. 3-11. The von Rosen splint has the advantages of being adjustable and durable, and the modified Craig splint is readily available, relatively inexpensive, and easy to clean. The latter is not well suited, however, for use with the very young infant because of limitations in available sizes. Some flexible abduction methods illustrated in Fig. 3-12 include the triple-diaper technique, the Frejka apron, and the Pavlik harness. The triple diapers are preferred for the newborn and neonatal period, and either the Frejka apron or Pavlik harness can be used in subsequent months as the child grows. The personal preferences of the physician will undoubtedly determine the particular device or devices used, and as long as the principles of treatment are followed the results will likely be equally effective.

Depending on the degree of instability demonstrated, the abduction apparatus can be used continuously or intermittently, with freedom permitted for baths and normal infant activity. In the large majority of instances, hip stability will be obtained within a few days or weeks. The patient should be gradually "weaned" from the device, but as a rule I do not discontinue it completely until the hip is normal, both clinically and roentgenographically. This may require nighttime use of the apparatus through the sixth month or even longer. Follow-up at various intervals must be carried out until the patient is fully ambulatory. The clinical and roentgenographic findings at this point govern the decision for future periodic evaluation (Fig. 3-13).

SUBLUXATION OF THE HIP IN EARLY INFANCY

As noted earlier, by an analysis of the statistical data alone it can be stated that untreated dysplasia of the hip will proceed to dislocation in about 10% of the cases. However, the behavior of the hip enroute to dislocation is not well understood, and there are very few reliable data from which to draw meaningful conclusions. I believe that even though progressive stability of the previously unstable (dysplastic) hip can be demonstrated by physical examination, some degree of capsular laxity and acetabular inadequacy undoubtedly must persist, thereby permitting the gradual development of a slight lateral and upward displacement of the femoral head. This leads to the anatomic and biomechanical factors that eventually produce an adduction contracture on the involved side. It is at this point, usually several weeks or months after birth, that the warning physical findings suggesting subluxation or an impending dislocation can most often be elicited.

Pathology

Pathologically, hip subluxation is considered to be a transitional state in the eventual progression to complete disloca-

Fig. 3-14. Five-year-old girl with bilateral dysplastic or subluxated hips, **A.** Later in life these may well represent those of this 35-year-old female whose dysplastic hip joint was discovered incidentally at the time of a lower spine examination, **B.** Six years later she developed disabling hip pain with obvious advanced secondary osteoarthritis, **C.** (Courtesy Dr. A. M. Okelberry.)

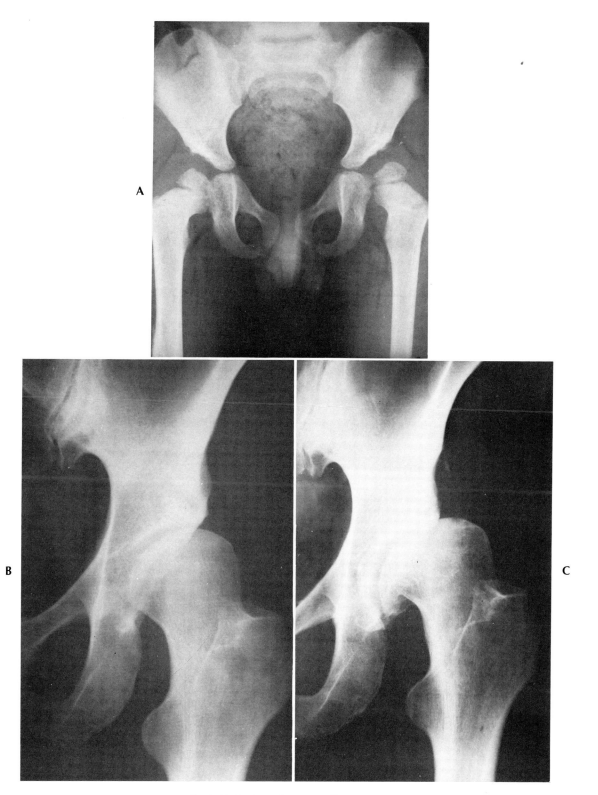

Fig. 3-14. For legend see opposite page.

tion, if untreated. Putti,[34] however, demonstrated that subluxation is an entity unto itself and that it may exist without ever progressing to dislocation. Many believe that it represents simply an advanced stage of dysplasia. From a therapeutic point of view, however, it means that a concentric reduction, if possible, must be obtained, because the head is not completely seated. For this reason it is appropriate to separate subluxation from dysplasia.

In subluxation the femoral head extrudes laterally from the acetabulum, but contact is maintained between their respective articular surfaces. The acetabulum is usually flattened and there is an increased obliquity of the cartilaginous roof. The perpendicular diameter of the socket is increased and the limbus is displaced upward.[17] Eventually the capsule thickens in the superior weight-bearing area.

Physical findings

In most cases of subluxation no abnormalities can be found on physical examination (Fig. 3-3). This ominous and worrisome situation explains why patients present themselves for the first time in late adolescence and adult life with painful hips that are the result of shallow, dificient acetabula and poorly covered femoral heads (Fig. 3-14). Often there will have been no identifiable clinical history of abnormality in childhood. The diagnostic physical findings will either have been totally absent or so subtle as to have been missed even by careful periodic examinations during later infancy and early childhood. The physical manifestations when present consist principally of an adduction contracture, *apparent* shortening, and asymmetric inguinal and thigh skin creases. There is almost always a stable hip, as can be determined by physical examination. In rare instances a positive subluxation-provocation test may be encountered during the first 6 weeks or 3 months of life; when this can be unequivocally demonstrated, an absolute diagnosis of a dislocatable hip can be made.

Roentgenographic changes

During these early weeks or months of life, the reliability and validity of the discernible changes in the infant's hip by radiography increases rapidly. When the physical findings exist as described earlier, significant alteration, as indicated on the film, will usually be evident so that a diagnosis of subluxation or "predislocation" can be made confidently. These abnormalities may include any one or all of the following: a delayed appearance of the capital femoral ossification center; an increased slope and abnormal configuration of the ossified acetabulum; and the lateral and upward displacement of the proximal femur (subluxation) (Fig. 3-15). Again, it is important to emphasize the need for a true anteroposterior view of the pelvis in order to make accurate evaluation of the hips possible.

Treatment

Because the femoral head still lies within the acetabulum and because the ultimate goal of treatment is the same as for newborn dysplasia, the treatment modalities are the same. The response to abduction treatment is usually prompt and predictable if undertaken in the period of early infancy (Fig. 3-16). However, the rapidity with which the hip corrects itself will depend a great deal on when or how early the diagnosis is made, on how earnestly the treatment was rendered, and, possibly, on whether or not a "primary" acetabular dysplasia exists. (The question of whether an acetabulum can have a "primary dysplasia" that is not secondary to dislocation is controversial

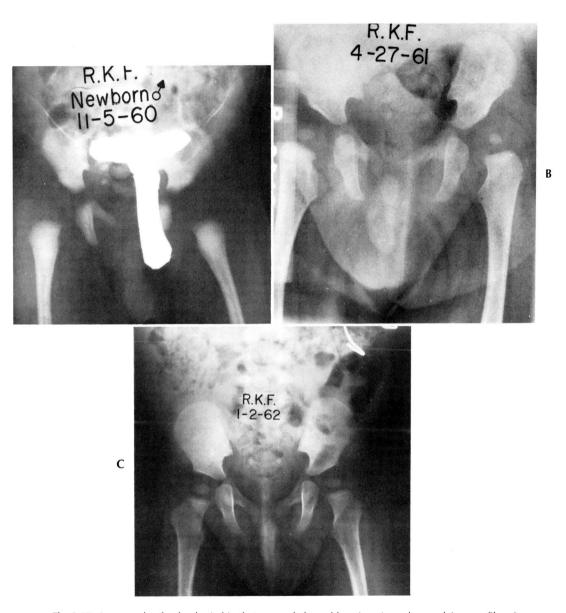

Fig. 3-15. An example of a dysplastic hip that proceeded to subluxation. A newborn pelvic x-ray film of a healthy male infant shows lateral displacement of the left hip, **A.** Both femora could be easily displaced from the acetabulum by manual manipulation. Recommended abduction treatment was refused. At 5 months of age an incidental follow-up x-ray film of the pelvis showed that the left hip was subluxated and that the right hip was clearly dysplastic, **B.** Clinically, both hips were stable and there were no diagnostic physical abnormalities at this time. Patient was hospitalized and placed in an abduction device for a period of 9 months. The result of such treatment is seen in **C.** Unfortunately, no further follow-up has been possible.

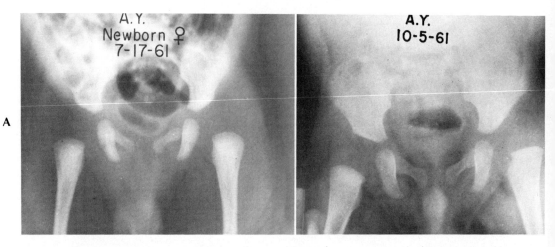

Fig. 3-16. Hip dislocation resulting from an untreated newborn dysplasia or subluxatable hip. The left hip could be easily passively subluxated shortly after birth, **A.** Subtle evidence of upward displacement on the left can be seen on the roentgenogram. Abduction treatment was recommended but refused, and on routine follow-up examination 3 months later the left hip was seen to be dislocated, **B.**

and has already been discussed in the section on etiology and pathogenesis in Chapter 2.)

I believe that such a condition as primary acetabular dysplasia does exist and, when found to be present, will not respond to the usual conventional measures of conservative abduction treatment.

NEONATAL DISLOCATION OF THE HIP

As noted earlier, the finding of a true, complete dislocation of the hip at birth is most unusual in the *otherwise normal* infant. Indeed, in contrast to dysplasia of the hip, I have seen only a few hips that were completely dislocated at birth that were not associated with other significant congenital abnormalities. When other significant musculoskeletal anomalies are present, such as myelomeningocele and arthrogryposis, a dislocated hip usually assumes a totally different profile and presents a different set of problems. For arbitrary and descriptive purposes these dislocations have been termed "teratologic."

Pathology

Thus, pathologically, two principal types of congenital dislocation of the hip can be defined: One includes the "typical" dislocation, which ordinarily manifests itself early in neonatal or postnatal life and is often not diagnosed before 3 months of age. The second (more rare) dislocation begins in utero and is usually associated with other abnormalities, both genetic and postural. This has been called the teratologic or "atypical" dislocation. Although some overlap may occasionally be encountered between these two conditions, it is helpful to employ this classification, especially from a therapeutic standpoint, because of the different set of problems usually presented by the atypical dislocation. It is for this reason that the teratologic dislocation will be discussed separately in Chapter 9.

The pathology of the typical dislocation will vary greatly depending on the age of the patient, but basically the essential problem is one of a complete dislocation such that the articular surfaces of the femoral head and acetabulum are not in contact. The mechanism by which the dislocation occurs is a much debated issue, and whether it occurs anteriorly, superiorly, or posteriorly has not been adequately or convincingly established. The most important issue, however, is not necessarily the direction by which the dislocation takes place, but rather the final location of the dislocated femoral head with respect to the acetabulum and the remainder of the pelvis. Hass[17] divided the condition into three basic groups—anterior, external, and posterior dislocations—with all demonstrating some degree of superior displacement. In 1939 McCarroll and Crego[28] reported ten patients with anterior dislocations; they believed that this was a distinct and separate entity. McCarroll again emphasized the importance of this particular dislocation in 1972.[29] Howorth and Smith[22] described a series of patients with anterior-superior dislocations, and later Farrell and Howorth[11] described another series having anterior dislocations. Hass[17] concluded that the process of dislocation involves a spectrum of behavior and that there are probably wide variations, not only from subluxation to dislocation, but also from anterior to posterior dislocation. These conclusions are compatible with mine.

It has been postulated that as the femoral head moves upward and outward beyond the limbus it deforms the limbus and pushes it upward. As the head continues to dislocate it slides above the limbus and tends to push the limbus back toward the acetabulum. On this hypothesis, the limbus, therefore, subsequently exerts a diminishing effect on the capacity of the acetabulum to receive the femoral head. This has led to the belief that the excision of the limbus is a necessary part of an open reduction. Putti,[35] on the other hand, concluded that the limbus played a part in preventing reduction only after the second or third year of life and only when a complete dislocation existed. It is my impression that the limbus can become infolded and can prevent reduction in rare instances, but as a rule it is not an essential part of the pathology.

In the young infant and child under 18 months of age, the dislocation will usually be simple and, except for a stretched and attenuated capsule and an elongated ligamentum teres, any other significant abnormalities in the cartilaginous skeleton will be rare. In older children more adaptive changes take place. The capsule becomes adherent to the outer wing of the ilium, and it undergoes considerable thickening in the superior weight-bearing area.[7] The inner surface of the capsule, which articulates with the femoral head, is smooth and glistening. Gradually in older children a constriction of the capsule takes place; this serves to obstruct efforts at reduction. The acetabulum becomes filled with a fibrofatty tissue, and additional more significant and potentially irreversible changes take place in the size and configuration of the acetabulum and femoral head. It is at this age that the challenge to the success of an attempted reduction becomes apparent.

Thus the pathology of dislocation is very complex and variable, largely reflecting the length of time the dislocation has persisted. Because of this, each age group presents its own special problems and challenges. For this reason the subsequent chapters are specifically oriented to different age groups.

Physical findings

When a dislocated hip is encountered at birth or during the neonatal period and is unencumbered by any associated abnormalities, the hip is usually easily reducible, and often it may be reduced on

68 Congenital dysplasia and dislocation of the hip

the examining table without anesthesia. This is especially true if the reduction is done gently and skillfully. The infant must be relaxed, preferably sucking from a bottle. Except for the dislocation that can be demonstrated by the Ortolani test, that is, the "jerk" of entry followed by a "jerk" of exit, there may be no other significant physical findings. In some patients, however, the usual findings associated with dislocation in the older infant are encounterd (Fig. 4-1). This means that the lower limb will actually be shorter (often difficult to demonstrate); there will be restricted abduction of the flexed thigh; the skin creases will be obviously asymmetric; and palpation of the hip area will reveal some asymmetry, *provided* that the dislocation is unilateral. In bilateral cases many of these findings will not be so apparent because they require comparison to the opposite hip in order to be conspicuous.

Roentgenographic findings

In contrast to *dysplasia* of the hip in the newborn, wherein a pelvic film may be completely normal, the pelvic roentgen-

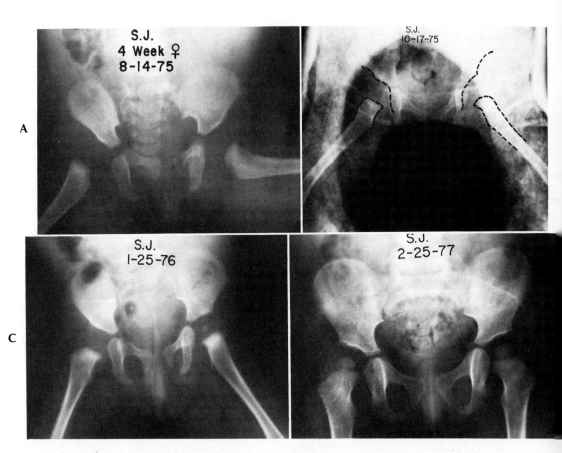

Fig. 3-17. This 4-week-old girl was found to have a dislocation of the right hip shortly after birth as seen in the pelvic x-ray film, **A.** The Ortolani sign was demonstrable on the examining table. After a preliminary period of skin traction, a closed reduction was accomplished without difficulty and a spica cast applied, **B.** Three and one-half months later a stable reduction had been achieved, although the femoral head ossification center had not yet appeared, **C.** One year later both hips were developing well, and the patient was fully ambulatory without a limp, **D.**

ogram will almost always be abnormal in instances of complete *dislocation.* The femoral metaphysis occupies a position upward and outward with respect to the acetabulum, the acetabular roof will *usually* have an increased slope, and other findings common to dysplastic hips will often be present (Fig. 3-17). Although there usually is very little doubt about the diagnosis, it is possible, nevertheless, that the film may not be diagnostic. Most often this depends on the manner in which the hip is positioned at the time the film is taken.

Treatment

There are two basic determinations that must be made in order to treat this condition appropriately during the neonatal period. The first is to determine the ease with which reduction can be achieved, and the second is to identify the degree of stability of the hip following reduction. It is also necessary to gain some idea of the reliability of the parents; the reason for this relates to the efficacy with which certain treatment programs can be expected to be carried out.

In those patients in whom the reduction can be easily accomplished, my preference for treatment of the truly dislocated hip in the neonate is the simple application of a hip spica cast, under very light general anesthesia. The femoral head should merely be "repositioned," and the anesthetic is administered only for the purpose of holding the child motionless while the cast is applied with the hip reduced. Under no circumstances should any forceful manipulation or extreme positions of the lower limb be utilized. The position of the lower limbs following reduction should be one in which there is no more than 45 to 60 degrees of abduction, as much flexion as is necessary for stability, and a relatively neutral rotation (Fig. 4-5). The cast remains in place for no more than 6 to 8 weeks, at which time there should be sufficient stability that a removable, flexible abduction device may be safely employed. My preference is the plastic abduction splint illustrated in Fig. 4-7; however, one may employ any of the devices that effectively maintain reduction, such as those used in the treatment of dysplasia. Customarily this second device is removed only for baths for another 6 weeks and, then, if both physical and roentgenographic findings confirm the maintenance of concentricity and the stability of reduction, the infant is gradually weaned from the splint. During the weaning process, usually the abduction device is utilized at naps and at night, then at night only, and finally, as the roentgenogram reveals progressive improvement in the development of the femoral head and acetabulum, the device is discontinued.

Another approach to the treatment of true dislocation in the neonate is the use of the Pavlik harness. In this method the device is employed as a gentle active-reduction mechanism (guided reduction) and is thereafter used to hold the hip reduced. MacEwen,[27] Ramsey and associates,[36] and Lovell[26] have found in reliable situations that this represents a very effective method and that it eliminates the need for a cast or for anesthesia. Because I believe that reduction should be accomplished as early as possible and that the femoral head should be concentrically reduced and held reduced, I prefer the former therapeutic approach. However, the Pavlik harness method does have some very attractive features.[27]

It is extremely important that faithful follow-up examinations be conducted at periodic intervals throughout the entire growth period of the patient. Intervals of 3 to 6 months are satisfactory for the first 2 or 3 years, and if appropriate development of the hip takes place these follow-up periods may be lengthened. At each visit a careful physical examination should be made, but roentgenograms are only taken as judgment dictates. The principal observations that need to be made in their order of relative importance are: the maintenance of concentricity of reduction; a progressive improvement in the acetabular ossification and femoral head coverage; the state of health of the capital femoral epiphysis, that is, a determination of whether it is ossifying properly and growing at a rate comparable to the normal side; the configuration of the proximal femur, specifically with respect to any angular or rotational abnormalities; and finally, the normality of the cartilage or clear space of the joint. As will be seen subsequently, any significant variation from normal in any of these parameters has considerable bearing on the subsequent anatomy and function of the hip joint. The significance of any of these adverse or undesirable sequelae will be discussed in Chapter 7.

By the age of 5 or 6 years, the adult bony configuration of the acetabulum should have been achieved, or at least continued improvement of the acetabular-femoral relationship should be evident. By the age of 13 years, an essentially normal adult hip should be present. This means that the femoral head and acetabulum are spherical and congruent; that the femoral head is normal in appearance and is well covered, having a C-E angle in excess of 20 degrees (preferably 30 degrees); that the cartilage space is normal; and that the configuration of the proximal femur is normal. Any significant deviation from these observations will almost surely result in some degree of future disability resulting from the development of secondary degenerative arthritis.

"IRREDUCIBLE" NEONATAL DISLOCATION

Occasionally a neonatal hip dislocation will be encountered that cannot be easily reduced or that is totally irreducible, even shortly after birth. Most of these will be antenatal, teratologic dislocations that present significantly greater problems in management. They must be approached in a highly individualized manner, and the need for preliminary traction and possible open reduction must be entertained. Ordinarily such difficult hips are best left unreduced for several months until the child becomes old enough to be considered for skin traction and probable open reduction. In these situations the approach to the problem is the same as for dislocations in the older infant and child, a subject that is discussed in Chapter 4.

REFERENCES

1. Andrén, L., and von Rosen, S.: The diagnosis of dislocation of the hip in newborns and the primary results of immediate treatment, Acta Radiol. **49:**89, 1958.
2. Barlow, T. G.: Early diagnosis and treatment of congenital dislocation of the hip, J. Bone Joint Surg. **44B:**292, 1962.
3. Burman, M. S., and Clark, C. H.: A roentgenologic study of the hip joint of the infant in the first twelve months of life, Am. J. Roentgenol. Radium Ther. Nucl. Med. **44:**37, 1940.
4. Caffey, J., Ames, R., Silverman, W. A., Ryder, C. T., and Hough, G.: Contradiction of the congenital dysplasia-predislocation hypothesis of congenital dislocation of the hip through a study of the normal variation in acetabular angles at successive periods in infancy, Pediatrics **17:**632, 1956.
5. Coleman, S. S.: Diagnosis of congenital dysplasia of the hip in the newborn infant, J.A.M.A. **162:**548, 1956.
6. Coleman, S. S.: Congenital dysplasia of the hip in the Navajo infant, Clin. Orthop. **56:**179, 1968.
7. Colonna, P. C.: Capsular arthroplasty for congenital dislocation of the hip, J. Bone Joint Surg. **35A:**179, 1953.
8. Colonna, P. C.: Care of the infant with congenital subluxation of the hip, J.A.M.A. **166:**715, 1958.
9. Cyvin, K. B.: Congenital dislocation of the hip joint: clinical studies with special reference to the pathogenesis, Acta Pediatr. Scand. [Suppl.] **263:**1, 1977.
10. Desche, P., Courtois, B., Carlioz, H., and Scott, P. J.: Symposium on an experience in screen-

ing dislocatable hips, Ann. Orthopediques de l'ouest, no. 9, 1977.
11. Farrell, B. P., and Howorth, M. B.: Open reduction in congenital dislocation of the hip, J. Bone Joint Surg. **17**:35, 1935.
12. Harris, W. H.: Personal communication.
13. Hart, V. L.: Primary genetic dysplasia of the hip with and without classical dislocation, J. Bone Joint Surg. **24**:753, 1942.
14. Hart, V. L.: Congenital dysplasia of the hip joint, J. Bone Joint Surg. **31A**:357, 1949.
15. Hart, V. L.: Congenital dislocation of the hip in the newborn and in early postnatal life, J.A.M.A. **143**:1299, 1950.
16. Hart, V. L.: Congenital dysplasia of the hip joint and sequelae, Springfield, Ill., 1952, Charles C Thomas, Publisher.
17. Hass, J.: Congenital dislocation of the hip, Springfield, Ill., 1951, Charles C Thomas, Publisher.
18. Hass, J.: Can congenital dislocation of the hip be prevented? N.Y. State J. Med. **58**:847, 1958.
19. Heublein, G. W., Bernstein, L., and Hubenet, B. J.: Hip lesions of infants and children seen at the Newington Home and Hospital for Crippled Children, Radiology **51**:611, 1948.
20. Hilgenreiner, H.: Zur Frühdiagnose und Frühbehandlung der angeborenen Hüftgelenkverrenkung, Med. Klin. **21**:1385, 1925.
21. Howorth, M. B.: The etiology of congenital dislocation of the hip, Clin. Orthop. **29**:164, 1963.
22. Howorth, M. B., and Smith, H. W.: Congenital dislocation of the hip treated by open operation, J. Bone Joint Surg. **14**:299, 1932.
23. Kleinberg, S., and Lieberman, H. S.: The acetabular index in infants in relation to congenital dislocation of the hip, Arch. Surg. **32**:1049, 1936.
24. Laurenson, R. D.: The acetabular index: a critical review, J. Bone Joint Surg. **41B**:702, 1959.
25. Levine, D. B.: Unpublished data.
26. Lovell, W. W.: Personal communication.
27. MacEwen, G. D.: Personal communication.
28. McCarroll, H. R., and Crego, C. H.: Primary anterior congenital dislocation of the hip, J. Bone Joint Surg. **21**:648, 1939.
29. McCarroll, H. R., Jr., and McCarroll, H. R.: Primary anterior dislocation of the hip in infancy, J. Bone Joint Surg. **54A**:1340, 1972.
30. Ortolani, M.: La lussazione congenital dell' anca, Bologna, 1948, Casa Editrice Licinio Cappelli.
31. Palmèn, K.: Preluxation of the hip joint, Acta Pediatr. [Suppl.] (Uppsala) **50**(129):1, 1961.
32. Perkins, G.: Signs by which to diagnose congenital dislocation of the hip, Lancet **214**:648, 1928.
33. Putti, V.: Congenital dislocation of the hip, Surg. Gynecol. Obstet. **42**:449, 1926.
34. Putti, V.: Early treatment of congenital dislocation of the hip, J. Bone Joint Surg. **11**:798, 1929.
35. Putti, V.: Early treatment of congenital dislocation of the hip, J. Bone Joint Surg. **15**:16, 1933.
36. Ramsey, P. L., Lasser, S., and MacEwen, G. D.: Congenital dislocation of the hip: use of the Pavlik harness in the child during the first 6 months of life, J. Bone Joint Surg. **58A**:1000, 1976.
37. Salter, R. B.: Etiology, pathogenesis and possible prevention of congenital dislocation of the hip, Can. Med. Assoc. J. **98**:933, 1968.
38. Salter, R. B.: Textbook of disorders and injuries of the musculoskeletal system, Baltimore, 1970, The Williams & Wilkins Co., p. 98.
39. Severin, E.: Arthrography in congenital dislocation of the hip, J. Bone Joint Surg. **21**:304, 1939.
40. Soutter, R., and Lovett, R. W.: Congenital dislocation of the hip: a study of 227 dislocations, J.A.M.A. **82**:171, 1924.
41. Stanisavljevic, S.: Diagnosis and treatment of congenital hip pathology in the newborn, Baltimore, 1963, The Williams & Wilkins Co.
42. von Rosen, S.: Early diagnosis and treatment of congenital dislocation of the hip, Acta Orthop. Scand. **26**:136, 1956.
43. von Rosen, S.: Diagnosis and treatment of congenital dislocation of the hip in newborns, J. Bone Joint Surg. **44B**:284, 1962.

CHAPTER 4

Diagnosis and treatment of congenital dislocation in the child under 18 months of age

Diagnosis
   Physical findings
   Radiographic features
   Pathology of dislocation
   Pathology of primary anterior dislocation
Treatment
   Traction and closed reduction
   Cast position
   Open reduction

DIAGNOSIS

If the diagnosis of hip dysplasia is not made during the newborn period, specific treatment will likely not be administered. The subsequent behavior of the dysplastic hip may result in either normal hip development, a persistent dysplasia, a subluxation, or a complete dislocation (see Chapter 3). As noted earlier, the physical and roentgenographic findings will vary widely depending on which of these conditions eventuate. As emphasized in the previous section, the earlier the diagnosis is made in either case, the more effective and less complicated will be the treatment.

Physical findings

Once a complete dislocation has occurred, the physical findings are nearly always diagnostic in the later months of infancy. The typical abnormalities will include true shortening, limited abduction of the flexed thigh, deeper and more numerous inguinal and thigh creases, shortening of the knee height with the flexed hip (Galeazzi), and occasionally an outward rotation attitude of the lower limb (Fig. 4-1). The findings will differ depending on whether the dislocation is unilateral or bilateral. During the first year of life there obviously will be no gait abnormalities to assist in the diagnosis. In the early months of life occasionally a hip that is clearly dislocated can be readily reduced on the examining table. The younger the infant and the more recent the dislocation, the greater the likelihood that this sign can be elicited. It is the reverse of the subluxation-provocation test and is the jerk of entry described by Ortolani.[9] In some young infants under 1 year of age, the previously existing limited abduction largely disappears when the hip is reduced by this maneuver. Then, when the thigh is again adducted, the femoral head can be felt and seen to exit from the acetabulum, demonstrating the so-called jerk of exit. This demonstration of instability and reducibility of the hip is the most reliable physical sign of dislocation, but unfortunately it can only be elicited in a minority of instances of the young infants in their early months of postnatal life.

Diagnosis and treatment in the child under 18 months of age

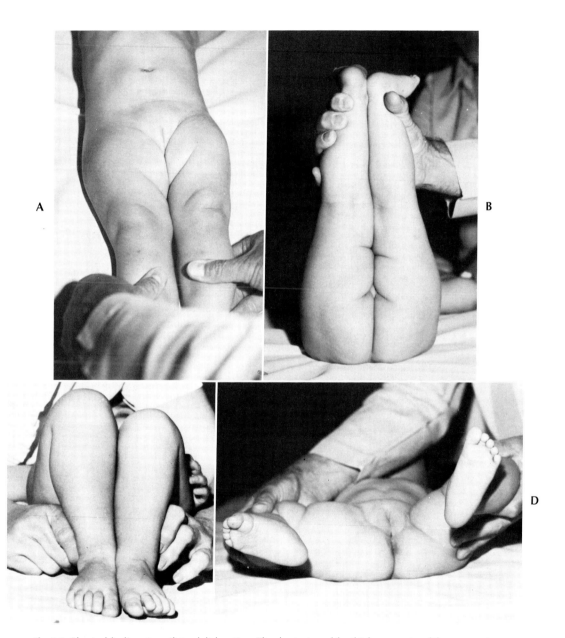

Fig. 4-1. Physical findings in unilateral dislocation. The shortening of the thigh segment and the asymmetry and deepening of inguinal and thigh creases on the left are well seen, **A.** These same manifestations are illustrated from the posterior view in **B.** Restriction of abduction of the flexed thigh is seen in **D,** and the knee level is seen lower on the left as shown in the Galeazzi test, **C.**

Radiographic features

As stated earlier, the pelvis undergoes its most rapid postnatal growth during the first year of life, and the changes seen on the pelvic x-ray film may show a considerable variation in the degree of abnormality throughout this period of growth. The dislocated femoral head usually ossifies much later than normal, and it occupies an upward and lateral position with respect to the acetabulum. The slope of the acetabular roof is higher than normal and the articular cortex is less well developed and may even be convex rather than concave as seen in normally developing hips. The ischiopubic synchondrosis is often delayed in its maturation, and the growing ossification centers of the pelvis will often be slightly retarded in their development (Fig. 4-2).

Pathology of dislocation

One of the classic reviews dealing with the pathology of congenital hip dislocation is that by Hass.[2] Most authors agree that the femoral head may be dislocated either anteriorly, laterally, or posteriorly, and always superiorly. In all instances the acetabulum, depending on the duration of the dislocation, manifests certain changes. The capacity is reduced, the pulvinar undergoes hypertrophy, the ligamentum teres becomes enlarged and elongated, the cartilage of the acetabulum thickens, and ultimately there is hypertrophy of the acetabular bony wall. Thus the socket becomes more shallow, the acetabular roof becomes more oblique, and ultimately, as Hass stated, "at a more advanced age, the acetabulum undergoes progressive involution, until finally it is transformed into a shallow depression, triangular in shape, and with an amorphous surface, with practically no resemblance to its former shape."[2]

The femoral head undergoes a reduction in size, and a gradual medioposterior flattening occurs. The femoral neck commonly exhibits increased coxa valga and occasionally coxa vara. Anteversion is also often increased, because of failure of the infant proximal femur to undergo its normal remodeling process in the direction of less anteversion. Variations in these abnormalities have been observed, however, depending on whether or not the dislocation was posterior, as is usually the case. In this situation the femoral

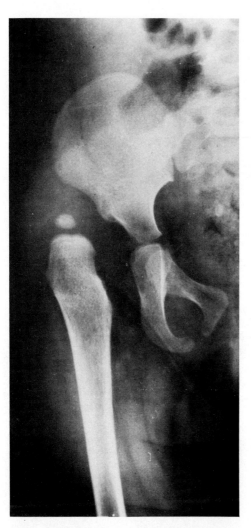

Fig. 4-2. Roentgenogram of complete dislocation of the hip in an 18-month-old child. The acetabulum is poorly formed and there is no significant shadow of articular cortex, indicating lack of effective articulation.

head is often well shaped and has a reasonably normal angle of anteversion.

Pathology of primary anterior dislocation

In a very small number of cases the femoral head lies anterior to the acetabulum and is usually accompanied by excessive anteversion. McCarroll and Crego[7] believed that it is important to identify this particular dislocation because of the need for a modification of treatment. Specifically, it is necessary to reduce the hip by traction and internal rotation of the thigh, followed by rotational osteotomy in order to correct the anteversion. I have seen only one such dislocation in an otherwise normal child (Fig. 4-12). Most anterior dislocations will be of the teratologic type, as seen in arthrogryposis.

TREATMENT
Traction and closed reduction

The great majority of patients in this age group can be treated by closed methods, utilizing a preliminary period of traction and a gentle closed reduction (repositioning), followed by appropriate immobilization in a hip spica cast (Fig. 4-3). Unless this effort fails there is no need to consider open reduction.

There has been and still exists a controversy regarding the relative values of skeletal vs skin traction preliminary to closed reduction. Arguments favoring skeletal traction include the following: (1) the ability to apply greater weight; (2) a reduced likelihood of skin problems (blister and tape reactions); (3) better control of rotation during traction; and (4) greater versatility for use in children of any age. Those favoring skin traction support it for the following reasons: (1) it is a noninvasive technique, thus pin tract and other complications of skeletal traction are avoided (epiphyseal plate injuries, etc.); and (2) it is easier to apply and implement.

I prefer skin traction for this age group. An arbitrary 2-week period of traction should precede any effort at gentle closed reduction under general anesthesia. The direction in which the traction exerts this effect is of some importance, but complete agreement on this issue has not been reached. In general, skin traction should not exceed 45 degrees of flexion or be less than 30 degrees of flexion. The reason for this is the fact that traction with the hip in full extension tends to tighten the hip capsule and as a result may compromise blood supply to the femoral head. On the other hand, if there is too much flexion, then the adductors and hip flexors (especially the iliopsoas) cannot be appropriately stretched. However, some believe that overhead flexion is the preferred route, because the hip is dislocated posteriorly and the goal of traction is to bring it anteriorly. Abduction should also not exceed 45 degrees, and this amount of abduction should be reached gradually. If the femoral head is upwardly displaced and the thighs abducted too early, it is conceivable (though not proved) that the limbus and/or portions of the superior joint capsule may be forced into the acetabulum during traction. Conceptually, it is attractive to attempt to maintain some degree of knee flexion during traction in order to relax the hamstrings[5]; however, I found this difficult to accomplish.

Care must be exercised to ascertain that the weight is not excessive and that the method of application of the skin traction is appropriate. Furthermore, in this age group it is best to place both limbs in traction because of the difficulty encountered in controlling the pelvis if traction is exerted on only one limb. Two to 4 pounds is about the maximum traction necessary and probably safe in children at this age; the skin pull should encompass the entire leg and thigh on both sides (Fig. 4-4). Application of some nonallergenic adhesive is very important. Over this a snug stock-

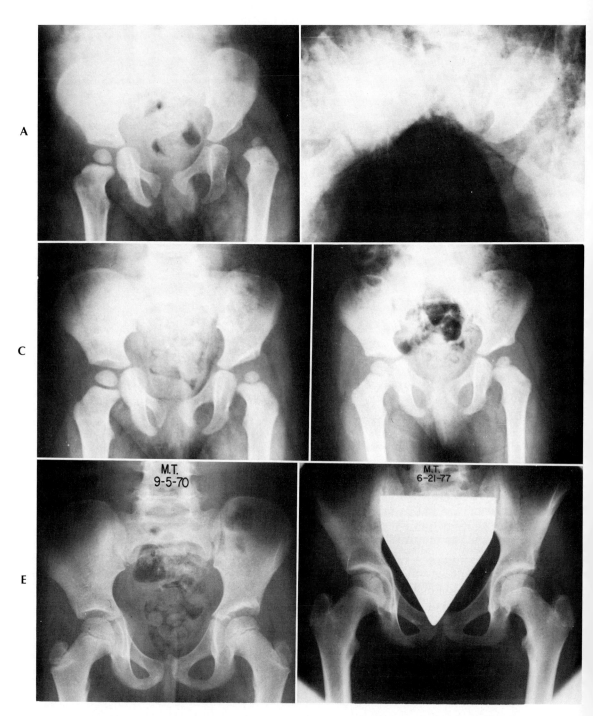

Fig. 4-3. Pelvic x-ray film of a 12-month-old female with dislocation of left hip, **A.** After 2 weeks of skin traction a closed reduction was accomplished, **B.** Seven months later the hip was stable and concentrically reduced, **C.** Roentgenograms taken at 2, 5, and 12 years of age reveal normal hip development, **D, E,** and **F.** The end result was a normal gait and physical examination.

Diagnosis and treatment in the child under 18 months of age 77

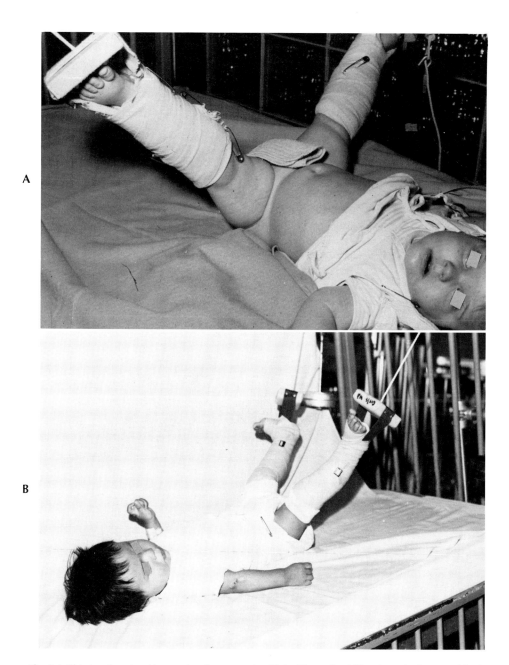

Fig. 4-4. Skin traction should extend well up onto the thighs. There should be about 45 degrees of flexion and comparable degrees of abduction of the thighs, **A** and **B.**

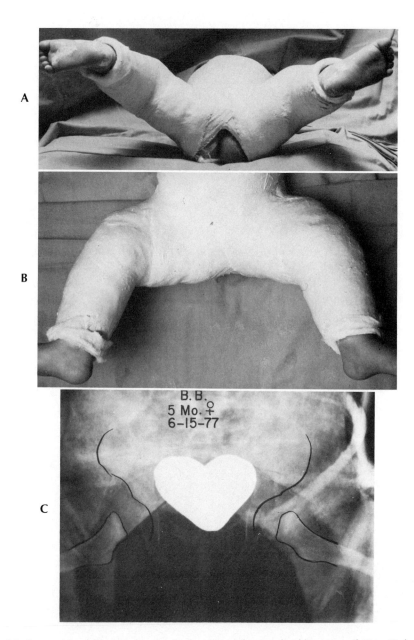

Fig. 4-5. Cast position following closed reduction. The abduction should not exceed 45 to 60 degrees, as shown in **A.** Thigh flexion should be provided according to requirements for stability, **B.** In the illustrations the perineal area of cast was subsequently cut out. Roentgenogram of this patient is seen in **C.**

inette is applied. Wide adhesive strips are applied over the surface of the stockinette and then wrapped with one or two snug layers of sheet wadding. This protects the bony prominences. An Ace bandage is then used to hold the adhesive strips on the limb, and the weights are placed on the adhesive tape as it extends from the foot as a stirrup.

The circulatory and neuromuscular status of the foot and toes should be checked several times a day by professional observers (nurses and/or the physician). If at any time there is any unexplained pain or a suggestion of circulatory or neurologic compromise, the traction must be discontinued immediately. This form of traction is not painful, and infants should not be fretful or fussy during the 2 weeks in which it is employed. During this traction period the surgeon may make attempts at reducing the hip, and often the femoral head can be repositioned easily if the child is temporarily removed from traction.

After the arbitrary 2-week period of traction, the patient is given a general anesthetic and the femoral head is gently

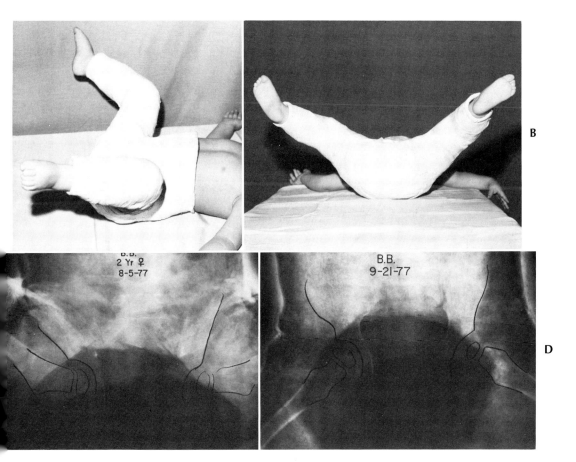

Fig. 4-6. The axillary or "human" position of hip spica plaster immobilization is illustrated in this patient. The thighs are flexed 10 or 20 degrees above a right angle, **A,** yet they are not abducted more than 50 degrees, **B.** The pelvic x-ray shows the flexed position of the hips, **C.** The limbs were subsequently brought downward as hip stability was achieved. The new position is seen in **D.**

repositioned into the acetabulum. No force should be used at any time. If a stable concentric reduction is achieved, then the same program is carried out as in the instance of neonatal dislocation. The hip spica cast is applied in the same manner, with the thighs held in 90 degrees more or less of flexion, but *no more* than 60 degrees of abduction (Fig. 4-5).

Cast position

Occasionally the reduced hip is stable only when the hips are flexed well above 90 degrees (Fig. 4-6). This is known commonly as the "axillary" position, presumably because of the proximity of the knees to the infant's axillae. This position of greater flexion causes no harm to the infant's hips *provided* that abduction does not exceed 45 to 60 degrees. In fact this flexed position has been called the human position by Salter and associates[10] because it simulates the normal healthy intrauterine fetal position of the thighs. Usually it is necessary to keep the thighs in this position for only 6 weeks, after which the position of the thighs is changed to a more conventional position of considerably less flexion. Thereafter, the elimination of the cast and initiation of bracing or splinting is an individual matter.

The initial cast is changed at 6 weeks and the thigh is brought down into less flexion and abduction. Roentgenographic verification of stability and concentricity of reduction must be made 1 week following the initial reduction and again at 6 weeks when the cast is changed. The second cast remains on for 6 more weeks; by this time the hip should be stable by physical examination and should be concentrically reduced by radiographic examination. An abduction device of the surgeon's choice may then be employed to maintain the thighs in modest flexion, abduction, and outward rotation (Fig. 4-7). The patient is gradually weaned from this device over the succeeding months. If the hip remains stable and the pelvic roentgenogram shows a satisfactory degree of reciprocal growth and development of the femoral head and acetabulum, then the device may gradually be discarded. Follow-up care must be rendered in the same fashion as described for open reduction in the following section.

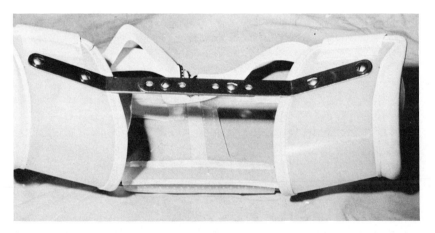

Fig. 4-7. Metal-reinforced, semirigid plastic abduction device. It is simple, easy to clean, and cannot abduct the thighs more than 60 degrees.

Open reduction

In the instance wherein concentric reduction cannot be achieved by an appropriate period of skin traction followed by gentle repositioning of the femoral head into the acetabulum, open reduction is indicated. Many factors enter into the decision to do an open reduction, and an equal number of variables exist governing the surgical approach that should be used. These controversies simply reinforce the highly individual and variable nature of the problems inherent in the treatment of congenital dislocation of the hip as well as emphasize the need for accurate definition of the problem prior to planning any therapeutic approach.

Operative treatment. Over the years significant developments in our surgical knowledge and technical expertise have occurred that provide improved guidelines for the surgical treatment of congenital hip dislocation. Our persisting challenge, as well as our dilemma, however, consists of the need for more clearly defined criteria to serve as indications for open intervention in congenital dislocation.

It has been argued that a properly performed open reduction of a congenitally dislocated hip may result in a reduced incidence of osseous and cartilage necrosis, a lesser likelihood of redislocation, and a better prognosis for ultimate and overall function of the hip. This is true for many children over 18 months of age, and it also holds true occasionally for children with a dislocated hip under 18 months of age. Thus as our knowledge of the highly individualized characteristics of congenital hip dislocation has increased, it has become established that in some situations operative treatment may be preferable to nonoperative, even though conceptually a successfully accomplished closed reduction offers greater advantages over open reduction.

Indications for open reduction. The primary indication for open reduction is failure to achieve a concentric, stable reduction by closed methods. In order to define "failure" and put it into perspective, it is essential to review the principles and concepts of closed reduction, as discussed earlier, and as herein summarized. First, preliminary skin traction for an arbitrary minimal period of 2 weeks is essential prior to an attempt at closed reduction; second, a general anesthetic should be given at the time of reduction, primarily to hold the infant quiet and immobile during application of the cast; third, the femoral head should simply be "repositioned" with no force at all being applied by the surgeon; fourth, the hip should be stable in a "physiologic" position. Finally, a postreduction x-ray film should be taken in order to show the hip to be concentrically reduced. If any one or more than one of these precepts are impossible to implement, or if they do not apply, then serious consideration should be given to open reduction. In summary, therefore, if the femoral head cannot easily be repositioned in a stable, physiologic position, or if a concentric reduction cannot be achieved, then open reduction should be considered.

As an extension of these rather general indications for open reduction in this younger age group, certain more specific indications can be listed. These are: (1) the irreducible hip, evident after an appropriate period of skin traction; (2) a hip that can be reduced closed but is grossly unstable in any position (in this instance, the femoral head is probably not well seated in the socket) (Fig. 4-8); (3) a hip that can be reduced satisfactorily, but that must be held in excessive abduction and forced internal or external rotation (an unphysiologic position that may compromise blood supply to the femoral head); and (4) finally, the hip that is not concentrically reduced ("stands out") fol-

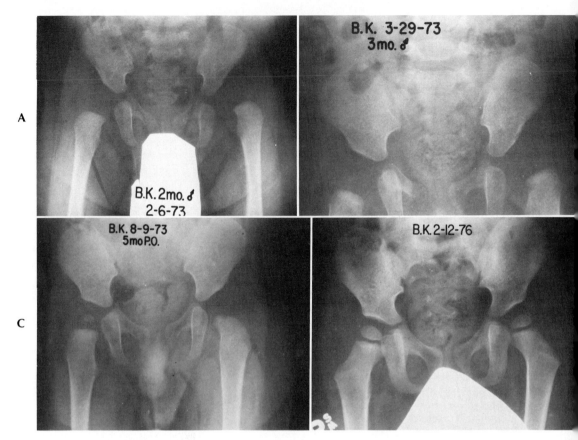

Fig. 4-8. Pelvic x-ray films of 2-month-old male with dislocation of left hip, **A.** An effort at closed reduction following preliminary traction failed, as evidenced by persistent dislocation 6 weeks later, **B.** A second effort at traction and closed reduction failed, and an open reduction via the medial (adductor) approach was accomplished. Five months postoperatively the hip was well reduced, **C**; 3 years later the hip was developing well, **D.**

lowing satisfactory closed reduction (Fig. 4-9).

The decision to accomplish an open reduction, however, must justify the added risks attendant on open reduction. These include the technical difficulties occasionally ascertained in the operation; the potential adverse effects of intra-articular scarring; possible mechanical damage to articular cartilage; and surgical infection. In the modern hospital and in the hands of an experienced pediatric hip surgeon, these potential problems can readily be justified in the presence of properly defined indications as listed in the preceding paragraph.

Methods of open reduction. The method of surgical approach must always be the surgeon's choice, based on the surgeon's own expertise and analysis of the problem. There are two well-established surgical approaches that can be utilized in open reduction of the infant hip. The one most commonly employed is the anterior approach, which is made through an iliofemoral incision or a variation of that incision. The second is that method originally described by Ludloff[4] and re-

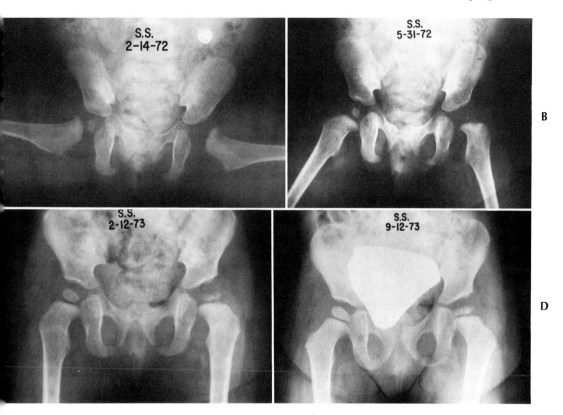

Fig. 4-9. Five-month-old female infant with dislocated left hip treated by closed reduction and abduction in plaster cast in "Lorenz" position, **A**. On removal of cast the hip remains subluxated ("standing out"), with metaphyseal changes suggesting femoral head necrosis, **B**. An open reduction via the medial (adductor) approach was accomplished, and satisfactory seating and development of the hip joint can be seen at 7 months and 15 months after surgery, **C** and **D**.

cently popularized by Mau[6] and Ferguson.[1] This approach to the hip joint is made via a medial (adductor) incision. Each has its advantages and disadvantages, which will be discussed subsequently after the technical details of both have been reviewed.

Technique of open reduction by the anterior (iliofemoral) approach. Through an incision placed over the anterior one third of the iliac crest and extending distally 2 or 3 inches over the proximal thigh, the lateral aspect of the ilium is exposed subperiosteally (Fig. 4-10). The apophysis is left undisturbed. The interval between the sartorius muscle and the tensor fasciae latae muscle is developed, and the sartorius muscle is sectioned at its origin from the anterior-superior iliac spine. The capsule of the hip joint is exposed directly beneath the overlying rectus femoris muscle. Tenotomy and upward reflection of the straight and reflected heads of the rectus femoris muscle aid in exposure of the capsule. At this point the iliopsoas muscle and tendon should be sectioned at or near their insertion on the lesser trochanter. This is helpful because it not only further exposes the anterior and inferior aspects of the capsule, but it also releases one of the most important structures commonly preventing con-

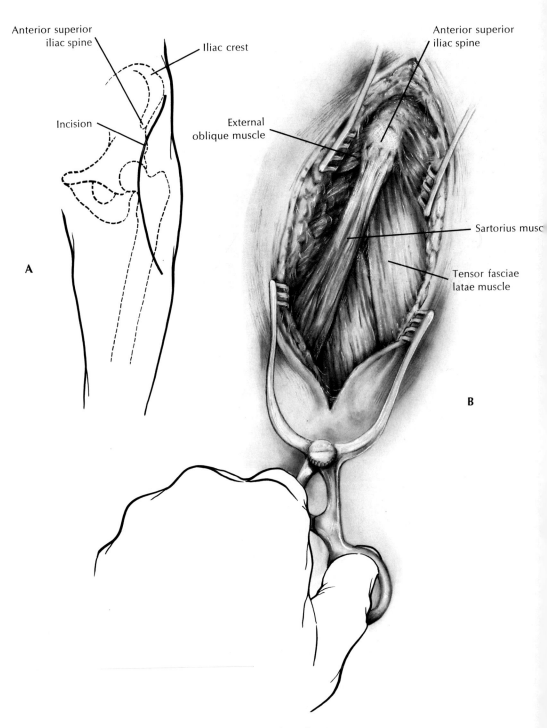

Fig. 4-10. For legend see p. 86.

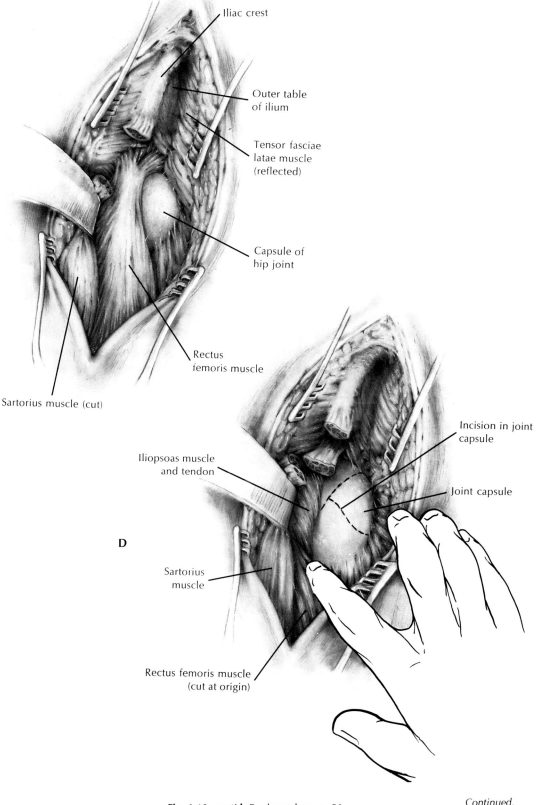

Fig. 4-10, cont'd. For legend see p. 86.

Continued.

86 Congenital dysplasia and dislocation of the hip

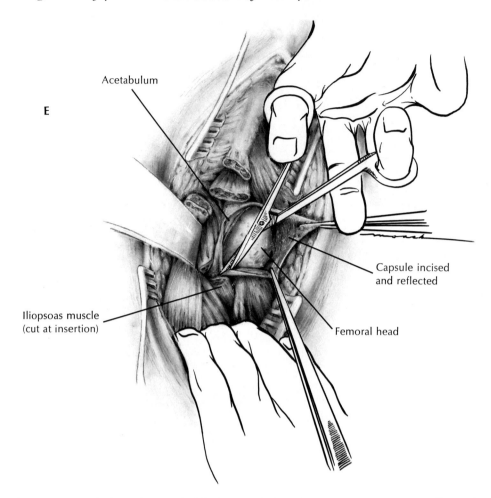

Fig. 4-10. Anterior iliofemoral approach to the hip is made through a generous anterior incision illustrated in **A.** The crest of the ilium and attached muscles and tendons are exposed, **B.** By reflection of the abductor muscles from the outer table of the ilium, the underlying hip capsule is exposed. The sartorius muscle is severed at its origin in order to enhance exposure, **C.** The rectus femoris muscle is detached from its origin and the anterior aspect of the capsule is further exposed. A T-shaped incision is made in the capsule to expose the femoral head, **D.** The iliopsoas muscle is then sectioned, along with the anterior and inferior aspects of the capsule, **E.** Removal of the ligamentum teres is optional, but the transverse acetabular ligament must be cut. The femoral head is reduced, the capsule is repaired by plication, and the wound is closed.

centric reduction of the congenitally dislocated hip (the iliopsoas tendon). At this juncture the hip capsule should be incised, with special attention being directed to releasing the anterior and inferior portions of the capsule as well as the transverse acetabular ligament. Great care should be exercised so that the cartilage on the femoral head is not damaged. The acetabulum is explored and cleaned of excess fat if necessary. Reduction usually is accomplished with ease. Most often the round ligament may have to be excised. Nearly always there is no evidence of appreciable blood supply seen in the cut end of the ligament.

After reduction is achieved an x-ray examination should be made in order to verify adequacy and concentricity of reduction. The capsule should be closed after any redundant portions have been excised. The iliopsoas tendon is not necessarily repaired, but all other tendons are reattached and the wound is closed. A one and one-half hip spica cast is applied with the hip being held in the most stable position. This is usually neutral or slight internal rotation with about 30 degrees of flexion and abduction.

The cast is retained for 2 or 3 months, depending on the child's age. If at that time x-ray and clinical examination reveal sufficient stability, the cast may be discontinued and the patient is allowed to regain hip ranges of motion, but without ambulation. A removable splint that holds the lower limbs in abduction and neutral rotation is employed day and night. Daily ranges of hip motion are performed under supervision of a therapist. The splint may be either the posterior half of the spica cast or an abduction bar attached to shoes. If, on the other hand, there is a question regarding stability, then another cast is applied for an additional 6 weeks. After this second period of immobilization, further casting is rarely necessary and the removable abduction splint can be safely utilized. Weight bearing may gradually be instituted. Thereafter, some type of nighttime retaining and positioning device, as described on p. 62, should be employed until a satisfactory range of motion is achieved and good hip stability is evident.

Technique of open reduction by the medial (adductor) approach. With the involved limb held in flexion, abduction, and external rotation, a longitudinal 3-inch incision is made over the proximal adductor region of the thigh, beginning with the adductor tubercle and extending distally over the course of the adductor longus tendon (Fig. 4-11). Alternatively, a transverse incision of similar length can be made over the adductor region just distal to the pubic tubercle. The adductor longus tendon is sectioned at its origin and reflected, thus exposing the underlying adductor brevis muscle. Using blunt digital dissection the interval posterior to the adductor brevis muscle is developed, and with the thigh held in flexion, abduction, and external rotation, the lesser trochanter can be easily palpated in this intermuscular interval. The iliopsoas tendon is then visualized and the fatty areolar tissue is removed about its insertion. A curved hemostat is placed beneath the tendon, and it is either lengthened by Z-plasty or sectioned transversely. The iliopsoas tendon and muscle are then reflected upward, exposing the underlying hip capsule. A curved retractor is placed over the neck and capsule of the femur, just beneath the iliopsoas tendon. The entire anterior, superior, and inferior portions of the capsule can be easily seen at this point, and the capsule is opened by a cruciate incision. The transverse acetabular ligament is then sectioned. The joint can be explored fairly well by this approach, but not quite so clearly or thoroughly as with the anterior method. The hip is usually easily reducible at this point, and often the elongated, somewhat hypertrophic ligamentum teres can be seen to lie redundantly within the socket. Unless it is a significant hindrance to reduction, the ligament need not be removed. Rarely excision of a limbus is necessary in order to accomplish reduction by this approach.

For stability, the femur is held in 30 degrees of abduction and flexion along with slight internal rotation. In this position the hip capsule cannot and should not be closed. The thigh must be held in this position during application of the spica cast.

During closure the adductor longus

88 Congenital dysplasia and dislocation of the hip

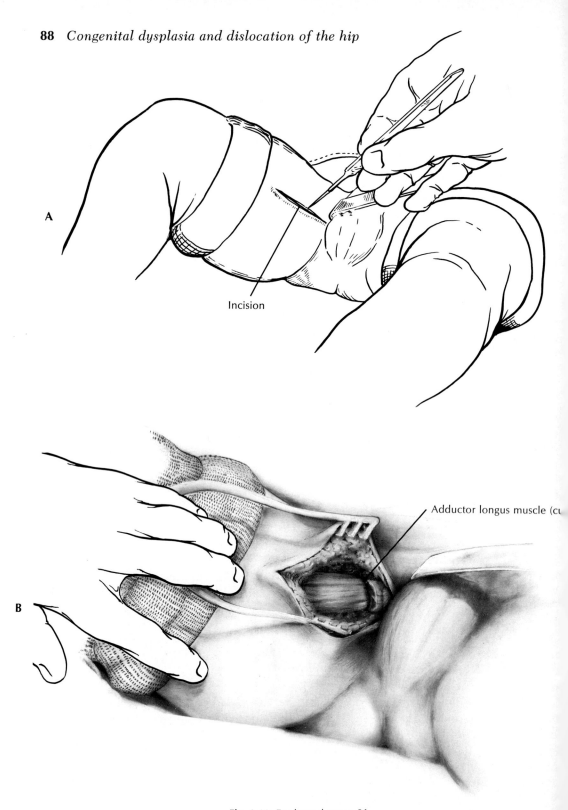

Fig. 4-11. For legend see p. 91.

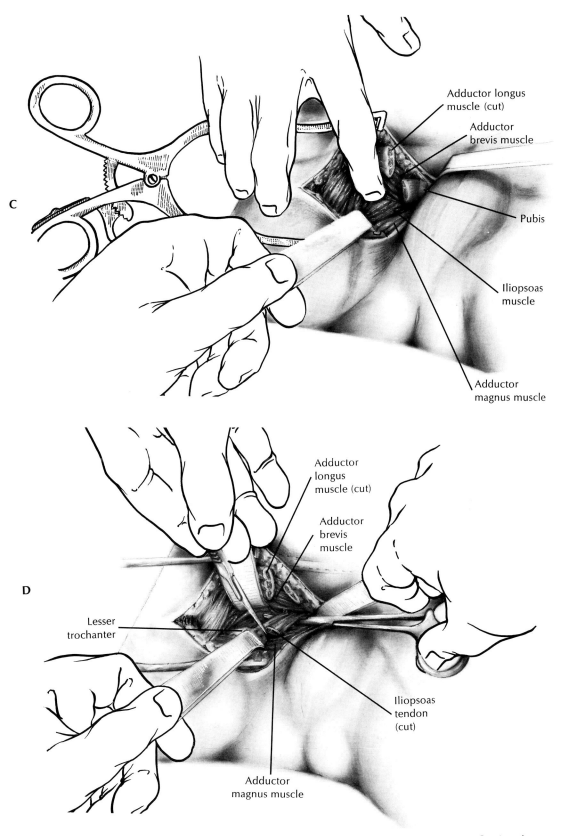

Fig. 4-11, cont'd. For legend see p. 91.

Continued.

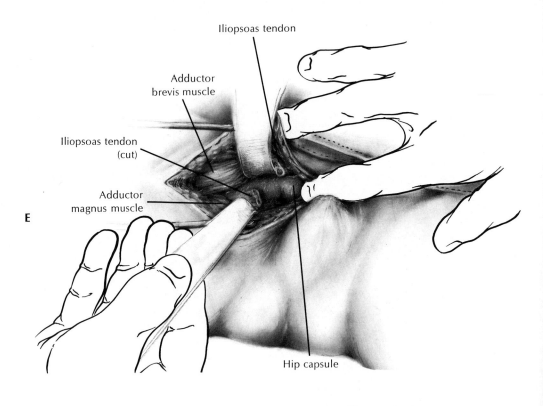
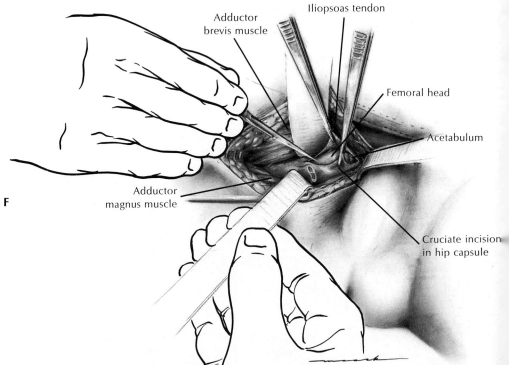

Fig. 4-11, cont'd. For legend see opposite page.

tendon may or may not be reattached, but it is usually not necessary to do so. No other deep repair is necessary, and after skin closure a 1½ hip spica cast is applied. During cast application pressure must be manually exerted over the greater trochanter, with the thigh being held in 30 degrees of abduction and flexion and a slight degree of internal rotation as mentioned previously. An x-ray film is taken to verify satisfactory reduction and position. The cast is left on for 3 months, and the postcasting care is the same as that for the anterior approach.

Advantages and disadvantages of different methods of open reduction. The selection of the anterior or the medial surgical approach involves more than just personal preference. There are distinct difference between the procedures, not only from the standpoint of the extent of surgical dissection required, but also from the point of view of versatility and appropriateness. The medial approach is simpler, involves less dissection, and represents the most direct attack on the major structures that are responsible for preventing reduction of the dislocation (iliopsoas tendon and constricted anterior inferior hip capsule). The anterior approach requires more anatomic dissection and as a result is a more extensive procedure; however, it provides greater versatility because (1) the joint can be explored more thoroughly and (2) simple extensions of the incisions or the dissection enables one to shorten the femur, if necessary, or to perform a pelvic osteotomy on the rare occasion when the indications justify it.

Certain hip dislocations in children under 18 months of age do not lend themselves well to the medial (adductor) approach, whereas the anterior approach, because of its versatility, will be more appropriate in these situations. These types of dislocation include instances of antenatal dislocation (Fig. 7-2); atypical or teratologic dislocations such as those encountered in myelodysplasia and arthrogryposis; highriding, rigid dislocations; and dislocations found in patients who have a grossly abnormal proximal femur or acetabulum. I also believe that *any* previously operated case should *not* be operated via the medial (adductor) approach.

Where these surgical approaches are indicated there is little challenge to the virtue of either one, but it is essential that the limitations and versatility of each be recognized. The location of the skin incision is important only to the extent that the goal and intended purpose of the operation are achieved. In this regard, only the perceptiveness and technical expertise of the surgeon can be combined to determine which operative approach is best suited for the problem. In general when performing an open reduction of the hip in a child under the age of 30 months and in the absence of the contraindications suggested above, I personally prefer the medial (adductor) approach because of its simplicity. However, if I consider that femoral shortening or pelvic osteotomy might possibly be required at the time of open reduction, or if there are other extenuating or complicated circumstances as mentioned on

---

Fig. 4-11. Adductor (Ludloff) approach. The incision is made in the proximal adductor region and extends upward as far as the pubic tubercle, **A.** The incision is deepened and the adductor longus muscle is sectioned at its origin, **B.** Blunt finger dissection posterior to the adduction brevis muscle exposes the lesser trochanter and iliopsoas tendon, **C.** The iliopsoas tendon is cut under direct vision, **D.** The iliopsoas tendon is retracted, exposing the hip joint capsule, **E.** The hip capsule is incised and reduction is accomplished, **F.**

p. 91, then I would select the anterior (iliofemoral) approach because of its versatility.

Tenotomizing vs lengthening of iliopsoas tendon and muscle. When the growth centers are healthy in the femoral head and trochanters, normal growth and remodeling of the proximal femur are a result of the normal, physiologic use of the hip joint. The two most important functions that influence the configuration of the upper femur are weight-bearing and muscle action. The effect of disturbances of these activities on the configuration of the upper femur has been demonstrated experimentally in animals by Hoyt and associates.[3] It is also very graphically reflected in the configuration of the proximal femur following such paralytic disorders as cerebral palsy, polio, and myelodysplasia. The issue of tenotomizing, lengthening, or transferring the iliopsoas tendon, therefore, assumes some degree of potential, if not actual, importance because muscle balance about the hip is altered by such surgery. At the present time, however, there is no good evidence to show that simple tenotomy of the iliopsoas tendon produces any disturbance in growth of the lesser trochanter or any alteration in configuration of the upper femur during subsequent growth. The probability is that the tendon reattaches in an elongated state in young children, and therefore the tenotomy is tantamount to lengthening. Therefore, although it is logical to lengthen or resuture the tendon, practically, it probably makes no difference.

Acetabular limbus in open reduction: anatomy and clinical significance. Excision of the acetabular limbus in open reduction has been a controversial issue in orthopedic surgery and deserves special mention. In order to discuss the role of the acetabular limbus in open reduction, it is essential to review the developmental, histologic, and gross anatomy of this structure as illustrated and described in Chapter 1.

The differences in concept between continental and American orthopedic surgeons concerning the importance of the limbus in open reduction of the hip are difficult to rationalize or explain. It is almost impossible to reconcile the expressions found in the literature that support equally good clinical and radiographic results of two totally different operations that are done for the same problem but are based on widely divergent concepts. This distressing situation exists, and will continue to exist, until all pediatric hip surgeons hopefully will achieve some general agreement on the following two very important issues: namely, (1) an understanding of the true pathology of the hip joint in congenital dislocation, and (2) a logical, technical solution to this problem, based on correction of the proved primary pathology. Until that agreement is achieved, one must assume that our understanding of the basic pathology in congenital dislocation of the hip is incomplete and not clearly defined. Current therapeutic programs must unfortunately, therefore, be based on what conceptually seems correct rather than on what has been undeniably proved to be right.

Excision of the limbus has been championed by many British and European surgeons. Their view is based largely on the belief that the major anatomic structure that prevents satisfactory reduction of the femoral head into the acetabulum is an enlarged and infolded limbus. By excising the limbus at its junction to the acetabular rim, Somerville[11] and Mitchell[8] have claimed that reduction can be effected easily, even in those instances of irreducibility. Ostensibly no effort is made to release the iliopsoas tendon or the inferior capsule or transverse acetabular ligament.

Most American surgeons give the

limbus little consideration when it comes to an open reduction of the hip in children under the age of 18 months. I have never excised an acetabular limbus in this age group, and other surgeons with comparable experience reflect the same observations.[12,13] Such a testimony does not necessarily constitute rightness; rather, it simply indicates that the importance of the limbus, as a deterrent to closed or open reduction, has not been yet demonstrated in the large majority of instances.

Disadvantages and complications of open reduction. Irrespective of the need for, or the method of, open reduction, there are certain disadvantages and complications associated with any open procedure, whether accomplished from the anterior or the medial approach. The greater likelihood for intra-articular adhesions, the increased possibility of mechanical damage to articular cartilage, and the remote possibility of surgical infection must all be considered when an open reduction is being considered. The potential for these problems emphasizes the need for critical attention to detail, from the standpoint of indications for the procedure as well as from the point of view of the technical accomplishments of the operation. Because of the many similar problems and complications that occur in all the age groups undergoing treatment of the differing manifestations of CDH, Chapter 7 has been devoted to these issues.

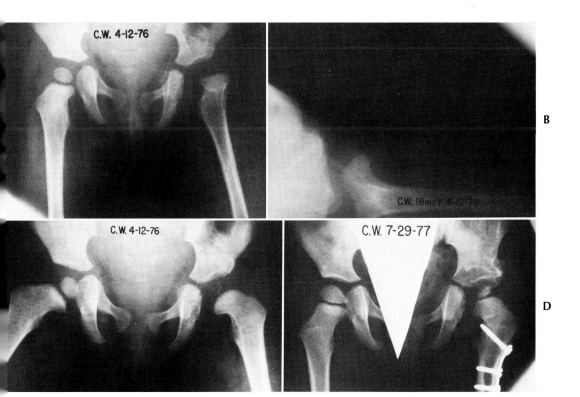

Fig. 4-12. An example of a primary anterior dislocation of the hip is seen in this pelvic x-ray film of an 18-month-old girl, **A** and **B**. Abduction internal-rotation film shows hip to be well seated, **C**, but there was nearly 90 degrees of anteversion. Therefore a combined open reduction, femoral shortening, and pericapsular pelvic osteotomy were accomplished, **D**.

Treatment of anterior primary dislocation. In treating anterior primary dislocation of the hip, the same concepts must be employed as for any of the "typical" dislocations. Usually, however, there is significantly increased anteversion in the affected femoral neck of these patients, and there is a high likelihood that proximal femoral rotational osteotomy will be required (Fig. 4-12). It should again be emphasized, however, that a femoral osteotomy *must not* be done until the femoral head is concentrically reduced and is stable in the position of inward rotation.

REFERENCES

1. Ferguson, A. B., Jr.: Primary open reduction of congenital dislocation of the hip using a median adductor approach, J. Bone Joint Surg. **55A:**671, 1973.
2. Hass, J.: Congenital dislocation of the hip, Springfield, Ill., 1951, Charles C Thomas, Publisher.
3. Hoyt, W. A., Troyer, M. L., Reef, T., and Sheik, S.: The proximal femoral epiphyses; experimental and correlated clinical observations of their potential, Proceedings of the AAOS, January 1966, J. Bone Joint Surg. **48A:** 1026, 1966.
4. Ludloff, K.: Zür blutigen Einrenkung der angeborenen Hüftluxation, Z. Orth. Chir. **22:**272, 1908.
5. MacEwen, G. D.: Personal communication.
6. Mau, H., Dorr, W. M., Henkel, L., and Lutsche, J.: Open reduction of congenital dislocation of the hip by Ludloff's method, J. Bone Joint Surg. **53A:**1281, 1971.
7. McCarroll, H. R., and Crego, C. H.: Primary anterior congenital dislocation of the hip, J. Bone Joint Surg. **21:**648, 1939.
8. Mitchell, G. P.: Problems in the early diagnosis and management of congenital dislocation of the hip, J. Bone Joint Surg. **54B:**4, 1972.
9. Ortolani, M.: La lussazione congenital dell'anca, Bologna, 1948, Casa Editrice Licinio Cappelli.
10. Salter, R. B., Kostuik, J., and Dallas, S.: Avascular necrosis of the femoral head as a complication of treatment for congenital dislocation of the hip in young children: a clinical and experimental investigation, Can. J. Surg. **12:**44, 1969.
11. Somerville, E. W., and Scott, J. C.: The direct approach to congenital dislocation of the hip, J. Bone Joint Surg. **39B:**623, 1957.
12. Westin, G. W.: Personal communication.
13. Williams, P.: Personal communication.

CHAPTER 5

Diagnosis and treatment of congenital dislocation in the child 18 months to 4 years of age

Diagnosis
   Physical signs
   Roentgenographic findings
Treatment in the child over 18 months
   Closed reduction
   Open reduction
Treatment of residual deformities following reduction
   Proximal femoral (intertrochanteric) osteotomy
   Distal femoral (supracondylar) osteotomy
Correction of acetabular deficiencies
   Pericapsular (Pemberton) osteotomy
   Innominate (Salter, complete) osteotomy
   Pericapsular (Pemberton) and innominate (Salter) osteotomies
   Combined operative procedures in young children
Treatment in the child over 4 years of age

DIAGNOSIS
Physical signs

The diagnostic physical findings encountered in congenital hip dislocation in the child over 18 months are usually very clearly defined and easy to identify. By age 18 months the child is invariably walking, and a characteristic limp or "waddle" will be apparent if the hip is dislocated. The limp will be especially evident in the patient with a unilateral dislocation because of the asymmetry of gait. In bilateral dislocation the disturbance in gait will be less obvious. This is one of the reasons why the diagnosis in patients with unilateral dislocation is often made sooner after walking begins than in those who have bilateral dislocation. The diagnosis of bilateral dislocation is often delayed until after age 18 months or 2 years or even longer. It is an interesting and significant observation, also, to note that the simple presence of either unilateral or bilateral dislocation, without any associated abnormalities, rarely is the cause of significant delay in ambulation in otherwise healthy children.

Other physical abnormalities will also vary according to whether the dislocation is unilateral or bilateral. In the unilateral dislocation one may compare the findings to an opposite normal hip, whereas in bilateral dislocation the abnormalities will be much the same on both sides. Thus in a unilateral dislocation the affected limb will be shorter, there will be an asymmetric limitation of abduction of the flexed thigh, the thigh and inguinal skin folds will be deeper and more numerous on the involved side, and the femoral head and greater trochanter will be palpated more posteriorly than on the opposite normal side. In addition there will be a distinctly positive Trendelenburg test on the involved side (Fig. 5-1).

In bilateral dislocation the major abnormalities consist of significant limita-

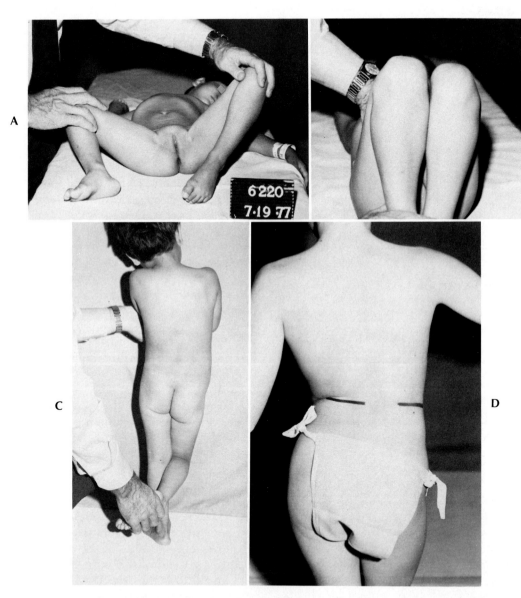

Fig. 5-1. In older children with unilateral CDH, not only will the involved flexed thigh be restricted in abduction, **A,** but the Galeazzi test will be positive, **B,** and the Trendelenburg sign will be positive, **C.** Another example of a positive Trendelenburg test is seen in this patient with a subluxating hip. The patient is unable to elevate or stabilize the opposite hemipelvis when standing on the affected limb, **D.**

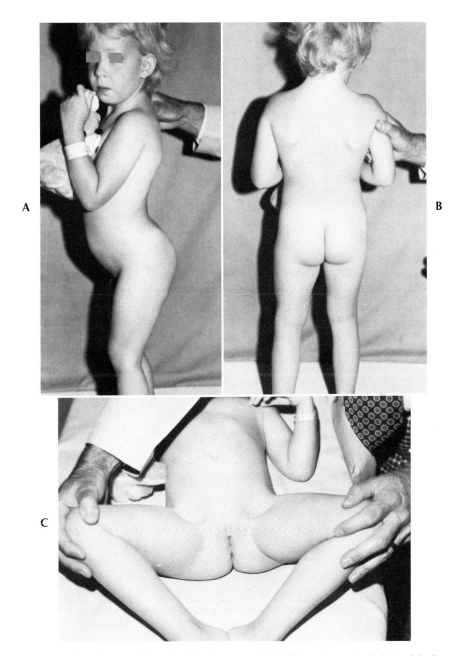

Fig. 5-2. Physical findings in bilateral CDH. Four-year-old girl illustrating typical physical findings of bilateral hip dislocation. The increased lumbar lordosis and prominent femoral heads presenting in the buttock are seen in **A.** The widened buttocks and perineum are seen in **B,** and the deep hollow in the femoral trigone on abduction of the flexed thigh is clearly evident in **C.** Note symmetric findings.

tion of abduction of the flexed thigh, a widening of the perineum, a greater prominence of the greater trochanter by palpation, increased lumbosacral lordosis when the patient stands, and deep hollows anteriorly in the inguinal regions where the femoral head is normally palpated. There will, of course, be no demonstrable shortening (although both limbs are truly shortened), and the inguinal and thigh skin creases will be symmetric (Fig. 5-2).

Variations in the rotational attitudes of the lower limbs, especially external rotation, have often been considered significant observations suggesting abnormalities of the hip. These deviations are most commonly postural in etiology and have little bearing on, or little significance in, the diagnosis of congenital hip disease. In most of these instances there will be a history that the child sleeps on the abdomen or back with outwardly or inwardly rotated lower limbs. Nevertheless, any significant lower limb torsional attitudinal abnormality in this age group deserves a very critical physical examination of the hips as well as an x-ray examination of the pelvis. (See High-risk group, p. 47.) It is important to emphasize that gentle examination of the child's hip with either unilateral or bilateral dislocation is generally always painless and provokes no unpleasant or untoward reaction in a child of this age. If painful symptoms are present, other possible hip disorders must be suspected.

Roentgenographic findings

In practically all instances of congenital dislocation of the hip in children of this age, the roentgenographic changes are positively diagnostic. By this time the ossification of the developing hip structures has proceeded to the point where an accurate determination of the dislocation can readily be made. The roentgenographic changes considered to be most helpful in the diagnosis of congenital hip dislocation are much the same as those described in Chapter 4.

TREATMENT IN THE CHILD OVER 18 MONTHS

When congenital dislocation of the hip is encountered in the child 18 months of age or over, in many instances it will require a surgical approach. The reasons for this are several: First, the soft tissues about the hip (tendons and capsular structures) have undergone so-called adaptive shortening secondary to the upward displacement of the hip. Second, the cartilaginous and ossified portions of the acetabulum, being without the normal stimulation and influence of the contained femoral head, have not developed in a normal fashion. Finally, because the femoral head has not been articulating with the acetabulum and as a result the musculature about the hip has not been utilized normally, alterations in the configuration of the growing proximal femur take place. The surgical and anatomic pathology of congenital hip dislocation is so variable that no one solution can possibly be suitable for all patients with this problem. When a surgeon contemplates treating a dislocated hip in a child over 18 months of age, these three considerations must be given careful and thorough consideration.

In all hip dislocations in this age group, the primary decision is to determine whether an open or a closed reduction should be accomplished. If an open reduction is planned, then the preferred surgical approach (anterior or medial) should be established, the character of the soft tissues about the hip must be assessed in order to determine the need for tenotomies and/or a femoral shortening procedure, the configuration of the proximal femur must be established, and the degree of development and contour of the acetabulum must be ascertained. It is essential that these considerations are fully defined before a logical and sensible program of treatment can be developed.

Closed reduction

It is possible in a significant number of instances to reduce a dislocated hip in a child over 18 months of age without doing an open reduction. An occasional hip that is unusually flexible and that telescopes easily can often be managed by closed reduction in children up to 24 or 30 months of age following an arbitrary 2-week minimum period of traction. The duration of traction required for successful reduction may vary from one individual to another. For example, Weiner and associates[45] have shown that in their hands the duration of traction must exceed 3 weeks in order to facilitate reduction and to keep femoral head necrosis to a minimum. Other observers have also shown that preliminary traction is important in reducing the incidence and degree of osseous necrosis in patients treated by closed reduction.[22,46] Intuitively, it seems logical to apply longitudinal traction on the limb as a preliminary treatment to closed reduction. Also, it seems appropriate to attempt to pull the femoral head down to the level of the acetabulum prior to an attempt at reduction. However, it is imperative that the following factors be given full consideration in determining how much traction should be used and for how long it should continue: the age of the child, the amount of upward displacement of the femoral head prior to treatment, whether the femoral head is brought down to the level of the acetabulum prior to attempted reduction, whether skin or skeletal traction is used, the ease of reduction, the position in which the hip is held following reduction (specifically relating to the dangers of any extremes of position), and, finally, whether percutaneous soft tissue releases (adductor tenotomy, etc.) are accomplished at the time of reduction. All of these factors are of considerable significance as they relate to the incidence and degree of femoral head necrosis following reduction. Because of the tremendous variability of these factors as they are encountered from one patient to another, any rigid approach to the duration or amount of preliminary traction does not seem justified. The objective that should be uppermost in the surgeon's mind is that the reduction is easily accomplished, that the reduced hip is stable, and that the hip can be held in a physiologic position that avoids any extremes of abduction or rotation.

During the past several years I have not used *skeletal* traction in the treatment of congenital dislocation of the hip at any age. The reasons are few and very easy to detail. First of all and most important in this deliberation, the use of skeletal traction implies a need for increased distraction force. This force, when discontinued following reduction, may result in increased pressure on the reduced femoral head. Second, there are several potential complications of prolonged skeletal traction, such as pin tract infections, epiphyseal plate injuries, and disuse osteoporosis. Finally, "decompression" resection osteotomy of the femur (see p. 100) provides a safer means of obtaining reduction in the high-riding femoral head that is difficult to reduce or is even "irreducible." Thus I agree with Westin[46] and many others that in the modern treatment of congenital dislocation of the hip at any age, *skeletal* traction is not necessary and may even be deleterious. As will be discussed subsequently, in many cases subtrochanteric femoral shortening at the time of reduction is more effective and probably safer than preliminary skeletal traction when an open reduction of congenital hip dislocation is being performed in a child over 30 months of age. Prior to that age, skin traction and appro-

100 Congenital dysplasia and dislocation of the hip

priate soft tissue releases will usually be effective in obtaining reduction.

Open reduction

Medial (adductor) vs anterior (iliofemoral) approach. In this age group the same considerations must be taken into account in deciding whether the hip joint should be approached from below (the adductor approach) or above (the iliofemoral approach) as were evaluated in treating the younger child under age 18 months. The same advantages and disadvantages to either approach also exist as were discussed in Chapter 4. The fact that these children will be older, sometimes will have been previously operated on, and will usually have more adaptive changes about the hip will make the iliofemoral procedure more appropriate in the majority of instances. Still, some children between the ages of 18 and 24 months may lend themselves to the medial (adductor) operation (Fig. 5-3).

Femoral shortening and open reduction of the hip. Ever since 1932 when

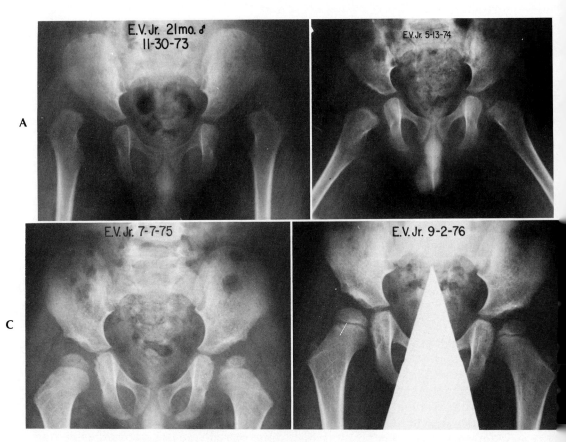

Fig. 5-3. A 21-month-old boy with bilateral dislocations of the hip, **A,** was treated by preliminary skin traction and bilateral open reduction of the hip via the medial (adductor) approach at separate operations, **B.** One year later the hips are stable but the acetabula are still sloping, **C.** Because Shenton's line is intact, pelvic osteotomy was not considered to be indicated at that time, and the hip joints 14 months later are seen in **D.** Pelvic osteotomy will likely not be necessary, but the patient will be watched closely through his growing years.

Ombrédanne[29] introduced and popularized the use of subtrochanteric shortening of the femur in open reduction of the hip, the operation has gained increasing acceptance in performing open reduction in children over the age of 30 months with hip dislocations. In a thorough and comprehensive review of the literature, Larsen[20] demonstrated that femoral shortening has been utilized in a variety of circumstances as well as in conjunction with other reconstructive procedures on the hip. I currently employ it whenever necessary in children over 24 or 30 months of age at the time of open reduction. The concepts behind the procedure were developed in children with the so-called irreducible or high-riding hip. By resecting a portion of the proximal femur, the resistance of the soft tissues (especially the adductor muscles) to reduction can be largely overcome. Furthermore, just as important, subsequent pressure on the reduced femoral head is decreased. This has led to employment of the term "decompression" osteotomy for this procedure by Westin.[46] In addition to the enhanced ability to gain reduction of the hip, any angular and/or rotational deformities of the proximal femur may be corrected simultaneously.

It is not simple to explain the precise mechanism by which the femoral resection assists in reduction of the hip, although once the surgeon experiences the results of the procedure it will be abundantly clear that it is very effective. As noted earlier, the pull of the adductor

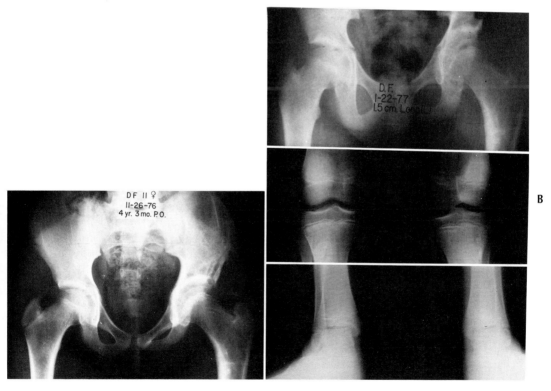

Fig. 5-4. An 11-year-old girl who underwent 2.0 cm of femoral shortening and Colonna arthroplasty for persistent dislocation at age 7 years, **A.** Currently she measures 1.5 cm longer on the operated side, **B.**

muscles and their associated fascial attachments is almost completely negated. Furthermore, all other muscles that cross the hip and insert on the femur and/or leg are functionally lengthened. The surprising ease with which the femoral head can be reduced into the socket following osteotomy is most impressive when compared with the difficulty one experiences during attempts at open reduction with the intact femur. An additional advantage occurs because the proximal fragment has greater mobility, which then makes dissection about the joint technically easier.

When this procedure is done in children in this age group there is very little alteration in limb length resulting from the osteotomy itself, because stimulation of growth (compensatory) of the femur by the surgical fracture produces sufficient increased length so that concern over a limb length inequality is vitiated, if not essentially negated. In one of my patients (Fig. 5-4) a surgical shortening of 2.0 cm ultimately resulted in an actual absolute increase in length of 1.5 cm on the involved limb.

Technique. Since it accompanies open reduction, the shortening procedure is best done by the anterior (iliofemoral) approach. The incision must be a generous one in order to accomplish both the open reduction and the shortening. It begins at the midpoint of the iliac crest and extends anteriorly to the anterior superior iliac spine and then distally over the proximal thigh for 2 or 3 inches paralleling the interval between the tensor fasciae latae and the sartorius muscles. It then curves posteriorly over the lateral aspect of the upper thigh, ending at the midlateral aspect of the proximal femur (Fig. 5-5). The incision is deepened and the open reduction is carried out in the same manner as described in anterior open reduction of the hip. The femoral head may be easily reduced in some instances, but in other circumstances either the head is reduced with difficulty or cannot be reduced at all. If the reduction is difficult a significant increase in pressure will be evident on the reduced femoral head, and in these instances a decompression femoral resection should be done. Correspondingly, in the irreducible dislocation, the osteotomy is done in order to facilitate reduction. Following the decision to perform the osteotomy, the lateral incision is then deepened and the tensor faciae latae muscle is cut transversely. This muscle is easily reflected laterally, thus exposing the underlying vastus lateralis muscle and the insertion of the gluteus maximus tendon. The lateral aspect of the femur is exposed by elevating the origin of the vastus lateralis muscle, beginning as close to the physeal plate of the greater trochanter as possible; however, care must be exercised so as not to damage the greater trochanteric growth center. Sufficient length of the femur is subperiosteally exposed circumferentially so that a small three- or four-hole plate can be applied. A "score" is made in the femur that parallels the longitudinal axis of the femur. The purpose of this score is to serve as an orientation for control of rotation after the femur has been cut and resected. The osteotomy is made just distal to the proximal one or two screws that will transfix the plate. The distal fragment is then stripped of its soft tissues for a distance of about 1 inch, and it is allowed to overlap as much as necessary for the reduction. At this point placement of the femoral head into the acetabulum may occur with impressive ease in the hip that previously was irreducible, and the reduced femoral head will have no evidence of excessive pressure. In some instances, however, especially in previously operated cases, additional dissection and soft tissue release will be needed before reduction can be effected. The amount of overlap of the femur required

Text continued on p. 109.

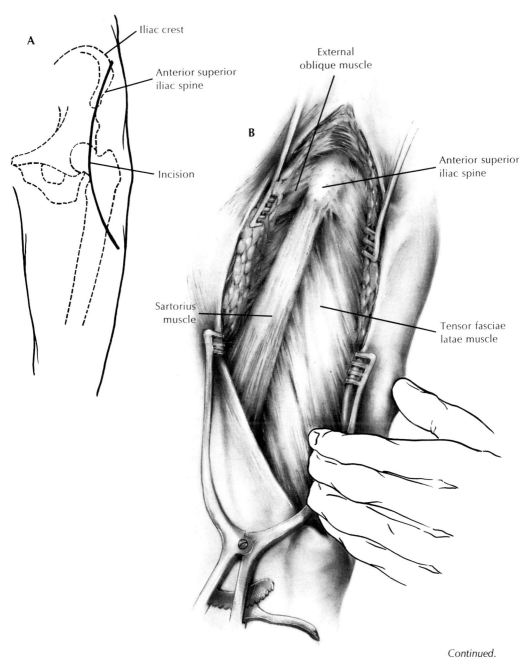

Fig. 5-5. Technique of open reduction and femoral shortening. Insert shows the generous iliofemoral incision. The crest of the ilium, and the sartorius and tensor fasciae latae muscles are exposed, **A** and **B**. The capsule of the hip joint is exposed, **C**, and opened in a T fashion, **D**. The distal end of the incision is extended and deepened, and the proximal femur is exposed, **E**. A longitudinal "score" is made in the proximal femur, and an osteotomy is accomplished, **F**. The fragments are permitted to overlap, and reduction is easily accomplished, **G**. The overlapping femur is then resected and a plate and screws are applied to stabilize the femur.

Continued.

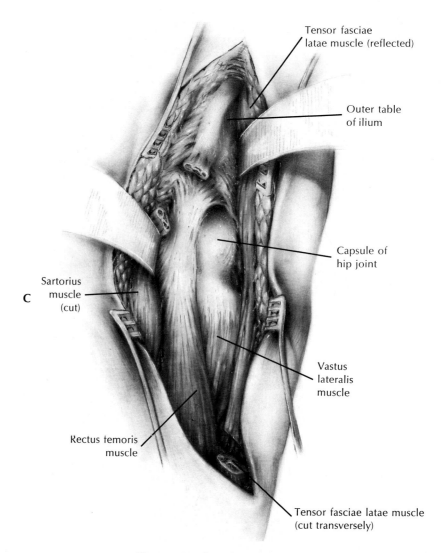

Fig. 5-5, cont'd. For legend see p. 103.

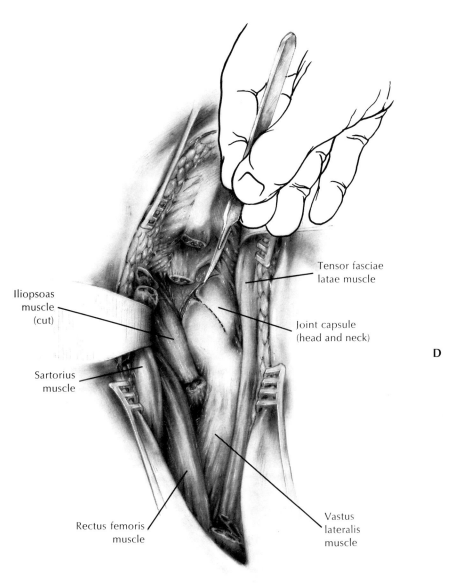

Fig. 5-5, cont'd. For legend see p. 103.

Continued.

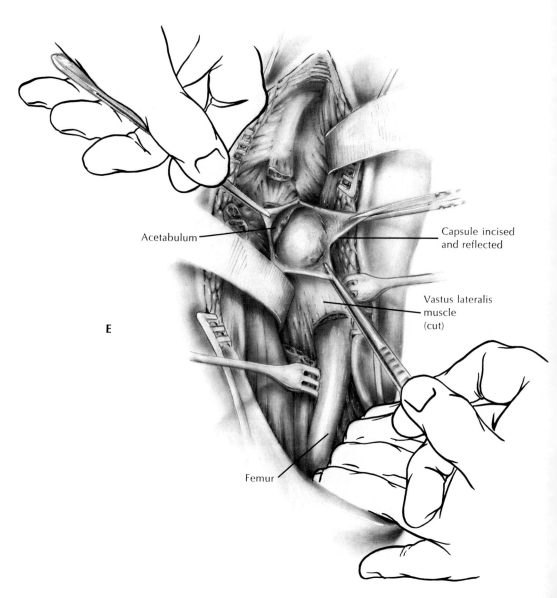

Fig. 5-5, cont'd. For legend see p. 103.

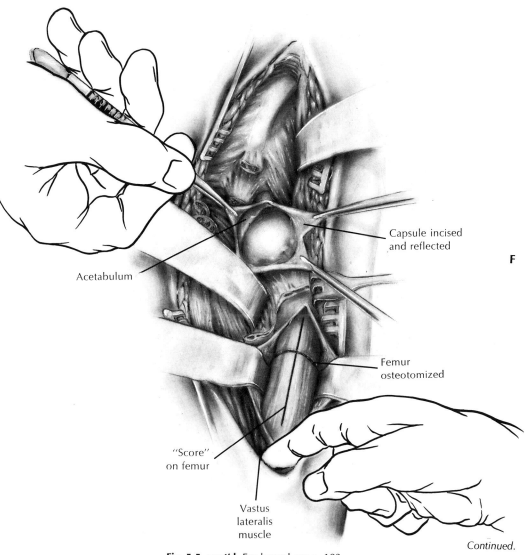

Fig. 5-5, cont'd. For legend see p. 103.

108 Congenital dysplasia and dislocation of the hip

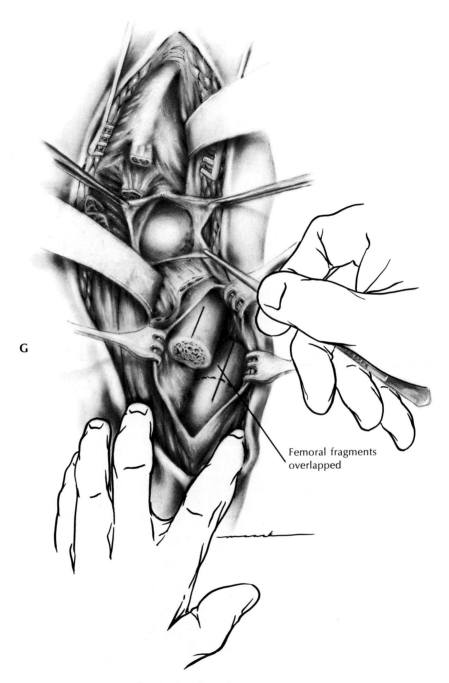

Fig. 5-5, cont'd. For legend see p. 103.

to permit easy reduction and to result in the required reduced pressure on the femoral head is then resected. This will vary from 1 to 3 cm, depending on the age of the child and the nature of the dislocation. The fragments are then reduced and the plate is applied. At this point any needed angular or rotational correction of the proximal femur can be easily achieved. After the plate is firmly fixed, one should be able to distract the femoral head manually from the socket for about 2 or 3 mm without difficulty, even with the thigh in full extension. This assures the surgeon that the femoral head has indeed been "decompressed." The resected bone is cut into small pieces and laid about the osteotomy site. Then, after the transverse cut in the tensor fasciae latae muscle is repaired, closure is effected in the same fashion as described in open reduction.

A pelvic x-ray film should be taken in order to evaluate concentricity of reduction, the position of the osteotomy, and placement of the internal fixation. A one and one-half hip spica cast is applied with the thigh held in the most physiologically stable position. This will usually be 30 degrees of hip flexion, 30 degrees of abduction, and neutral or slight internal rotation. Another pelvic x-ray film should be taken following application of the cast to assure maintenance of reduction. A representative patient undergoing femoral shortening is shown in Fig. 5-6.

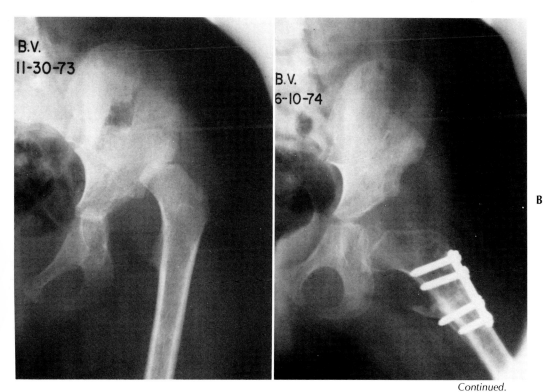

Continued.

Fig. 5-6. A 4-year-old female with untreated congenital dislocation of the hip, **A.** Without prior skeletal traction an open reduction with 2.0 cm of femoral shortening was accomplished, **B.** At age 5 years an innominate osteotomy was considered essential after a satisfactory range of hip motion was achieved, **C.** The result 2 years later is seen in **D.**

110 Congenital dysplasia and dislocation of the hip

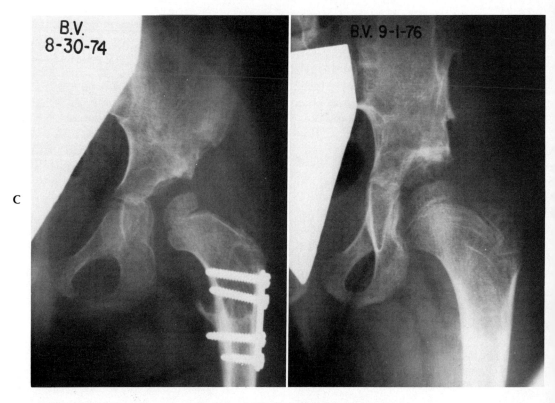

Fig. 5-6, cont'd. For legend see p. 109.

Postoperative care following open reduction with or without femoral shortening. The cast is left on for a minimum period of 8 weeks. An x-ray film of the pelvis should be again taken during the early postoperative period, primarily to ascertain the position of the femoral head with respect to the acetabulum. When the cast is removed both physical and x-ray examinations of the hip should be conducted. If the hip is stable and concentrically reduced, guarded range of motion may be started utilizing a removable external appliance as described in the previous chapter. Either the posterior half of the original spica cast or a newly created posterior shell may be used. Alternatively an abduction bar attached to the shoes may be utilized. Ordinarily the subtrochanteric osteotomy, if done, will have healed by this time. However, if there is doubt about the union, hip motion without weight bearing may be safely started as long as the internal fixation is in good position. It is the added safety and stability provided by the plates that has encouraged my use of the plate in contrast to simple transfixion pins or wires. Such wires or pins occasionally have to be removed prematurely and nearly always have to be extracted when the cast is removed. With the retained plate added protection of the osteotomy is provided. In contrast to the technique of shortening with the overlap technique, it is possible also to maintain continuity of the medullary canal when the plate is used. In older children this is especially advantageous if the possibility of subsequent total hip arthroplasty exists. Of course there is a disadvantage to the plate in that it has to be removed. However, this minor drawback appears to be justified in view of the greater safety and the other advantages that the plate provides.

In some instances the hip may not appear sufficiently stable following the initial 8 weeks of cast immobilization to permit a program of motion; in this situation a one and one-half hip spica cast should again be applied for an additional 4 to 6 weeks. The decision regarding the need for a second cast is a highly individual one and is largely made by intuition.

Over the succeeding 6 weeks a gradual weight-bearing program is begun, provided that the osteotomy (when done) has healed satisfactorily. Children at this age usually need little encouragement to walk unless there have been extenuating circumstances occasioned by complications or prolonged immobilization. Also, in most instances formal physical therapy is largely unnecessary during convalescence.

Throughout the following years periodic clinical and x-ray examinations must be conducted. During the first postreduction year evaluation should be carried out at least every 3 months. Thereafter, the follow-up intervals may be lengthened to 6 months or 1 year depending on the observations listed below. These follow-up examinations are mandatory in order to make the following important determinations: (1) the concentricity of reduction; (2) the development of the acetabulum; (3) the growth and configuration of the upper femur; and (4) the viability of the femoral head.

Concentricity of reduction. The most important single determinant to establish during follow-up examinations is the concentricity and stability of the reduction. Unless this has been achieved and maintained, the hip is doomed to major compromise in function with probable ultimate failure. If the reduction is not maintained, immediate efforts at achieving this all-important goal must be started. This is such an important issue that it is discussed in depth in Chapter 7. In determining "concentricity of reduction" it is essential that the three basic roentgenographic evaluations on p. 144 be made. Besides these conventional anteroposterior, abduction–internal rotation, and groin lateral views, arthrography should be used if necessary. Arthrography, however, is not necessary on a routine basis, despite the fact that some believe that it is a required study.

Arthrography. It is difficult to explain the controversy that exists regarding the indications for and value of arthrography in congenital dislocation of the hip. On the one hand some authors believe that arthrography is indicated in virtually all instances of dislocation prior to and following reduction. Others believe that arthrography is rarely indicated, and they reserve it for those special problems that cannot be adequately defined by conventional x-ray evaluation. I adhere to the latter philosophy wherein arthrograms are only taken in special circumstances and under specific indications.

If a concentric reduction is readily demonstrated by clinical and conventional roentgenographic examination, I believe there is no reason to perform an arthrogram. If open reduction is indicated because of obvious failure to obtain a concentric reduction, I do not perform an arthrogram. The arthrotomy will provide far more information than the arthrogram, and the latter would therefore be largely superfluous. However, when there is doubt about a concentric reduction as evidenced on the routine roentgenogram and when the outcome of the arthrogram may provide valuable evidence in favor of or against an operative procedure, then I believe that an arthrogram has real value. An example of a good indication for an arthrogram is seen in Fig. 5-7.

If the reduction remains concentric

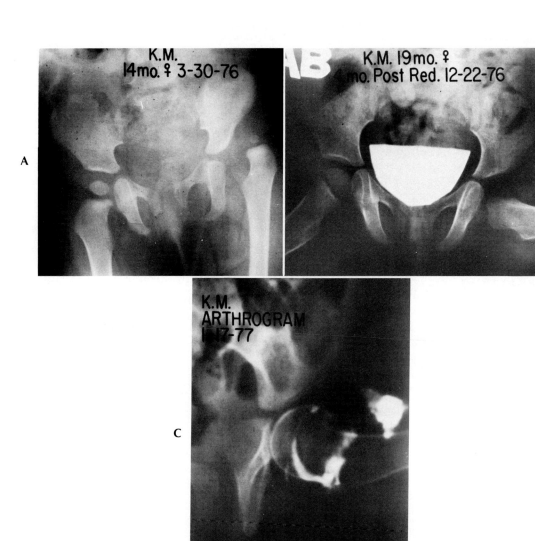

Fig. 5-7. Indication for arthrogram. Pelvic x-ray film of a 14-month-old girl with dislocation of the left hip, **A.** Four months postreduction the pelvic films showed some question of concentricity of reduction, **B,** even though clinically the hips appeared well reduced and stable. An arthrogram confirmed the concentric reduction with an asymmetry of femoral head ossification, **C.** (Courtesy Dr. Leon Krueger.)

during these periods of observation, but the hip demonstrates any degree of instability (subluxation) with various positions of the thigh, a stabilizing procedure may be indicated. Usually the cause of the instability will be a deficient acetabulum, but in some instances the proximal femur may have a deformity such as excessive valgus of the neck-shaft angle or excessive anteversion that contributes to the instability. In rare circumstances, both abnormalities may exist. These represent the second and third determinants mentioned on p. 111.

Development of acetabulum. Depending on the age at which the reduction is accomplished, the acetabulum has a variable capacity to remodel and resume normal growth with the ultimate development of a reasonably normal socket. In children treated at 18 months of age, many of the acetabula will respond to concentric reduction and a perfectly satisfactory acetabulum will result in the great majority of instances. However, in children over 2 or 3 years of skeletal age, this capacity for significant remodeling becomes progressively compromised and many acetabula will not remodel sufficiently well to result in a stable, satisfactory hip. In these circumstances an innominate osteotomy, either the incomplete, pericapsular (Pemberton) or complete, innominate (Salter), may be necessary in order to provide a satisfactory acetabulum. It is the frequently anticipated need for pelvic osteotomy in this age group that has prompted many surgeons to accomplish the pelvic correction simultaneously with open reduction. This highly individualized and important issue will be discussed in greater depth shortly.

As will be detailed in the section covering the treatment of dysplasia in the older child and adolescent, the indications for either of the innominate osteotomies require not only the presence of a deficient socket, but also a demonstration that normal, spontaneous correction of the acetabulum will likely not occur. Once these indications have been unequivocally identified *and* the all-important prerequisites have been satisfied, then either of these procedures on the innominate bone should be accomplished. Again, the choice of the procedure at this age should be based on the surgeon's preference and technical expertise. The details of these operations are discussed later in this chapter.

Growth and configuration of proximal femur. It has already been shown (p. 92) that configuration of the proximal femur is dependent on at least three important factors: (1) the viability of femoral head and its growing articular cartilage; (2) the viability or state of health of the physeal plates of the greater trochanter and femoral epiphyses, and (3) the degree of normal function exerted on these sensitive and responsive growth centers, especially relating to muscle balance and weight bearing. One could add to that the poorly identified and controversial issue of primary "dysplasia" of the hip (see Chapter 2). In these latter circumstances a primary deformity of the acetabulum, the proximal femur, or both exists, resulting presumably from some heritable and congenital defect in normal growth.

The most significant concern involves any compromise in the viability of the femoral head epiphysis or its associated physeal plate. Ischemia of the femoral head and its sequelae are not always preventable, and signs suggesting this untoward change must always be watched for. Failure of the femoral head to grow and remodel because of necrosis represents a major therapeutic problem because of the deformities that can result. Again, this important issue will be discussed in greater depth later in this section as well as in Chapters 7 and 8.

Deformities of proximal femur. The

two abnormalities often seen in the proximal femur in congenital hip dysplasia are excessive anteversion and angular deformities of the neck-shaft angle. The latter can be seen as either excessive coxa varus or excessive coxa valgus. Since there is such a wide range of normal in these determinations and because the exact degree of anteversion is so difficult to identify roentgenographically, it is almost impossible to put a numerical figure on the term "excessive." The decision has to be made on the basis of clinical judgment, as determined by the three standard x-ray films alluded to earlier. In addition, there have been several sophisticated roentgenographic methods developed that are designed to measure anteversion more accurately, and these may be used if necessary.

Evaluation of proximal femoral deformities. Several techniques for determining the angle of declination of the femoral head in the live child have been developed during the past 25 years. Most are based on the same concept, namely, the employment of both anteroposterior and cross-table or groin lateral views of the hips.[18] The true angle of declination (anteversion, retroversion, or torsion) is then computed utilizing trigonometric formulas.

Anatomically the angle of declination (anteversion) is defined as the angle that is subtended between the long axis of the femoral neck and the dicondylar axis of the femur (Fig. 5-8). In the adult this angle averages 15 degrees, as determined by studies on cadaveric femora. In the newborn infant the angle is considerably greater, averaging 40 degrees[35] and more until 16 years of age, when there is a gradual reduction of this angle to the adult value (Fig. 5-9). Fundamentally this angle may be the result of anteversion or retroversion of the femoral neck, torsion of the femoral shaft, or a combination of both. In concept it is attractive to separate these different anatomic relationships, and in the femur, which can be dissected and studied throughout its entire length, this is possible. However, in the live child, utilizing currently available roentgenographic techniques, this is neither possible nor necessarily practical. In other words it is feasible to establish with a moderate degree of accuracy the angle of anteversion (declination) or retroversion that exists in a clinical situation, but it is currently not possible to identify

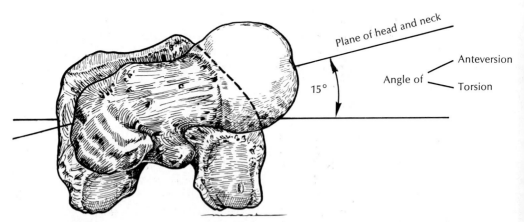

Fig. 5-8. Diagrammatic representation of the angle of declination of the femoral head and neck as related to the dicondylar axis of the femur. This angle, also known as the angle of anteversion, is equivalent to the angle of femoral torsion. Normally in the adult this is about 15 degrees.

which specific anatomic factors (anteversion, torsion, or both) account for this angle. Fortunately, this frailty does not materially alter the ultimate clinical significance of the determination.

The radiographic techniques for determining femoral torsion or anteversion (or retroversion) described by Magilligan[24] and by Dunlap and Shands[11] have been helpful because of their relative ease and simplicity of accomplishment. The techniques require only two roentgenograms of the hip, and these can be taken with standard x-ray equipment. The procedure described by Dunlap and Shands[11] requires a special positioning device, but this device is easy to obtain or construct and ostensibly provides accuracy of measurement. Both techniques require measurement of the apparent angle of inclination (the neck-shaft angle) and the apparent angle of anteversion or femoral torsion (angle of declination). These values are then subjected to special trigonometric formulas in order to calculate the true angle of inclination and the true angle of torsion or declination. Both of these authors have compiled graphs that simplify the calculations. For details of these procedures the reader is referred to the original publications, because I do not utilize either of these techniques.

More accurate measurement has been demonstrated by Hubbard and Staheli[16] using the axial tomograph, but the technical difficulties and increased cost inherent in this technique appear to outweigh the value of the procedure. This is especially true in view of the fact that no hard and fast data are available that define excessive anteversion.

All of these techniques provide a means of numerically quantitating the angle of anteversion of the hip. However, more and more surgeons are beginning to rely on the simple three basic x-ray views mentioned on p. 144, without resorting to specialized methods. When one realizes the frailty of establishing the need for accurate calculations in dealing with the problem of femoral anteversion, it is easy to understand why these computations are assuming less critical importance.

Viability of femoral head. Necrosis of

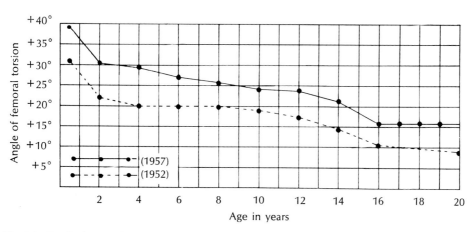

Fig. 5-9. Graph showing femoral torsion in normal children. The solid line on the graph (1957 study) represents the average values in 238 children with roentgenograms made with the hips in 10 degrees of abduction. The broken line represents the average degree of femoral torsion determined in 215 normal children in 1952, when the roentgenograms were made with the hips in 35 degrees of abduction. The 1952 determinations are less accurate and their values are from 5 to 9 degrees lower than those in the 1957 study. (From Shands, A. R., Jr., and Steele, M. K.: Torsion of the femur, J. Bone Joint Surg. **40A:**803, 1958.)

the femoral head has rarely if ever been seen in instances of hip dysplasia or dislocation unless treatment has been administered. For practical purposes, therefore, osteonecrosis of the femoral head must be considered largely iatrogenic. The possible causes of bone necrosis following treatment consist of the following: (1) forcible reduction of the dislocation; (2) undue pressure on the femoral head following reduction; (3) extreme positions of internal rotation, external rotation, or abduction of the thigh either in the treatment of dysplasia or following reduction; (4) injudicious severance of the femoral head vasculature at the time of open reduction; and finally, (5) complications of surgery such as infection (septic necrosis).

The sequelae of necrosis are very far-reaching and include not only the deformities of the upper femur (p. 194) but also gross deformities of the femoral head such as coxa plana and "bilabiation." The latter occurs when a combination of necrosis and subluxation (or inadequate reduction) occurs. As the necrotic femoral head is compressed against the acetabular rim a "furrow" in the head is created that divides the head into two "labia" (Fig. 5-10). Finally, the same factors producing osteonecrosis may also lead to cartilage necrosis, with resultant stiffness and the inevitable, subsequent development of osteoarthritis. Clearly, the surgeon must exercise all efforts relentlessly toward avoidance of any of these occurrences, because femoral head necrosis has been one of the most serious and, heretofore, most common complications of treatment of dysplasia and congenital dislocation of the hip.

In order to prevent or minimize the likelihood of occurrence of femoral head necrosis, great care must be exercised during reduction of the femoral head and in the positioning of the thigh after reduction. Reduction, as emphasized earlier, should be described as a gentle "repositioning" maneuver in which the only purpose for the anesthetic is to hold the infant or child motionless during application of the cast. Pressure on the femoral head must be minimized by use of preliminary traction in young infants and children, by muscle, tendinous, and capsule-releasing procedures during open reduction, or by femoral-resection ("decompression") osteotomy in older children. The limb must be immobilized in a "physiological" position that avoids any extremes of rotation or abduction. Salter and associates[34] have made a strong plea for employment of the "human" position during immobilization, which accentuates the salubrious effects of flexion and neutral rotation of the thigh following reduction. It is significant that all studies to date have resulted in unanimous condemnation of the so-called frog-leg position. For example, a recent review of 110 patients treated by plaster immobilization in the flexed, abducted, and externally rotated (frog-leg) position in the Salt Lake City area revealed an incidence of 65% of femoral head necrosis, either partial or complete. This position and that of forced internal rotation have been shown by Ogden[27] to compress branches of the medial and lateral circumflex arteries, thereby contributing to ischemia of the femoral head (Fig. 5-11). Also, Ogden and Southwick[28] have demonstrated that forced abduction of the hip can compress the lateral epiphyseal artery against the posterior rim of the acetabulum. Thus, from a practical clinical point of view as well as from experimental data, the deleterious effects of extreme positions of hip immobilization are well established. All efforts, therefore, either nonoperative or operative, must be directed toward avoidance of this pitfall.

Unfortunately, but realistically, occasional instances of necrosis of the femoral head will likely continue to occur follow-

Diagnosis and treatment in the child 18 months to 4 years of age 117

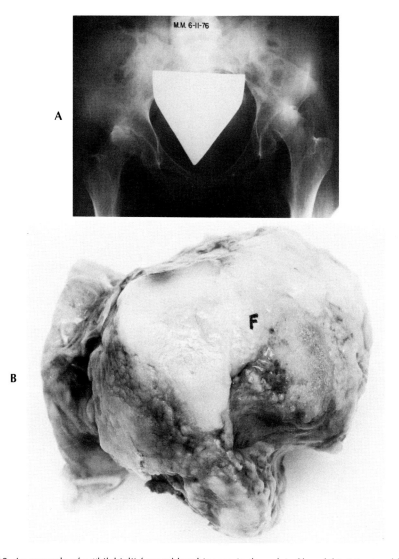

Fig. 5-10. An example of a "bilabial" femoral head is seen in the pelvic film of this 13-year-old girl, **A**. Osseous necrosis and chondrolysis are responsible for the collapse and "bilabiation" seen in the removed femoral head, **B**. The furrow, F, can be easily seen.

118 *Congenital dysplasia and dislocation of the hip*

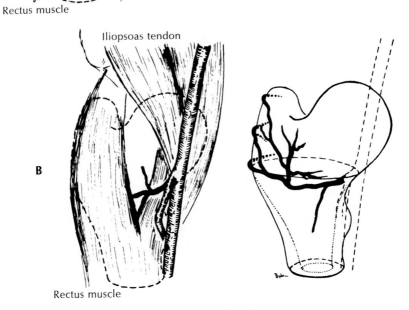

Fig. 5-11. Drawing to show relationship of the circumflex femoral vessels to the adjacent musculature, illustrating how taughtness of these muscles produced by forced positions of rotation may compress these important blood vessels supplying the femoral head. (From Ogden, J. [Ferguson, A. B., ed.]. In Orthopedic surgery in infancy and childhood, ed. 4. Copyright © 1975, The Williams and Wilkins Co., Baltimore.)

ing treatment of congenital dislocation of the hip despite all conscientious and knowledgeable efforts directed toward its prevention. Because of the importance of this complication and its occasional unavoidable incidence, the treatment of the sequelae and consequences of necrosis as a complication will be discussed in Chapter 7.

TREATMENT OF RESIDUAL DEFORMITIES FOLLOWING REDUCTION

After a concentric reduction of the femoral head has been achieved and all of the foregoing determinants have been assessed, it is necessary that consideration be given concerning the need for correction of any residual deformities in either the proximal femur, acetabulum, or both. The approach to this problem has become and remains somewhat controversial, depending on where the major deformity is considered to reside. Thus some authors have believed that corrections on the femoral side are more likely to produce the best hip, whereas others have thought that the pelvic side deserves the greatest attention and will most appropriately solve the problem. Some, of course, reason that it may be one or the other or both sides of the hip joint that deserve correction. I believe that it is essential to define the problem as accurately as possible and to accomplish that procedure or combination of procedures that most directly corrects the identifiable deformity, irrespective of where it is.

Proximal femoral (intertrochanteric) osteotomy

I believe that the indication for proximal femoral osteotomy in congenital dysplasia or dislocation consists of a *well-defined* deformity of the proximal femur that, when corrected, enhances the stability of the hip joint. Conversely, it does not appear appropriate to create a deformity of a bone that has *normal* configuration, in an effort to provide stability of a joint, when the cause for the instability most likely is in the configuration of the acetabulum or in the laxity of the capsule and ligaments of the joint. Undeniably, there are instances where the proximal femur will be the primary problem or major contributing site of the problem, and in these instances a well-executed corrective proximal femoral osteotomy is essential. In older children it may even be combined with pelvic osteotomy when the acetabulum is considered inadequate.

Evolution of proximal femoral osteotomy. During the past 3 decades there has been an increasing awareness of the concept that certain deformities of the proximal femur may play a significant role in contributing to the instability of the hip joint. Several basic and clinical studies have alluded to this issue. These include contributions by Lorenz,[21] Badgley,[3] Muller and Seddon,[26] MacKenzie and associates,[23] and Langenskiöld.[19] All seem to agree, irrespective of the etiologic factors involved, that excessive anteversion and/or valgus of the proximal femur contribute to hip joint instability and retardation of normal acetabular development. Conversely, correction of these deformities at an early age (3 to 4 years or earlier) was believed to enhance hip stability and to stimulate normal acetabular growth and development. This, therefore, led to the employment of a varus rotational femoral osteotomy designed to correct the deformities. It was used in 1953 by Platou[32] and Somerville[37] and in 1955 by Chuinard.[6] They all employed it as a primary procedure and usually in combination with open or closed reduction of the hip. Platou[32] preferred to perform an open or closed reduction and place the hip in the most stable position, which usually was found to be 40 to 90 degrees of inward rotation

120 Congenital dysplasia and dislocation of the hip

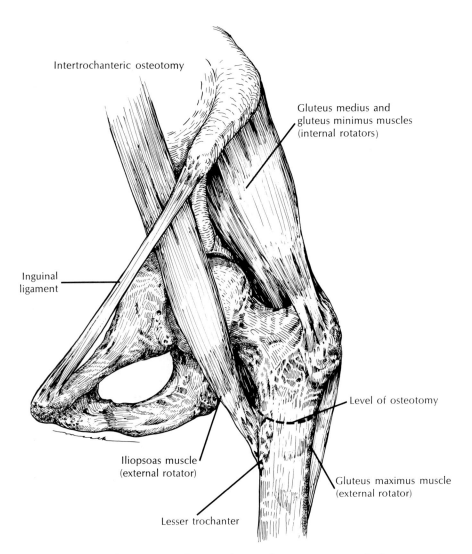

Fig. 5-12. Diagram of preferred anatomic location of intertrochanteric osteotomy. The iliopsoas attachment to the lesser trochanter and the gluteus maximus insertions are below the osteotomy, and the gluteus minimus and medius muscles (internal rotators) are above the osteotomy.

of the thigh. After removal of the cast, he then determined the amount of anteversion present by taking multiple x-ray views with the hip in varying degrees of inward rotation. The amount of inward rotation required to obtain the best position of the head and neck in the acetabulum then determined the amount of rotation to be corrected, which was then accomplished by subtrochanteric osteotomy.

Somerville[37] originally identified the need for derotational osteotomy after performing a series of open reductions and arthrograms. He frequently observed excessive anteversion of the femoral neck and believed that if the deformity were not corrected following reduction, the anterior capsule would stretch out, allowing subluxation or redislocation to occur. He also believed that if the capsule gives way less force will be transmitted through the femur and that as a result there will be less tendency for the excessive anteversion to correct with growth. This led Somerville[38] in 1957 to postulate a spectrum of disease that included "persistent fetal alignment." This was Somerville's effort to explain persistent anteversion of the femur, which caused an attitude of inward rotation of the entire limb beginning at the thigh.

Chuinard emphasized the importance of varus rotational osteotomy as early as 1955.[6] He believed that skeletal traction was essential for the reduction of the dislocated hip and that if anteversion were uncorrected, it would result in instability and poor hip development. He also believed that the *intertrochanteric* osteotomy was preferred, specifically above the level of the lesser trochanter and above the insertion of the gluteus maximus muscle. I also prefer this location because this osteotomy reduces the outward rotating power of the iliopsoas and gluteus maximus muscles, yet it preserves the inward rotating strength of the adductor and other pelvifemoral muscles (Fig. 5-12). Subsequently Chuinard[6,8] strengthened his conviction regarding the value of this osteotomy, which provides dynamic and static muscle forces that help maintain stability of the reduction and stimulate normal acetabular development. He also observed that the varus component of the osteotomy usually corrected with growth. I believe that correction of the varus position occurs very slowly after age 5 or 6 years and does not occur predictably if the capital epiphysis and physeal plate are not healthy. Therefore, in children over 6 years of age or in the presence of significant femoral head necrosis, varus osteotomy must be done very cautiously. Based on studies of the groin lateral (Laage) x-ray views, Chuinard[7] has also recommended that some degree of extension should be added to the osteotomy, in order to enhance stability of the hip in those instances where the femoral head tends to extrude anteriorly.

Prior to performing femoral osteotomy, Chapchal[4] insisted on accurate demonstration that a satisfactory position of the femoral head within the acetabulum could be obtained with inward rotation and abduction. He also believed that femoral osteotomy could be combined with innominate osteotomy when the latter was indicated. He stated that the corrective effect of the femoral osteotomy on acetabular growth and development became vitiated after age 3 years; therefore, he preferred to perform an intertrochanteric osteotomy only as a means of correcting specific deformities of the femur after the age of 3 years.

Monticelli[25] supported Chapchal's indications and goals of varus intertrochanteric osteotomy, and Tönnis[43] emphasized the following very important prerequisites, with which I wholeheartedly agree: there must be a concentric reduction of the femoral head in the acetabulum, and there must be a satisfactory range of hip motion prior to surgery. These issues are further discussed in the following section.

The technique that I prefer for performing proximal femoral rotational and/or angulation osteotomy is the intertrochanteric osteotomy as popularized by Chuinard (p. 121). The site of the osteotomy is critical since it is placed above the lesser trochanter as well as above the insertion of the gluteus maximus tendon. Furthermore, at the intertrochanteric level, angular corrections are also accomplished much more effectively. An example of a patient treated by intertrochanteric osteotomy is seen in Fig. 5-13. Any corrective osteotomy in the upper femur must be accurately held by some form of internal fixation, external fixation, or transfixion until satisfactory healing has occurred. The choice of devices is not so important as the purpose that they serve. My preference is some form of internal fixation utilizing a plate and screws (Fig. 5-14, A), or a two-piece nail-plate device (Fig. 5-14, B). Unfortunately these internal fixation devices must be removed at some subsequent time after healing has occurred, and this represents a distinct disadvantage because of the necessity of a second operative procedure. However, I believe that the protection offered by the internal fixation devices during the healing phase and during the recovery of range of motion and the early period of ambulation offsets this disadvantage. An alternate method of fixing the osteotomy is by transfixion pins that exit through the skin and are fixed in a plaster spica cast or in a Roger-Anderson device. I have found that these

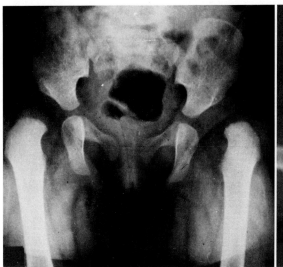
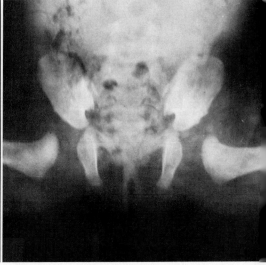

Fig. 5-13. An 11-month-old girl with dislocation of left hip and subluxation of the right, **A.** Frog-leg lateral view shows apparent excessive anteversion, **B.** Six months later the hips appear reduced, but with excessive anteversion, **C.** Intertrochanteric rotational-varus osteotomies were accomplished at age 2 years when it was shown that greater stability was present with the thighs held in abduction and internal rotation. The appearance 3 months after surgery is seen in **D.** Note evidence of femoral head necrosis. Five years later the heads are ossifying well and the acetabula are improved, **E.** At age 12 years the hip joints are well developed and stable; however, the right acetabulum covered the head less well, **F.** The appearance of the hip joints at age 15 years, 2½ years after innominate (Salter) osteotomy, is seen on the right, **G.** The plates should have been removed earlier.

Diagnosis and treatment in the child 18 months to 4 years of age

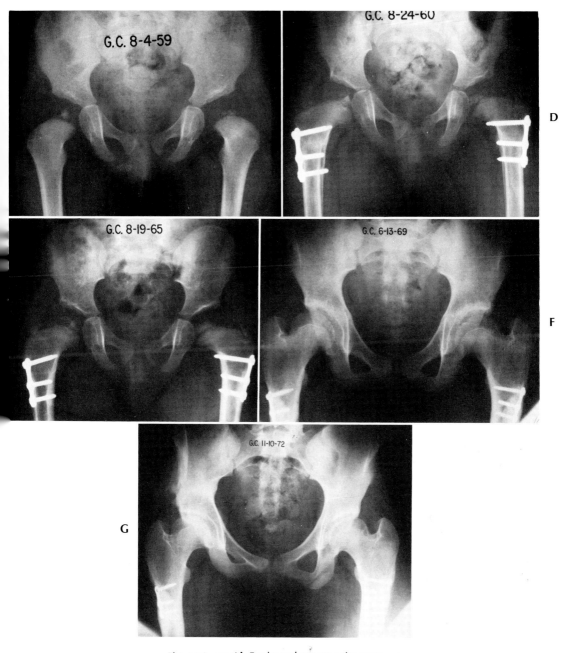

Fig. 5-13, cont'd. For legend see opposite page.

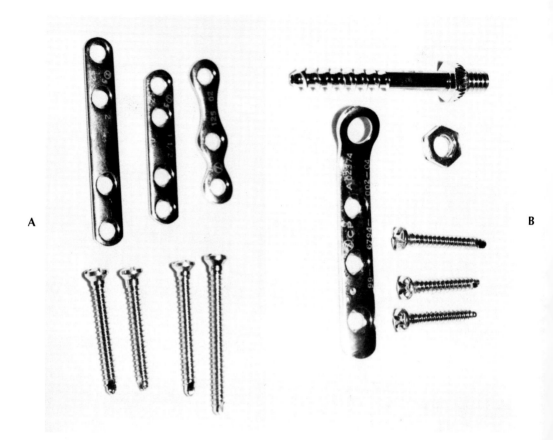

Fig. 5-14. Ordinary surgical steel plates shown in **A** are very satisfactory in young children under 36 months, whereas the Coventry screw and plates, **B**, are preferred for older children over 3 years.

are technically more difficult to use, that they expose the osteotomy site to the exterior, and that they sometimes may have to be removed before solid bony healing has occurred. In my experience the disadvantages of the transfixion pins exceed any technical advantage they might have.

Prerequisites. After the need for proximal femoral osteotomy has been determined, it is critical that certain prerequisites be met in order to avoid disappointment and failure following its accomplishment. The first and foremost prerequisite is, naturally, a clear definition of the configuration of the proximal femur in all three planes. Second, the femoral head must be stable and concentrically seated in the acetabulum when the femur is placed in abduction and internal rotation. Finally, there must be a "satisfactory," well-documented range of motion. If the configuration of the proximal femur is not well defined, there is no way to determine how much and which type of correction to achieve. If the femoral head is not concentrically reduced and stable in abduction and internal rotation, it will be subluxated and just as unstable after osteotomy as it was before. If the range of motion is not satisfactory, a deformity in attitude of the lower limb will be created as a result of the osteotomy. For example, if there is no internal rotation possible, or if abduction is restricted, then either external rotational osteotomy, varus osteotomy, or both will result in an externally rotated and/or adducted attitude of the hip.

Contraindications and complications. Clearly when the indications or prerequisites are not satisfied, a contraindication to osteotomy exists. Technical complications of femoral osteotomy include overcorrection, undercorrection, and technical failure in the use of internal or transfixion devices.

Distal femoral (supracondylar) osteotomy

The use of rotational supracondylar osteotomy has been recommended in the past for young children who have excessive anteversion. It is obvious that only rotational deformities can be corrected by this method. Furthermore, this osteotomy offers no major advantage over intertrochanteric osteotomy except that it can be done with a tourniquet; however, this rather minimal advantage does not outweigh the greater versatility and anatomic advantages of the intertrochanteric osteotomy discussed earlier. Thus I rarely if ever perform supracondylar femoral osteotomy for proximal femoral deformities in congenital dislocation of the hip, *unless* it is done simply to correct an internal rotational contracture of the thigh or hip created by prolonged cast immobilization in that position during treatment.

CORRECTION OF ACETABULAR DEFICIENCIES

Acetabular abnormalities are far more significant in congenital hip dysplasia and dislocation than are femoral deformities. It is to this particular problem that many surgeons in the past have addressed themselves. The evolution of our current techniques in the correction of acetabular deficiencies represents a fascinating saga in children's hip surgery; in order to understand the value of our present methods, the following brief historical review is essential.

Correction of residual acetabular deficiencies has been attempted in a variety of ways, based on diverse concepts. Early surgeons such as Albee[1] turned down a flap of bone and articular cartilage from the outer wing of the ilium, just above the acetabulum. Into the gap created by the flap, he placed tibial bone struts for support. Other surgeons* later developed modifications of the Albee procedure. All were designed to form a superior buttress for the femoral head utilizing various grafting techniques. Subsequently, Heyman,[15] and more recently Wilson,[47] developed further modifications of the "shelf" procedure. All of these operations have become relegated either to the historical archives or to the category of salvage procedures (see Chapter 8).

In 1955 Chiari[5] initiated pelvic osteotomy as a means of correcting acetabular deficiencies in congenital dislocation. He originally conceived of this operation as a definitive reconstructive procedure. However, for a variety of reasons discussed in Chapter 8, the Chiari pelvic osteotomy is now considered essentially a salvage operation. Salter[33] and Pemberton[30] independently developed corrective pelvic osteotomies that had two important concepts in common; namely, (1) the osteotomy rotated part or all of the acetabular roof forward and outward over the femoral head; and (2), in contrast to the Chiari osteotomy, the normal articular cartilage of the acetabulum was preserved as a weight-bearing surface. This latter accomplishment is the principal reason why these two procedures are considered reconstructive rather than salvage operations.

The pericapsular (Pemberton) osteotomy requires the presence of a triradiate cartilage for its effective execution; the

---
*See references 9, 10, 13, and 14.

innominate (Salter) osteotomy requires a mobile and flexible symphysis pubis in order that satisfactory rotation of the inferior pelvic fragment can be accomplished. This may be very difficult to achieve in young adults; as a result, this technical problem led to Steel's[39] development of the triple innominate osteotomy. This procedure relies on osteotomies of the ilium, ischium, and pubis to increase the mobility of the inferior or acetabular fragment. The acetabular fragment is rotated outward and forward in the same manner as with the innominate osteotomy of Salter, and it is transfixed in a similar fashion. Later Sutherland and Greenfield[41] accomplished acetabular rotation by performing an iliac osteotomy as well as an osteotomy through the superior and inferior pubic rami just lateral to the symphysis pubis. Rotation of the acetabulum by performing a periarticular osteotomy of the entire pelvis has been developed by Eppright,[12] Wagner,[44] and Kawamura.[17] This procedure, known as a dial osteotomy, also preserves the articular cartilage and, therefore, technically qualifies as a reconstructive procedure. Because these latter procedures described by Steel,[39] Sutherland,[40,41] and Eppright[12] are usually done in older children and adolescents, they will be discussed in Chapter 6. At the current state of our technical expertise, therefore, it appears appropriate to conclude that acetabular deficiencies can be corrected by two basic methods. One technique preserves the acetabular articular cartilage and simply rotates the acetabulum over the femoral head in order to improve the weight-bearing surface. The other method utilizes capsule-covered bone as the increased buttress for the femoral head, and the increased weight-bearing surface does not utilize articular cartilage. From a practical standpoint the former techniques are called "reconstructive" and the latter "salvage" (see Chapter 8).

The most well-accepted current methods of correcting acetabular deficiencies in congenital dysplasia of the hip in children include either the pericapsular (Pemberton) osteotomy or the innominate (Salter) osteotomy. Though somewhat similar in their principle, as noted on p. 125, they are technically considerably different in the means by which they are accomplished. Both are based on the concept that the major defect is an abnormality either in the configuration or the orientation of the acetabulum. The femoral head is considered to be improperly covered in the anterior and superior or superolateral portions. The osteotomies are both devised to remedy that defect. In the pericapsular (incomplete) osteotomy, the anterior two thirds of the entire acetabulum are hinged forward, outward, and downward, utilizing the triradiate cartilage as the fulcrum. In the innominate (complete) osteotomy, the innominate bone is sectioned completely, and the entire acetabulum is redirected forward, outward, and downward with the fulcrum or axis of rotation being located at the symphysis pubis. Details of the techniques of the two procedures follow.

Pericapsular (Pemberton) osteotomy

Through an anterior (iliofemoral) incision the lateral aspect of the ilium is exposed subperiosteally by reflection of the tensor fasciae latae and the gluteus medius muscles (Fig. 5-15). The sartorius muscle is sectioned at its origin and reflected distally. An assistant places a sharp rake retractor on the iliac apophysis; utilizing an elevator, the surgeon reflects the apophysis medially at its osteochondral junction. The iliacus muscle is then reflected subperiosteally from the inner table of the ilium, thus completely exposing the anterior two thirds of the ilium. The anterior aspect of the ilium is cleaned of soft tissue, and the straight and

Diagnosis and treatment in the child 18 months to 4 years of age 127

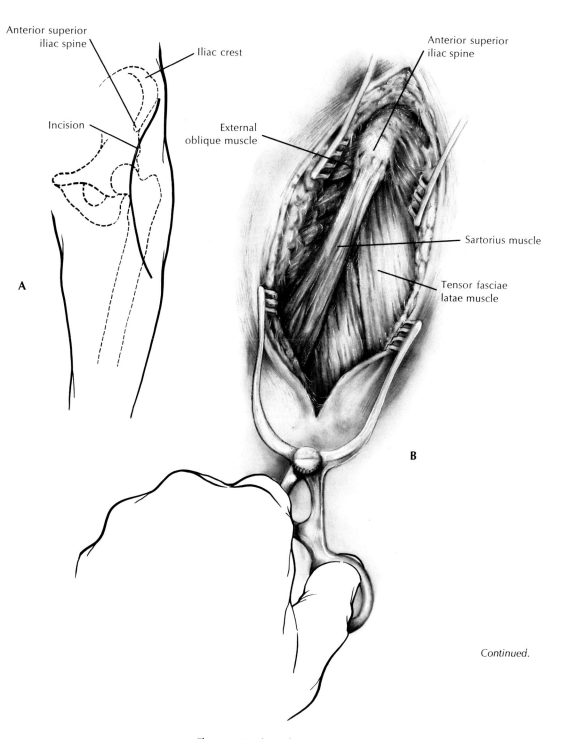

Fig. 5-15. For legend see p. 128.

Continued.

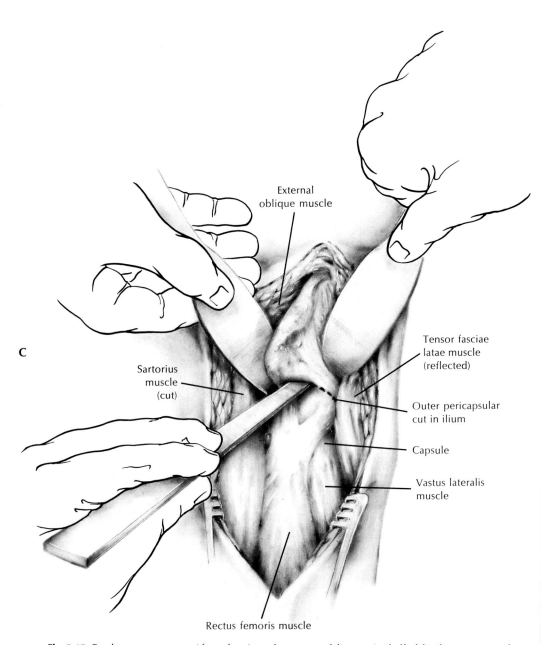

Fig. 5-15. Pemberton osteotomy. After subperiosteal exposure of the anterior half of the iliac crest, **A** and **B,** and with retractors placed into the sciatic notch on both sides of the pelvis, a curved pericapsular osteomtomy is made into the outer table of the ilium, **C.** A similar osteotomy is then made on the inner wall that parallels the outer table osteotomy. It is, however, made at a more inferior (distal) level, **D.** A generous-sized, triangular graft is obtained from the anterior crest of the ilium, **E,** and this graft is placed into the gap created by downward displacement of the inferior fragment created by the previously made osteotomy, **F.**

Diagnosis and treatment in the child 18 months to 4 years of age

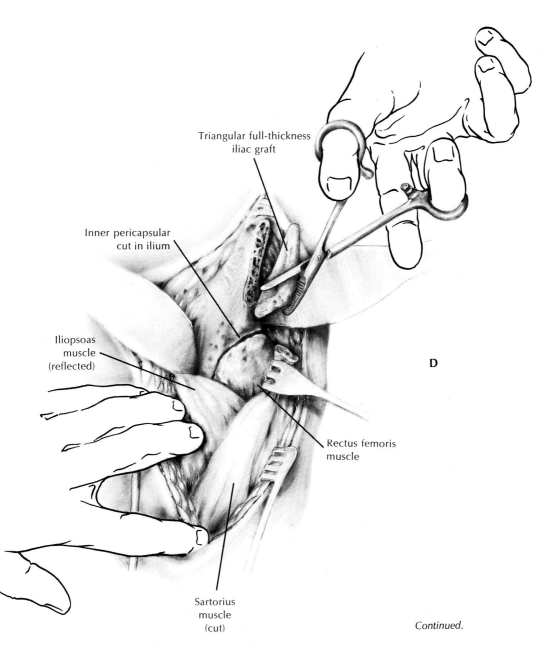

Fig. 5-15, cont'd. For legend see opposite page.

Continued.

130 *Congenital dysplasia and dislocation of the hip*

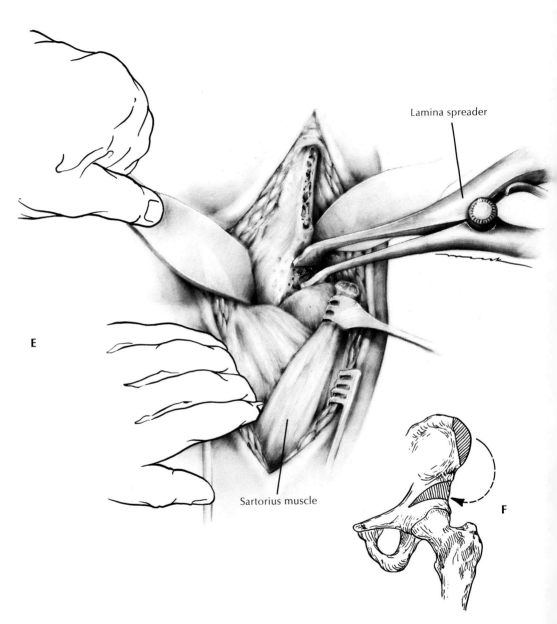

Fig. 5-15, cont'd. For legend see p. 128.

reflected heads of the rectus femoris muscle are exposed along with the capsule of the hip joint. At this point arthrotomy and joint exploration may be done if indicated. A retractor is placed subperiosteally into the sciatic notch on either side of the ilium. At this time it is advisable in older children to tenotomize the tendinous portion of the iliopsoas muscle. Care must be exercised to protect the femoral nerve during this procedure.

The osteotomy in the ilium is first made in the outer table. A curvilinear osteotomy, paralleling the capsule of the hip joint, is made initially. The osteotomy begins at the level of the anterior-inferior iliac spine, just above the reflected head of the rectus femoris muscle, and extends posteriorly and inferiorly toward the posterior arm of the triradiate cartilage. The most posterior and inferior portion of the osteotomy is the most difficult to accomplish, since it must be done largely without direct visualization and must be accurately placed anterior to the sciatic notch, yet posterior to the hip joint margin. A similar cut is made on the inner table of the ilium. Depending on the need for greater or lesser lateral extension of the osteotomized fragment, the outer osteotomy should be made either more superiorly or more nearly parallel, respectively, to the inner cut. Both inner and outer table osteotomies are then joined by means of a curved osteotome, and the full thickness of the ilium is sectioned as far posteriorly and inferiorly as the triradiate cartilage. The inferior segment is then levered forward, outward, and downward and held there by means of a lamina spreader. Grooves are made in the opposing cancellous surfaces of the osteotomy. These grooves are designed to receive and help stabilize the graft from the ilium. The iliac crest is cleaned of any remnants of cartilage and periosteum and a triangular, full-thickness graft is removed from the crest. It is inserted into the space between the osteotomized fragments and firmly impacted into place. When the lamina spreader is removed, the graft should be both rigidly held and inherently stable. No internal fixation is necessary. The sartorius, tensor fasciae latae, and iliacus muscles are sutured to each other and the wound is closed. A one and one-half hip spica cast is applied, which is removed after 6 weeks; if healing is evident by x-ray examination, graduated weight bearing is permitted. An example of a patient treated by a Pemberton osteotomy is seen in Fig. 5-16.

Advantages and disadvantages. The incomplete osteotomy leaves the posterior and inferior portions of the acetabulum relatively undisturbed; therefore, the osteotomy is sufficiently stable so that internal fixation is not required. Also, since the fulcrum of rotation (the triradiate cartilage) is closer to the area of correction, a lesser degree of rotation and angulation of the acetabular fragment is necessary, as compared to the complete innominate osteotomy, in order to gain the desired correction. Finally, except for the placement of retractors, no instrumentation in the sciatic notch is required; therefore, there may be less likelihood of damage to the neurovascular structures in the notch. This latter advantage, however, is offset by one of the disadvantages; that is, the most posterior and inferior portion of the osteotomy is largely done blindly because of the difficulty in visualizing the triradiate cartilage from the anterior exposure.

Another disadvantage of the pericapsular osteotomy is the fact that the configuration of the acetabulum must be changed somewhat, simply because the osteotomy is incomplete. This is perhaps the most serious criticism of the procedure. In my opinion this significant issue dictates that the operation should

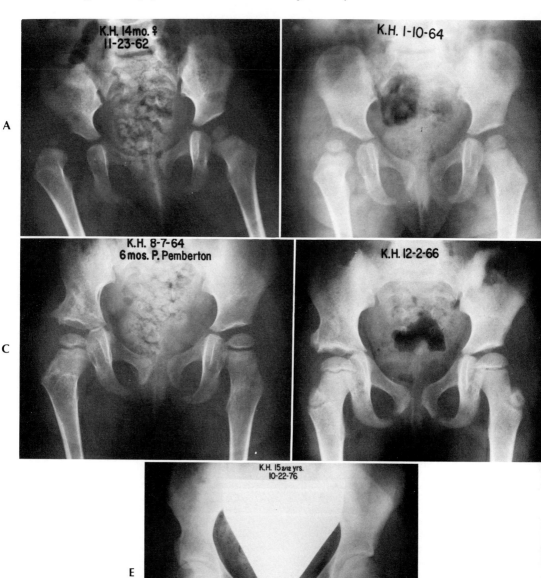

Fig. 5-16. An example of pericapsular osteotomy. A 14-month-old girl with dislocation of right hip is seen in **A**. At age 28 months the hip is reduced, but the acetabulum is oblique, the lateral rim is irregular, and the femoral head tends to be somewhat lateral, **B**. With abduction-internal rotation and groin-lateral views, the hip was well centered; therefore, a pericapsular osteotomy was accomplished, **C**. The appearance of the hip is seen 2 years later, **D**, and 12 years later, **E**. The patient is asymptomatic with no limp and with a normal range of motion.

be utilized only in children who have considerable remodeling capacity (biologic plasticity) of their acetabulum and femoral head. As a general rule this osteotomy should be reserved for children who are skeletally under 7 years of age. Also, unless the triradiate cartilage is open, the procedure cannot be done as originally described; this imposes a major restriction with respect to the age when the operation is done. Even if one wished to do the pericapsular procedure, this would be very difficult, if not impossible, to accomplish in a child over 10 or 12 years of age. A final disadvantage has to do with the technical difficulty of the operation. Because of the technical demands for precisely placing the cuts in the ilium, this osteotomy is more difficult to accomplish satisfactorily than is the complete innominate osteotomy. Unless the surgeon has done this procedure under supervision on more than one occasion, it would be wiser not to attempt the pericapsular osteotomy.

Innominate (Salter, complete) osteotomy

The ilium is exposed in the same fashion as described in the pericapsular osteotomy (Fig. 5-17). The iliac apophysis may be reflected in one of two ways. Either the apophysis can be split vertically and half is reflected both laterally and medially or the apophysis can be reflected in the same manner as described in the pericapsular osteotomy. When the capsule is exposed, arthrotomy and joint exploration may be carried out *if indicated*. In older children the tendinous portion of the iliopsoas muscle should be sectioned just as in the pericapsular osteotomy.

Retractors are placed subperiosteally into the sciatic notch, both inside and outside the innominate bone, and a Gigli saw is placed in the sciatic notch. This is best done by placing a guiding finger into the notch on the lateral side of the ilium and inserting a curved kidney-pedicle clamp into the notch from the medial (inner) side. The Gigli saw can be easily passed around the notch with the clamp. The osteotomy is then made from behind, moving forward, and the Gigli saw exits just above the anterior inferior iliac spine. The plane of the osteotomy should ordinarily be made so that the lateral cut is higher than the inner cut. Thus when the inferior fragment is rotated forward, outward, and downward, the cut surfaces become relatively parallel in the frontal plane. It is extremely important that the inferior fragment be *pulled* forward by either a towel clip in younger children or a bone hook (inserted into the posterior aspect of the inferior fragment) in older children. The hip is then placed forcibly into flexion, abduction, and external rotation, and, with forward traction on the lower fragment, it will be rotated forward so that the anterior portion of the osteotomy is open and the posterior aspect of the osteotomy is closed. In older children and adolescents I find that a lamina spreader placed anteriorly *in conjunction* with the bone hook in the inferior fragment assists in gaining the desired correction.

A triangular, full-thickness graft taken from the iliac crest is then inserted into the opening between the fragments. The two fragments of the osteotomy and the graft are then transfixed by one or two threaded Steinmann pins. Stability should be tested manually, and a pelvic x-ray film should be taken to verify the placement of the pins. Closure is accomplished and the cast application and aftercare are the same as with the pericapsular osteotomy. In older children the time of cast immobilization may be extended to as long 8 weeks (Fig. 5-18).

Advantages and disadvantages. In this procedure the entire acetabulum is rotated and redirected forward and outward, with the fulcrum or axis of rotation

Text continued on p. 138.

134 Congenital dysplasia and dislocation of the hip

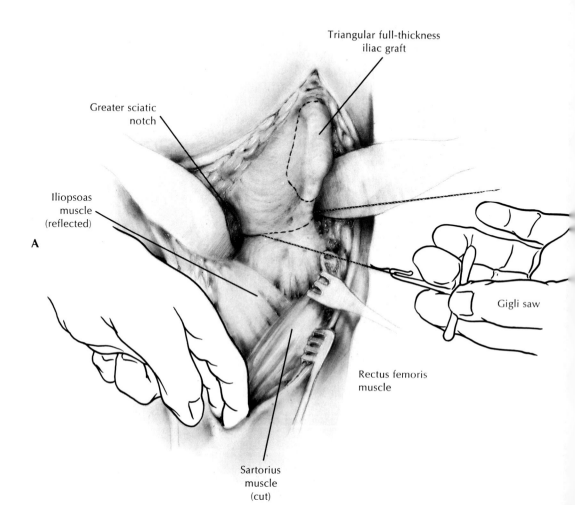

Fig. 5-17. After the anterior half of the ilium has been subperiostally exposed (as in the pericapsular osteotomy), a Gigli saw is passed through the sciatic notch, **A.** The ilium is cut completely through, with the angle of the osteotomy such that the outer cut is higher (more cephalad) than the inner cut. A bone hook is then placed into the posterior aspect of the distal fragment and this inferior fragment is pulled forward and outward, rotating it so that the anterior aspect of the osteotomized fragments is opened widely, but the posterior aspect is closed, **B.** A triangular graft taken from the ilium is then placed (not driven) into the triangular gap created between the two fragments, and this graft and the two fragments are transfixed with two threaded Steinmann pins, **C.** (Adapted from Salter, R. B.: Innominate osteotomy in the treatment of congenital dislocation and subluxation of the hip, J. Bone Joint Surg. **43B:**518, 1961.)

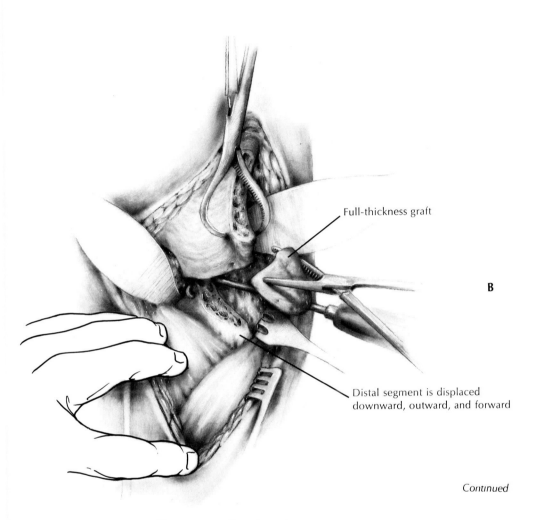

Fig. 5-17, cont'd. For legend see opposite page.

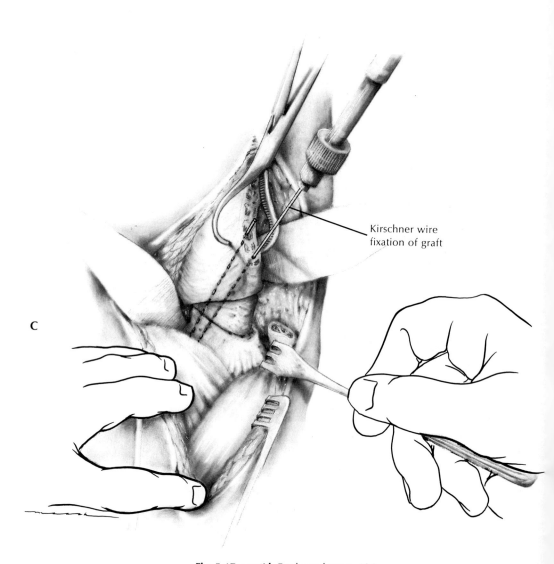

Fig. 5-17, cont'd. For legend see p. 134.

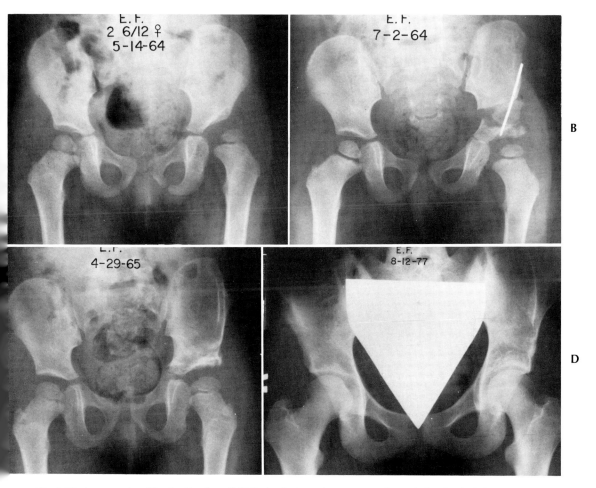

Fig. 5-18. An example of the "redirectional" (Salter) osteotomy in treatment of acetabular dysplasia in a young child. Pelvic roentgenogram following closed reduction of a unilateral dislocation of the left hip in a 2½-year-old female is seen in **A**. Note the broken Shenton line, blunting of lateral acetabular rim, and other features suggesting an inadequate acetabulum. A redirectional pelvic osteotomy was accomplished 6 weeks later, **B**. Over 1 year later the hip joint was much improved, **C**, and 13 years later an essentially normal hip resulted, both clinically and roentgenographically, **D**.

being at the symphysis pubis. Thus no change in the shape of the socket occurs, and the acetabulum is simply "redirected," resulting in a change in its attitude. This procedure has greater versatility than the incomplete osteotomy because it can be used at any age through skeletal maturity. It technically is less difficult to perform than the pericapsular procedure, and when properly done can provide adequate femoral head coverage in all childhood age groups. Its major disadvantage is the fact that there is some inherent instability of the fragments, thus dictating the need for internal fixation (Steinmann pins), which must be placed precisely and accurately across the two fragments *without* penetrating the pelvis or hip joint. An x-ray examination at the time of surgery is essential in order to document the placement of the pins. Also, the pins must be removed at a subsequent operative procedure. This, however, is obviously a relatively unimportant disadvantage. A final, also rather insignificant, technical disadvantage is the fact that a greater degree of acetabular rotation must be utilized in order to accomplish a comparable degree of correction done by the pericapsular method. This is because the fulcrum (symphysis) is further removed from the site of desired correction (acetabulum) than in the pericapsular osteotomy. Though technically easier than the pericapsular osteotomy in some parameters, there is one aspect of the operation that represents a major pitfall, and that is the previously noted fact that the osteotomy is inherently *unstable*. This has led to many catastrophic failures in Salter osteotomies done by inexperienced surgeons (see Chapter 7).

As is evident, each of these procedures has certain advantages and disadvatages when compared to each other. The surgeons' responsibility is to choose the procedure that in *their hands* will most effectively and safely accomplish the acetabular correction desired.

Pericapsular (Pemberton) and innominate (Salter) osteotomies

Indications. In keeping with the goal of the procedures, that is, to correct a persistent defect in the acetabulum, especially in the anterior and superolateral portion, it is obviously essential that this defect clearly exist in order for either procedure to be indicated. Although such an indication seems on the surface rather simple, demonstration and documentation of this abnormality is difficult to do on young children whose cartilaginous acetabula have not become completely ossified. Furthermore, reliable three-dimensional roentgenographic evaluation is difficult to achieve in the acetabulum in the young child between 18 months and 5 years of age by means of ordinary x-ray examination. Also, contrast arthrography, which conceptually should enable one to visualize the true cartilaginous configuration of the joint, has many shortcomings, especially as it relates to assessment of the joint in the cross-table or groin lateral view of the hip. Finally, any single x-ray examination made during the first 5 years on a growing and developing hip joint will not necessarily reveal the potential that exists for subsequent normal development (Figs. 5-19 and 5-20).

Ideally, therefore, a method of determination is needed that can accurately identify and quantitate the acetabular abnormality and that can predict with some degree of reliability which acetabula will eventually develop normally and which ones will not. Until that method of evaluation is developed and its validity proved, the indications for either pericapsular osteotomy or innominate osteotomy in the child under 5 years of age will remain rather nebulous and somewhat arbitrary. Unfortunately, that is our cur-

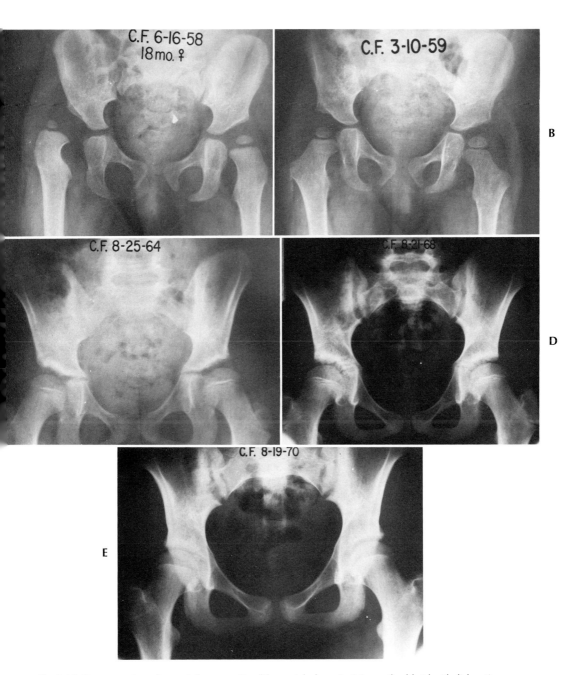

Fig. 5-19. Demonstration of remodeling capacity of the acetabulum. An 18-month-old girl with dislocation of right hip and dysplasia of the left hip, **A,** was treated by closed reduction and cast immobilization, **B.** Five years later the hips were well reduced, but the acetabula were still slightly sloping, **C.** No treatment was administered, and the appearance of the hips was seen 4 years later, **D,** and 6 years later, at age 14 years, **E.** Notice satisfactory femoral head coverage with completely normal Shenton lines. The patient was asymptomatic and had no limp and normal ranges of hip motion.

140 *Congenital dysplasia and dislocation of the hip*

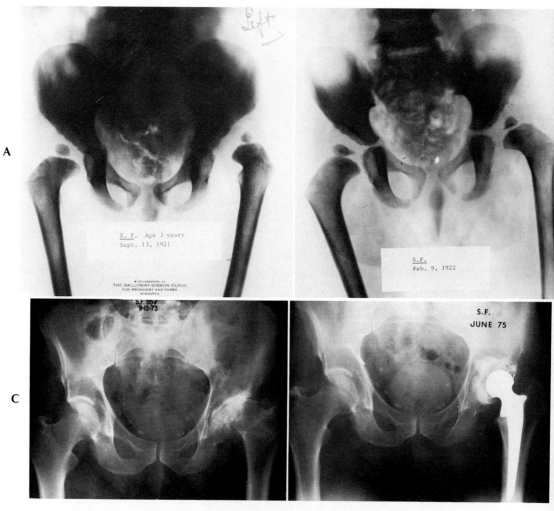

Fig. 5-20. Long-term follow-up to show remarkable capacity of the acetabulum to remodel. **A,** The pelvic x-ray film of a 3-year-old boy having a dyplastic hip on the right and a dislocated hip on the left. The pelvic film, **B,** was taken 6 months later after open reduction of the left hip. Note persistence of dysplasia on the right. Fifty-two years later, without any further treatment, the right hip is completely normal, whereas the hip subjected to open reduction has developed far-advanced osteoarthritis, **C,** necessitating total hip arthroplasty, **D.** (Courtesy Reckling, F. W.: Fifty-five–year follow-up of a patient with bilateral hip disease: dysplasia of one hip and dislocation of the other, J. Bone Joint Surg. **58A:**897, 1976.)

rent state of knowledge with respect to this issue in children whose skeletal age is under 5 years.

Despite these presently existing frailties, there are certain radiographic determinants available that, when coupled with judgment and clinical experience, can produce a reasonably defensible indication for either of these procedures. Most of these criteria are of a temporal nature. It is essential, therefore, when innominate osteotomy for a young child is being considered, that the surgeon has a series of sequential x-ray films taken periodically over a period of at least 12 to 18 months, or longer if possible, in order to document the growth and development of the acetabulum. The radiographic data most useful and most reliable can be listed and illustrated as follows: (1) failure of the ossified portion of the acetabular roof to reduce its slope *after* reduction has been achieved; (2) a persistent and *unchanging* break in the Shenton line (utilizing comparable femoral rotation); (3) persistent or progressive extrapelvic protrusion of the ossified femoral head (Fig. 5-21); (4) persistent blunting and convex configuration of the lateral portion of the acetabular roof (Fig. 5-22); and (5) finally, and most importantly, a composite evaluation of all the roentgenographic data, after they have been placed into perspective with the clinical history and physical examination.

Prerequisites. Once the indication for performing either of these procedures has been identified, it is mandatory that three prerequisites be met before proceeding with surgical correction. Unless these prerequisites are fulfilled, failure will most likely ensue.

The most important prerequisite for either the innominate or the pericapsular osteotomy is that the femoral head be concentrically reduced in the acetabulum. This relationship can best be demonstrated by an anteroposterior view of the pelvis with the femora held in abduction and internal rotation. If satisfactory congruity and/or concentric reduction is not achieved, then an absolute contrain-

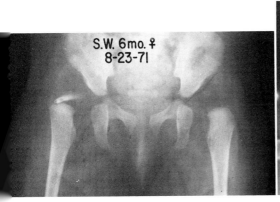
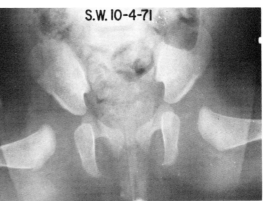

Continued.

Fig. 5-21. Pelvic film of a 6-month-old patient with bilateral dislocation treated by preliminary traction and closed reduction, **A** and **B**. Eighteen months later the femoral heads are well reduced but the acetabula are not well remodeled and the Shenton line remains broken, especially on the right, **C**. Two years later and 4 years later the same failure of normal remodeling is evident, **D** and **E**. An abduction-internal rotation film shows the femoral heads to be well seated, **F**, and, therefore, bilateral pericapsular osteotomies were accomplished, **G**.

142 *Congenital dysplasia and dislocation of the hip*

C

E

G

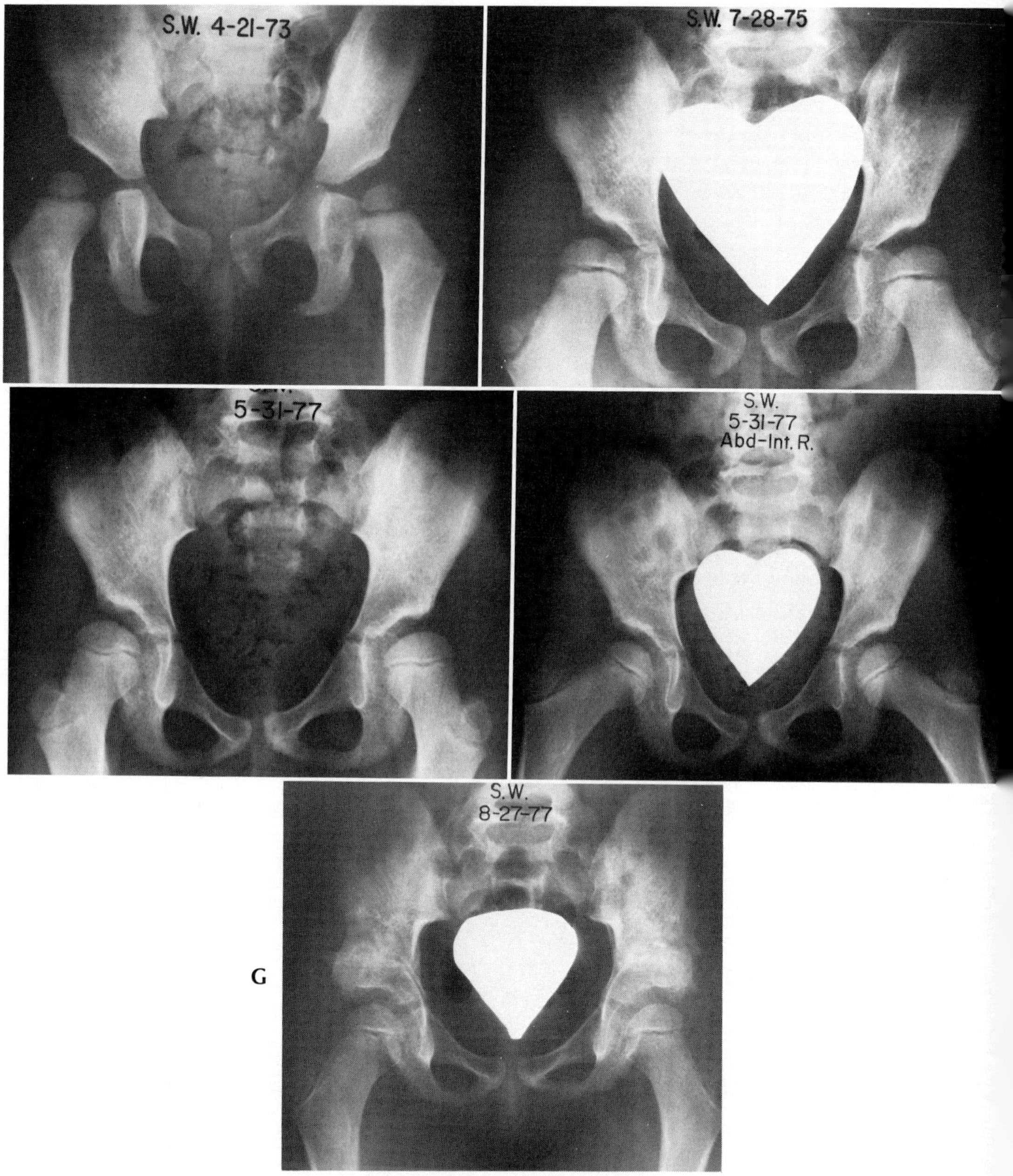

Fig. 5-21, cont'd. For legend see p. 141.

dication to pericapsular or innominate osteotomy exists (Fig. 5-23).

The second most important prerequisite is that a satisfactory range of motion of the hip must be present prior to acetabular surgery. When intra-articular adhesions exist, when major contractures of the hip joint are present, or when there is appreciable reduction in hip motion, an acetabular osteotomy may actually contribute to and accentuate any prior joint restriction of motion.

Finally, evidence of good cartilage space and congruity of the articulating joint surfaces is most desirable. In young children considerable potential for remodeling and adaptation of either the femoral head or the acetabulum is present, and one must use judgment with respect to the width of the cartilage space and the absolute degree of congruity necessary, as long as concentric reduction has been achieved. Clearly, the more congruous the head and acetabulum, the greater likelihood of success and the lesser likelihood of failure. To what extent this prerequisite is adhered to will depend on many of the aspects discussed on p. 148.

Complications. It must be emphasized that the goal of either of these procedures is to correct a defect in the acetabulum. Neither was designed to "gain reduc-

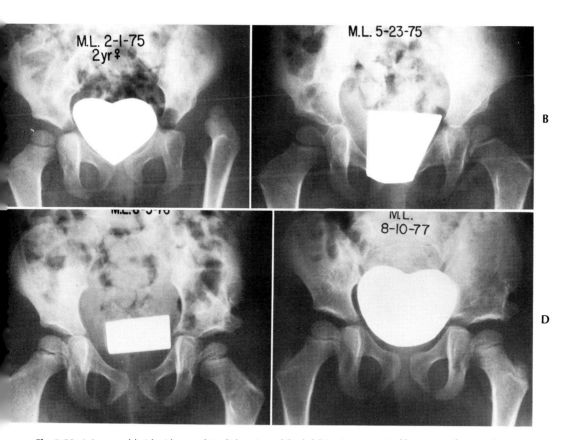

Fig. 5-22. A 2-year-old girl with complete dislocation of the left hip, **A,** was treated by open reduction via the medial approach. Because of a persistent break in the Shenton line and blunting of the lateral acetabular roof, **B,** a pericapsular innominate osteotomy was accomplished as seen in **C,** a film taken 1 year postoperatively. The result 1 year later is seen in **D.**

144 Congenital dysplasia and dislocation of the hip

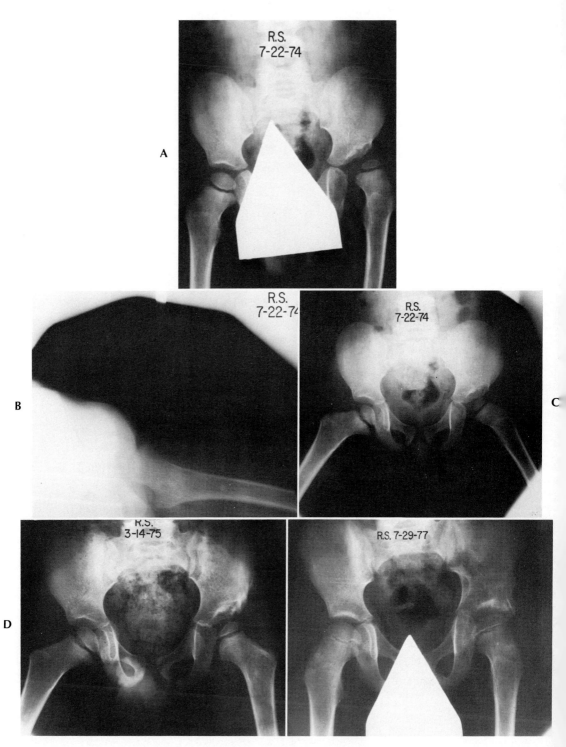

Fig. 5-23. For legend see opposite page.

tion." This simple statement of the objectives sounds superfluous and redundant, but many of the failures of both of these procedures can be traced to an evident misunderstanding of their purpose. Thus complications such as incomplete correction, persistent subluxation, and redislocation are largely the result of not having insisted on a concentric, congruous reduction *before* proceeding with pelvic osteotomy. These particular complications will be discussed in greater detail in Chapter 7.

When done for childhood dysplasia of the hip, the most frequent complications include displacement of the osteotomy, failure to gain adequate correction of the deformity, penetration of the hip joint by the transfixion pins, reduced range of hip motion (usually temporary), and pin tract infections (rare). Each of these results largely from errors either in judgment or in the technical accomplishment of the procedure. A more detailed discussion of these complications and their treatment will be found in Chapter 7.

Combined operative procedures in young children

Rarely in children under 18 months of age will an open reduction of the hip require additional reconstructive procedures on either side of the joint. Acetabular rotational or proximal femoral osteotomy is seldom indicated prior to 18 months of age because of the great ability of the skeleton to remodel and undergo adaptive changes, once a concentric reduction is achieved and maintained. Only if satisfactory subsequent remodeling of the acetabulum and upper femur fail to occur should operative procedures on these structures be required. The age of 18 months is purely an arbitrary division, however, and should not be used as a rigid criterion in determining the specific types of operative treatment in borderline situations.

On the other hand it is well established that the older the child is at the time of open reduction, the greater will be the likelihood of a need for combined procedures. This is because of the increased probability that adaptive bony and cartilaginous abnormalities will have developed in either the acetabulum or femur (or both) as a result of the greater duration of the dislocation. Understandably, the longer the femoral head is dislocated from the acetabulum the longer the stimulus to normal reciprocal development of these two structures will have been missing. Thus whether an acetabular or femoral deformity requiring operative correction exists at the time of open reduction will vary considerably from patient to patient, depending largely on the patient's age and the duration of the dislocation.

Open reduction and pelvic (pericapsular or innominate) osteotomy. In some patients over 18 or 24 months of age at the time of open reduction, there will be a need for additional or simultaneous surgery on the acetabulum. The deliberations involved in determining the need for such procedures and the wisdom with which such a decision is made are extremely important. Conceptually, the decision to accomplish a pelvic osteot-

---

Fig. 5-23. Minimal number of plain x-ray films include an anteroposterior view of the pelvis with the femora in neutral rotation, **A,** a cross-table groin lateral view of the hip, **B,** and an anteroposterior view with the thighs in abduction and inward rotation, **C.** This hip does not appear concentrically reduced, and arthrography would likely be helpful in delineating the problem. Pelvic osteotomy was considered contraindicated without open reduction. An open reduction was accomplished and the appearance of the hip 8 months later is seen in **D.** Because of failure of the acetabulum to remodel, a pericapsular pelvic osteotomy was done, **E.**

omy at the time of open reduction implies that the surgeon has the following three pieces of information:
1. That a concentric reduction of the femoral head in the acetabulum has been achieved
2. That the acetabulum is sufficiently inadequate that it cannot provide stability of the femoral head at the time of reduction
3. That the acetabulum will not undergo sufficient remodeling following concentric reduction so as to result eventually in a stable, normal-appearing joint

Evidence that a concentric reduction exists is a *prime* prerequisite for performance of either the pericapsular or innominate osteotomy. If this cannot be verified by direct observation and by roentgenographic examination if necessary, then simultaneous pelvic osteotomy is contraindicated. If concentric reduction is achieved, but because of an inadequate or abnormally directed acetabulum the hip is unstable, then improvement of stability by pelvic osteotomy is justified. And, finally, if in the judgment of the surgeon there is inadequate potential of the acetabulum for remodeling, then one may implement the acetabular osteotomy as a means of avoiding a second operative procedure. Clearly, this latter issue must be very highly individualized. It requires mature judgment on the part of the surgeon, because unfortunately no clear-cut or specific guidelines for making this decision are currently available. Some specialized situations may exist that clearly indicate the need for the combined procedure. For example, a case of congenital hyperthermia may occur (Fig. 5-24), or in some circumstances the follow-up on a child may be lost on the part of a derelict parent (Fig. 5-25). In such cases the combined procedure is likely a better solution in contrast to staging the operation. As the results of many simultaneous open reductions of the hip and pelvic osteotomies have been assessed, however, both Tachdjian[42] and MacEwen[22] have joined me in exercising great concern over the increased incidence of complications encountered when this combined procedure has been done by inexperienced

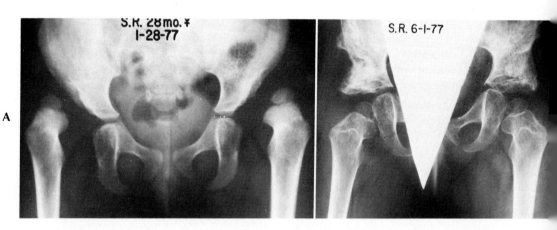

Fig. 5-24. Pelvic x-ray films of 28-month-old girl with bilateral dislocation of the hip, **A.** She had a strong family history for congenital hyperthermia, thus it was believed that as much should be accomplished at one operation as possible. Bilateral open reduction and simultaneous pericapsular osteotomies were accomplished without incident, **B.**

surgeons. It is agreed that many innominate osteotomies result in complications of one sort or another that actually make further restorative and reconstructive surgery much more difficult. When this observation is added to the dilemma about our yet poorly established indications for reconstructive pelvic osteotomy in children under age 4 or 5 years, the issue of routinely performing the two operations simultaneously is one that can and must be seriously challenged.

In this consideration it is extremely important to emphasize the goals and purposes of the osteotomies (pericapsular and innominate). These were conceived and developed to serve as reconstructive acetabular and stabilizing procedures in order to *maintain* reduction and *not* as a method of *obtaining* a concentric reduction. In many of the identified failures of these operations it has been abundantly clear that their original intent and purpose were not clearly understood. As a

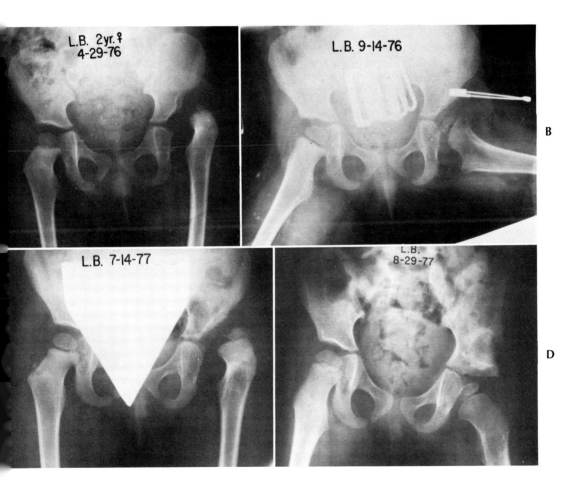

Fig. 5-25. This 2-year-old Navajo girl with dislocation of the left hip, **A,** was successfully treated by closed reduction and could be held reduced in an abduction device, **B.** The mother discontinued the splint, and the hip promptly redislocated, **C.** In this case, because of lack of reliable follow-up care, an early pelvic osteotomy done simultaneously with closed (or open) reduction may have prevented this complication. She was readmitted, and open reduction accompanied by a pelvic osteotomy was accomplished, **D.**

result, most failures of either procedure can be traced to their having been employed for inappropriate indications and misconceived purposes, that is, as a means of *gaining* reduction rather than as a means of *stabilizing* the reduction. Under no circumstances, therefore, should either the pericapsular or innominate osteotomy be employed in conjunction with open reduction until the femoral head has been concentrically reduced in the acetabulum. Instances that emphasize the results of failure to adhere to this principle will be illustrated and discussed in detail in Chapter 7.

The decision to perform an acetabular osteotomy simultaneously in order to provide greater stability to the reduced femoral head requires a *preoperative* evaluation of the configuration of the acetabulum by x-ray examination as well as an *intraoperative* appraisal of the stability of the reduction. Thus a poorly ossified acetabulum with increased obliquity of the acetabular roof as seen by x-ray examination *preoperatively* may well indicate the need for innominate or pericapsular osteotomy. Correspondingly, at the time of reduction, observations that suggest a significant deficiency of the anterior and superior portions of the acetabulum or clear-cut instability of the acetabular-femoral relationships can also justify performing the acetabular procedure simultaneously with open reduction.

When performing an acetabular procedure in conjunction with open reduction of the hip, it is essential that all measures be taken to avoid creating any excessive pressure on the femoral head when the acetabulum is rotated, either in a forward or downward direction. This necessitates that the iliopsoas tendon and muscle, or at least the tendinous portion of that muscle, be either sectioned or lengthened in all instances. Also, serious consideration must be given to femoral shortening. This is especially indicated in children over the age of 2 or 3 years or in children with unusually high-riding and more rigid dislocations in which reduction might be more difficult to achieve. In some cases of open reduction, therefore, especially in older children and children with high-riding dislocations, open reduction may require procedures on both sides of the joint done at the same operation. This combination of procedures, however, will practically never be indicated or necessary in children under 18 months of age.

Arthrotomy at the time of reconstructive pelvic osteotomy. Some surgeons, notably Sutherland[40] and Pemberton,[31] routinely perform arthrotomy of the hip at the time of performing an isolated reconstructive pelvic osteotomy. In other words the hip is or has been reduced and the indication for the osteotomy is simply a dysplastic acetabulum. The justification for the routine arthrotomy seems rather nebulous to me, because of its questionable value. Unless the hip is dislocated by the surgeon at the time of arthrotomy, then the interior of the joint cannot be examined or explored. This does not seem to be appropriate. Furthermore, a decision to perform a reconstructive pelvic osteotomy must be predicated on the presence of a concentric reduction. Possibly one can argue that an arthrotomy carefully done cannot cause any harm, but I believe that routine arthrotomy at the time of pelvic osteotomy in the presence of *concentricity of reduction* is totally unnecessary. Naturally, however, if there is strong doubt about reduction, then either arthrography, arthrotomy, or both, are indicated.

Open reduction and combined pelvic osteotomy and femoral shortening. This technically demanding operative procedure requires the surgeon to reach several conclusions both *preoperatively* and *intraoperatively* prior to proceeding with all aspects of the operation.

Preoperative determinations include an assessment of the configuration and attitude of the acetabulum, an evaluation of the degree of upward displacement of the femoral head, some estimate of the flexibility (or rigidity) of the dislocation, and a determination of the presence of any significant angular or torsional deformity of the upper femur. In order to make this assessment, the minimum x-ray evaluation outlined on p. 144 must be conducted and some concept of the mobility of the hip should be gained by appropriate preoperative physical examination.

Intraoperative determinations include evaluation of the stability of reduction, the concentricity of reduction, the degree of coverage of the reduced femoral head, the estimated amount of pressure on the reduced femoral head, and any significant angular or rotational deviations from the normal configuration of the upper femur.

On the basis of these preoperative and intraoperative observations, a reasonably reliable decision can be made as to whether or not this combination of procedures is indicated. The experience of the surgeon clearly enters strongly into the decision as to whether it is indicated and justified. One must consider all of the advantages of doing the procedures simultaneously and weigh them against the disadvantages. The advantages of doing all procedures at the same operation are obvious; namely, only one operation is required, only one period of immobilization is necessary, and, therefore, the total recovery period is shorter. Obviously, if drawbacks to this combination operation did not exist, one could hardly argue against doing the procedure even when there might be doubt about some of the specific determinations mentioned earlier. On the other hand, there are disadvantages and negative aspects to combining these procedures. Whenever the number of variables is increased, there will be an increased possibility of untoward results. Thus, reducing the hip, correcting the acetabular deficiency, and shortening (and altering the configuration of) the femur at one time essentially triples the potential source of complications and problems such as redislocation, intraarticular adhesions with resultant stiffness, cartilage necrosis, bone necrosis, and so forth. One must, therefore, weigh carefully all of these distressing possible sequelae against the very attractive advantage of solving surgically all major problems at one sitting. To make that decision calls for clinical judgment, which results only from extensive experience in children's hip surgery.

The technical details of each of these procedures have been described in earlier sections, and it is obvious that any one or all of these can be acomplished through the same incision, or an extension thereof. The postoperative management of a patient undergoing this combined procedure follows the same basic format and embraces the same considerations as for any of the operations. Thus the length of plaster immobilization approximates 6 to 8 weeks, followed by appropriate splinting or bracing and a progressive range of motion and weight-bearing program. In this latter regard individual consideration must be given to satisfactory maintenance of concentric reduction, to the stability of the reduction, to the degree of bone healing, to the state of health of the capital femoral epiphysis, and to the integrity of the joint. If intraarticular stiffness, cartilage necrosis, or bone necrosis develops, then a delayed weight-bearing activity program may be imposed. Also, if either the femoral or iliac osteotomy is delayed in healing, then weight bearing must be delayed. If any evidence of subluxation or instability occurs, then appropriate steps must be taken to correct them before weight-bearing activities are begun.

TREATMENT IN THE CHILD OVER 4 YEARS OF AGE

Children who are skeletally over 4 years of age represent a distinct challenge with respect to treatment of a congenital dislocated hip. By this time a considerably greater alteration has taken place in the configuration of the acetabulum and the femoral head, and the soft tissues have become further adapted to the foreshortened character of the limb. The exact time beyond 4 years of age when one should decline efforts at reducing the hip is not known, but it will vary according to the following significant factors: (1) whether the dislocation is unilateral or bilateral; (2) the skeletal age of the patient; (3) whether the dislocation is high-riding and rigid or whether it telescopes easily; (4) whether there has been any previous surgical treatment; (5) the presence or absence of other abnormalities; and (6) racial and ethnic considerations.

It is justifiable to attempt reduction of the *unilateral* dislocation of the hip at almost any age, provided the surgeon is sufficiently facile technically to cope with the various problems that can present themselves at the time of surgery. The hip of a younger child, ages 4 to 7 years, can often be reduced by measures mentioned earlier in this chapter. This includes open reduction and femoral shortening, with or without preliminary skeletal traction.[2] The older the child, the greater the probability of major alterations in size and configuration of the head or acetabulum, and thus the greater the likelihood of incongruity of the articular surfaces. When significant incongruity exists, there will be an increased probability of localized increased pressure on the articular surfaces when the hip is reduced, resulting in cartilage necrosis and stiffness. In such cases and in those wherein a satisfactory reduction cannot be achieved because of incongruity, I believe that Colonna arthroplasty in conjunction with femoral shortening is the desired procedure (Chapter 8). Thus a surgeon undertaking an open reduction of the hip in a child in this age group must

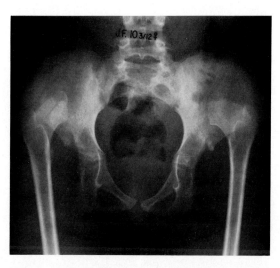

Fig. 5-26. A 10-year-old white girl had bilateral complete dislocations of the hip, known since early childhood. Treatment had been refused on philosophic grounds. The high-riding dislocations with poorly formed acetabula in a 10-year-old child should probably not be treated.

be equipped to handle the most complicated and sophisticated reconstructive procedures in children's hip surgery.

A reduced hip that has fair to good motion is better than a unilateral complete dislocation when it comes to accomplishing procedures such as total hip arthroplasty. Not only will the bone stock be better and the hip musculature better developed, but the technical aspects of a total hip procedure will be rendered much safer and easier. Thus one may look on reducing the dislocated hip of an older child as the first stage of a probable two-stage procedure. If it fails a fusion may still be done during adolescence without burning any bridges.

On the other hand, in the case of bilateral dislocation, the problem becomes much more complicated. In these instances one must be reasonably confident that the hips will not be made unattractively stiff by an open reduction, and thus the upper limit for considering open reduction and femoral shortening in bilateral cases must be around ages 5 to 7 years. This decision must again be modified either upward or downward, depending on the factors alluded to earlier. Bilateral stiff hips in a young patient in

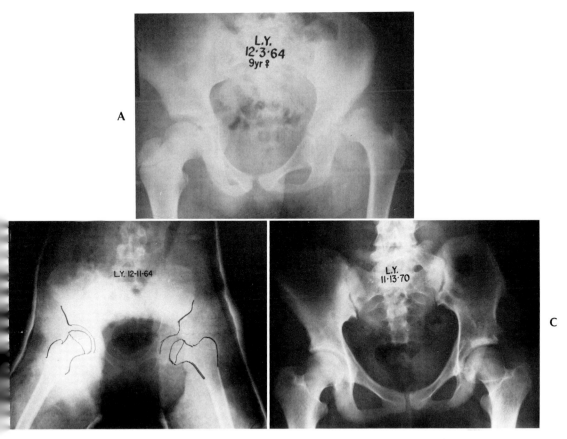

Fig. 5-27. This 9-year-old Navajo girl with a unilateral untreated dislocation of the left hip, **A**, underwent successful open reduction and pericapsular pelvic osteotomy without femoral shortening, **B**. This satisfactory result, **C**, would be unlikely in a white patient of this age. For details of her complete course see Fig. 7-11.

whom fusion, because of bilaterality, and total hip surgery, because of age, are contraindicated, produce a severe disability. In such circumstances the hips are better left unreduced during childhood and adolescence (Fig. 5-26).

Clearly, a high-riding, rigid dislocation may make a reduction technically impossible, or the reduction will produce such pressure on the head of the femur that cartilage and bone necrosis are inevitable. Also, most of these will be antenatal dislocations, in which there has been far advanced adaptive change on both sides of the joint, and thus, in effect, the anatomic circumstances similar to a much older dislocation are evident. It takes mature judgment and experience to decide that the safety and efficacy of a surgical procedure in such instances justify its performance. Conversely when the dislocated hip has great mobility as demonstrated by push-pull films and when, therefore, the femoral head can be brought down near the acetabulum by firm manual traction, one may consider performing open reduction at an older age than outlined earlier. This is especially true when the bony acetabulum appears well formed on x-ray examination.

The history and sequelae of prior surgical procedures can have a profound influence on any effects of reduction of dislocation. In these instances iatrogenic deformities often exist, and there is often considerable periarticular scar tissue present. In most cases any endeavors at surgical correction will largely fall into the salvage group. These problems and their solutions are discussed fully in Chapter 8.

Other musculoskeletal and soft tissue abnormalities must also be considered when contemplating reduction of a dislocated hip in a child over age 4 years. Such considerations must include restriction of joint motion in the hip and knee, any neurologic manifestations, any cutaneous manifestations, such as dermatomyositis or scleroderma, the presence or absence of certain syndromes such as the Down syndrome, and so forth.

Racial and ethnic differences in the response to treatment of congenital dislocation of the hip represent fascinating and provocative issues. It has been clearly demonstrated in my experience that Navajo Indian children at any age respond much more favorably to operative procedures on the hip joint than do white children of similar ages undergoing the same operation. This has been reasonably well established in a computerized study of members of both races who were treated at the Intermountain Unit of the Shriners Hospital.[36] The explanation for such differences in response to surgical treatment remains obscure, but it has encouraged me to consider open reduction in Navajo children at a somewhat older age than in white children (Fig. 5-27). Whether similar differences exist in other racial and ethnic groups is not clear to me.

The foregoing discussion is designed to emphasize the tremendously individualized character of the problem in treating older children with congenital dislocation of the hip. Fortunately, the condition in this age group is rare and will undoubtedly become more so in the United States as our medical sophistication increases. Hopefully, this particular portion of this text will become obsolete in the near future.

REFERENCES

1. Albee, F. H.: The bone graft wedge: its use in the treatment of relapsing, acquired, and congenital dislocation of the hip, N.Y. State J. Med. **102**:433, 1915.
2. Ashley, R. K., Larsen, L. J., and James P. M.: Reduction of dislocation of the hip in older children: a preliminary report, J. Bone Joint Surg. **54A**:545, 1972.
3. Badgley, C. E.: Correlation of clinical and anatomical facts leading to a conception of the etiology of congenital hip dysplasia, J. Bone Joint Surg. **25**:503, 1943.

4. Chapchal, G. J.: Intertrochanteric osteotomy in treatment of congenital dysplasia of the hip, Clin. Orthop. **119:**54, 1976.
5. Chiari, K.: Ergebnisse mit der Beckenosteotomie als Pfannendachplastik, Z. Orthop. **87:**14, 1955.
6. Chuinard, E. G.: Early weight bearing and correction of anteversion in the treatment of congenital dislocation of the hip, J. Bone Joint Surg. **37A:**229, 1955.
7. Chuinard, E. G.: Femoral osteotomy in the treatment of congenital dysplasia of the hip, Orthop. Clin. North Am. **3:**157, 1972.
8. Chuinard, E. G., and Logan, N. D.: Varus-producing and derotational subtrochanteric osteotomy in treatment of congenital dislocation of the hip, J. Bone Joint Surg. **45A:**1397, 1963.
9. Compere, E. L., and Phemister, D. B.: The tibial peg shelf in congenital dislocation in children, J. Bone Joint Surg. **17:**60, 1935.
10. Dickson, F. D.: The shelf operation in the treatment of congenital dislocation of the hip, Surg. Gynecol. Obstet. **55:**81, 1932.
11. Dunlap, K., Shands, A. R., Hollister, L. C., Gaul, S. Jr., and Streit, H. A.: A new method for determination of torsion of the femur, J. Bone Joint Surg. **35A:**289, 1953.
12. Eppright, R. H.: Unpublished data.
13. Ghormley, R. K.: Use of the anterior superior spine and crest of ilium in surgery of the hip joint, J. Bone Joint Surg. **13:**784, 1931.
14. Gill, A. B.: Plastic construction of an acetabulum in congenital dislocation of the hip—the shelf operation, J. Bone Joint Surg. **17:**48, 1935.
15. Heyman, C. H.: Long term results following a bone-shelf operation for congenital and some other dislocations of the hip in children, J. Bone Joint Surg. **45A:**1113, 1963.
16. Hubbard, D. D., and Staheli, L. T.: The direct radiographic measurement of femoral torsion using axial tomography: technic and comparison with an indirect radiographic method, Clin. Orthop. **86:**16, 1972.
17. Kawamura, B.: Dome osteotomy, Congenital Dysplasia of the Hip Symposium, Royal Oak, Michigan, 1974.
18. Laage, H., Barnett, J. C., Brady, J. M., and associates: Horizontal lateral roentgenography of the hip in children, J. Bone Joint Surg. **35A:**387, 1953.
19. Langenskiöld, F.: On the transposition of the iliopsoas muscle in operative reduction of congenital hip dislocation, Acta Orthop. Scand. **22:**295, 1952.
20. Larsen, L. J.: Surgical treatment of congenital dislocation of the hip in the older child, Abbott Lecture, 1975, Abbott Proc. **6:**1, 1975.
21. Lorenz, A.: Über die Behandlung der irreponiblen angeborenen Hüftluxationen und der Schenkelhals pseudoarthrosen mittels Gabelung (Bifurkation des oberen Femurendes), Wien. Klin. Wochenschr. **32:**997, 1919.
22. MacEwen, G. D.: Personal communication.
23. MacKenzie, I. G., Seddon, H. J., and Trevor, D.: Congenital dislocation of the hip, J. Bone Joint Surg. **42B:**689, 1960.
24. Magilligan, D. J.: Calculation of the angle of anteversion by means of horizontal lateral roentgenography, J. Bone Joint Surg. **38A:**1231, 1956.
25. Monticelli, G.: Intertrochanteric femoral osteotomy with concentric reduction of the femoral head in treatment of congenital acetabular dysplasia, Clin. Orthop. **119:**48, 1976.
26. Muller, G. M., and Seddon, H. J.: Late results of treatment of congenital dislocation of the hip, J. Bone Joint Surg. **35B:**342, 1953.
27. Ogden, J. A.: Changing patterns of proximal femoral vascularity, J. Bone Joint Surg. **56A:**941, 1974.
28. Ogden, J. A., and Southwick, W. O.: A possible cause of avascular necrosis complicating the treatment of congenital dislocation of the hip, J. Bone Joint Surg. **55A:**1770, 1973.
29. Ombrédanne, L.: Précis clinique et opératoire de chirurgie infantile, ed. 3, Paris, 1932, Masson & Cie Editeurs.
30. Pemberton, P. A.: Pericapsular osteotomy for congenital dislocation of the hip: indications and techniques. Some long-term results, J. Bone Joint Surg. **47A:**437, 1965.
31. Pemberton, P. A.: Personal communication.
32. Platou, E.: Rotation osteotomy in the treatment of congenital dislocation of the hip, J. Bone Joint Surg. **35A:**48, 1953.
33. Salter, R. B.: Innominate osteotomy in the treatment of congenital dislocation and subluxation of the hip, J. Bone Joint Surg. **43B:**518, 1961.
34. Salter, R. B., Kostuik, J., and Dallas, S.: Avascular necrosis of the femoral head as a complication of treatment for congenital dislocation of the hip in young children: a clinical and experimental investigation, Can. J. Surg. **12:**44, 1969.
35. Shands, A. R., Jr., and Steele, M. K.: Torsion of the femur, J. Bone Joint Surg. **40A:**803, 1958.
36. Snider, R.: Unpublished data.
37. Somerville, E. W.: Open reduction in congenital dislocation of the hip, J. Bone Joint Surg. **35B:**363, 1953.
38. Somerville, E. W.: Persistent foetal alignment of the hip, J. Bone Joint Surg. **39B:**106, 1957.
39. Steel, H. H.: Triple osteotomy of the innominate bone, J. Bone Joint Surg. **55A:**343, 1973.
40. Sutherland, D. H.: Personal communication.

41. Sutherland, D. H., and Greenfield, R.: Medial pubic osteotomy in difficult Salter procedures, Proceedings of the Western Orthopedic Association, October 1974, J. Bone Joint Surg. **57A:**135, 1975.
42. Tachdjian, M. O.: Personal communication.
43. Tönnis, D.: An evaluation of conservative and operative methods in the treatment of congenital hip dislocation, Clin. Orthop. **119:**76, 1976.
44. Wagner, H.: Osteotomies for congenital hip dislocation. In Proceedings of the fourth open scientific meeting of The Hip Society, St. Louis, 1976, The C. V. Mosby Co., p. 45.
45. Weiner, D. S., Hoyt, W. A., and O'Dell, H. W.: Congenital dislocation of the hip: the relationship of premanipulation, traction and age to avascular necrosis of the femoral head, J. Bone Joint Surg. **59A:**306, 1977.
46. Westin, G. W.: Personal communication.
47. Wilson, J. C., Jr.: Surgical treatment of the dysplastic acetabulum in adolescence, Clin. Orthop. **98:**137, 1974.

CHAPTER 6

Diagnosis and treatment of residual dysplasia in the older child or adolescent

Nonoperative treatment of hip dysplasia in infancy and childhood
Operative treatment of hip dysplasia in childhood and adolescence
   General considerations
Surgical procedures involved in treatment of acetabular dysplasia
   Operative procedures on the acetabular side
   Operative procedures on the femoral side
   Combined acetabular rotation and proximal femoral osteotomy

As noted in Chapter 4, abnormal physical findings in residual dysplasia of the hip are almost totally wanting. Occasionally, dysplasia of the hip in later infancy and early childhood does manifest itself by means of subtle degrees of limited hip abduction, but *more often* it cannot be detected by physical examination alone. Indeed, most instances of hip dysplasia in the latter months of infancy and in childhood are discovered incidentally by x-ray examination. The x-ray changes are characterized by a shallow, sloping acetabulum and an inadequately covered femoral head (Fig. 6-1). The Shenton line is usually broken, but there is a concentric relationship between the femoral head and acetabulum, and the head can be well seated in the socket with the thigh held in abduction and internal rotation. Additionally, there may be angular (varus or valgus) and/or rotational (excessive anteversion) deformities of the proximal femur. These femoral deformities, especially excessive anteversion and valgus, may further contribute to reduced femoral head coverage by the inadequate acetabulum (Fig. 6-2). Although basically stable, the biomechanical situation in such a hip represents a *potentially* unstable situation, and, unless corrected (either spontaneously or by definitive treatment), these hip deformities will undoubtedly result in the development of premature secondary osteoarthritis sometime during adult life (Figs. 6-3 and 3-14). The capricious and sinister nature of this particular sequel of newborn dysplasia is, therefore, quite evident. On the one hand it very often offers no detectable abnormalities on physical examination at a time when correction can be effected, but on the other hand it represents a potentially disabling problem in later life when only a salvage procedure can be offered.

Because there is no sure way of identifying hip dysplasia in later infancy and childhood by physical examination, because routine x-ray films of the pelvis are not taken unless an abnormality is otherwise suspected, and, further, because dysplasia is not symptomatic at this age, it is quite clear that a certain number of children with dysplasia of the hip will

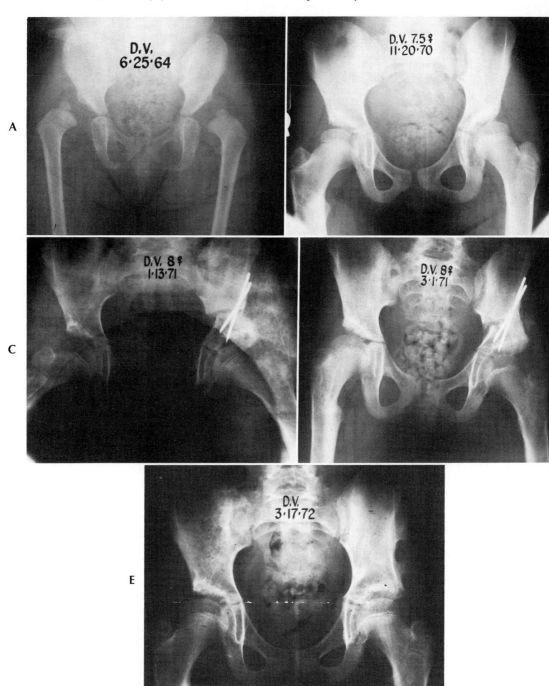

Fig. 6-1. A 2-year-old girl with bilateral dislocation of the hip, **A**, was treated by closed reduction. Five and one half years later the acetabula remained slightly oblique and the Shenton line was disturbed, the left hip more so than the right, **B**. The C-E angle measures 12 degrees on the left hip. A redirectional (Salter) pelvic osteotomy was accomplished as shown in **C** and **D**. At age 10 years the hip had a normal range of motion and the child was asymptomatic and walked without a limp, **E**.

Residual dysplasia in the older child or adolescent 157

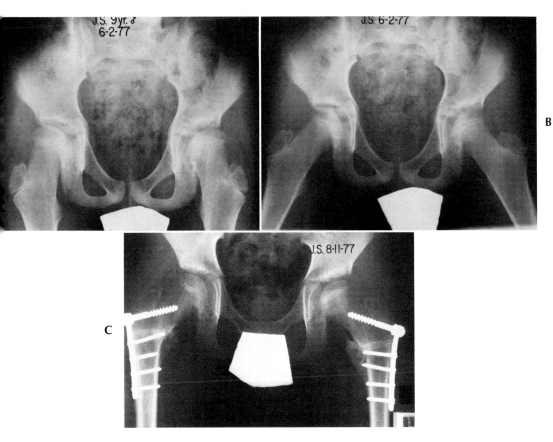

Fig. 6-2. This 9-year-old boy was treated by closed reduction for bilateral dislocation of the hips at age 18 months. His pelvic x-ray film at age 9 years showed moderately severe coxa valga, **A.** An abduction-internal rotation film showed the acetabula to be normal and the femoral heads to be well seated, **B.** Bilateral varus-rotational osteotomies were accomplished at the same operation, **C.**

proceed undetected into adult life. Some may be indentified incidentally, but most will likely not be detected at all until they develop symptoms of osteoarthritis later on.

NONOPERATIVE TREATMENT OF HIP DYSPLASIA IN INFANCY AND CHILDHOOD

Since the femoral head is usually concentrically reduced in the socket in the dysplastic hip and since the hip is basically somewhat stable, all therapeutic efforts should be directed toward restoring the anatomy of the acetabulum and upper femur to as close to normal as possible. To what extent conservative measures (splinting, bracing, etc.) can be effectively employed during the later months of infancy and early childhood is not easy to document, and the efficacy of such treatment must be weighed against the tendency for some hip dysplasias to correct spontaneously. Nevertheless, since nonoperative treatment is innocuous, I believe that the use of some form of external appliance is justified and indicated at least through age 2 years, or as long as radiographic improvement in the hip can be observed. The device should

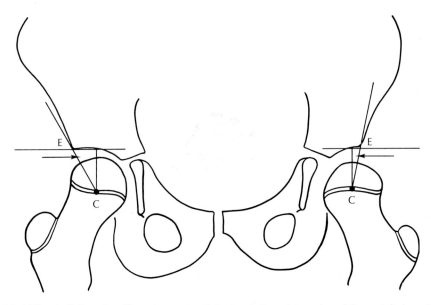

Fig. 6-3. Wiberg's C-E angle utilizes the center of the head, C, and the edge of the acetabulum, E, as reference points. A vertical line is drawn upward from the center of the head to intersect with a horizontal line. Then a line is drawn that connects points C and E. The angle subtended by those two lines is then known as the C-E angle. If this angle is less than 20 degrees, the acetabulum is considered dysplastic when applied to children over 5 years of age and the likelihood of degenerative arthritis developing in early adult life is great.

consist of some form of abduction mechanism that tends to thrust the head of the femur concentrically into the acetabulum and to correct any adductor muscle tightness that might be present. The issue governing the nature of the device employed centers about the question of whether the femur should be internally rotated and extended or externally rotated and abducted. Surprisingly, there is little evidence currently available that strongly supports one method or another. This can largely be explained by the earlier observation that quantitation of the results of any form of nonoperative treatment is unreliable. In treatment of this condition I prefer the simple abduction mechanism pictured in Fig. 4-7, but other methods are probably just as effective. Important in the implementation of these external devices is the principle of *physiologic positioning*. Since infants and children at this age are very active and are ambulatory in most instances, the splint should be worn only during naps and sleeping; therefore, it must be a removable device in order to permit ambulation and normal functional use of the muscles and bones and joints. For this reason, rigid cast immobilization is not only unnecessary but is *contraindicated*.

If improvement in the radiologic appearance of the hip joint gradually occurs, then the device should continue to be employed until maximum clinical and radiologic improvement of the hip has occurred. Obviously the duration of treatment may vary depending not only on the age at which the diagnosis is made and the treatment begun, but also on the severity of the dysplasia. If no change can be seen in the radiographic appearance of the hip as observed over a sufficient period of treatment (minimum, 9 to 12 months) or if inadequate correction is achieved, nonoperative measures will likely prove fruitless and consideration should be given to operative correction of the deformities. I believe, however, that one should observe the hip until age 4 or 5 years, as long as the hip remains stable, before a decision is made for corrective surgery. The reasons for this point of view are discussed below.

OPERATIVE TREATMENT OF HIP DYSPLASIA IN CHILDHOOD AND ADOLESCENCE
General considerations

Several subtle and yet unproved postulates must be considered in the deliberations regarding operative correction of residual dysplasia in this age group. First of all, it is very important to emphasize that the ultimate clinical and developmental behavior of a dysplastic hip, as encountered during early childhood, *cannot* be accurately predicted. Some cases may spontaneously improve and others may gradually become more dysplastic, developing subsequently symptoms of pain, restriction of motion, and disability even in early adolescence. Second, one has to deal with the controversy of whether or not surgical alteration of the proximal femur (varus rotational osteotomy) can effectively change the configuration of the acetabulum in these children over age 3 or 4 years. There are no well-documented controlled studies that support the concept that proximal femoral osteotomy can reliably or *predictably* alter the eventual shape of the acetabulum in children over 4 or 5 years of age, although Chuinard[1] and Somerville[5] have demonstrated that in the first 2 to 3 years of life this may well occur. Third, there are no irrefutable radiographic or clinical data that clearly outline the indications for an operation on the acetabulum in children 4 or 5 years old. Even though arthrography may be helpful in outlining the cartilaginous configuration and relationship of the femoral head and acetabulum, and despite the fact that a broken Shenton line suggests a defective acetabular roof, no radiographic discipline can accurately predict the future behavior of the acetabular cartilaginous anlage.

Indications. In establishing indications for operative treatment in residual hip dysplasia, the surgeon must make an assumption that if progressive improvement in the radiographic appearance of the acetabulum in a three-dimensional evaluation does not take place in an extended period of observation, the acetabulum will possibly remain dysplastic. What the surgeon does not know, however, is (1) the exact length of time necessary for such an observation in order to be reliable, and (2) what constitutes valid criteria by which failure of the acetabulum to improve is established. Also, there are no long-term studies yet available that can unequivocally and with certainty show that any operative procedure on either the proximal femur or on the acetabulum will materially alter the ultimate adult behavior of the treated childhood dysplastic hip. On the other hand there is a great deal of biomechanical and retrospective clinical evidence to support the concept that improved coverage of the adult hip is more likely to provide lasting wear,[11] but clear-cut criteria dealing with quantitation and qualitation of the amount of femoral head coverage essential *during this age group* are not so clear. It is evident, therefore, that currently accepted indications for surgical treatment of dysplasia of the hip in early childhood must be accepted with some reservation. However, the following two basic indications have been established that most surgeons accept: (1) a persistent deficiency in the acetabulum and (2) a clearly defined deformity of the proximal femur. Both, of course, may exist in the same hip at the same time. This section will deal with those procedures that are currently considered applicable to these residual dysplastic deformities. When discussing each of these operations, the indications that I utilize will be emphasized, and the prerequisites, contraindications, and complications will be outlined.

Radiographic evaluation. In order to define the problem accurately in dysplasia of the hip, at least three roentgenographic determinations are required. These include a conventional AP view of the pelvis with the patellae pointing directly forward, an AP view of the pelvis with the femora in abduction and internal rotation, and a cross-table or groin lateral view[4] of the hip taken with the patella pointing forward. These views provide the following data: (1) two views of the acetabulum and its femoral relationships, (2) the angular configuration of the proximal femur (varus or valgus), and (3) a reasonably accurate evaluation of the degree of anteversion (or retroversion, if it exists) of the femoral neck. Without these determinations, a surgical procedure on the hip cannot be accurately planned or executed. The need for arthrography to define the problem further is a highly individualized issue, and I reserve that procedure for those instances where there may be some uncertainty about the concentricity of reduction or the congruity of the femoral head and acetabulum (Fig. 5-7). In dysplasia of the hip, when concentricity of reduction can be satisfactorily demonstrated by the plain films, an arthrogram will rarely be needed (see Chapter 5). Wiberg's[11] retrospective roentgenographic study showed that hip joints demonstrating reduced coverage of the femoral head were the ones most likely to develop early osteoarthritis. He found that it was possible to determine, with a reasonable degree of accuracy, how much of the femoral head was not covered, using a simple calculation. He identified the exact center of the femoral head (C) and the edge of the acetabulum (E) and then drew a line between those two points. The angle subtended by that line and a perpendicular line from the center point was called the C-E angle (Fig. 6-3). He was able to show that when this angle after age 5 years is less than 20 degrees, the femoral head is inadequately covered, and, therefore, a reconstructive procedure on the hip is probably justified. On the other hand one must be very *careful* to verify that during the radiographic examination the femur is in its normal weight-bearing position with the patellae pointing straight forward. Misleading values have resulted from x-ray films taken with the femur in either internal or external rotation. A potential pitfall in the C-E determination also exists when one attempts to use this method in very young children. I believe that this calculation has no reliable validity in hip joints of patients under the age of 5 years and that, conversely, the older the patient the more reliable the determination.

Physical examination. In addition to the x-ray determination, a careful physical examination should be done with special reference to ranges of motion and to any limb length inequality. Documentation and evaluation of the ranges of motion of the hip are essential prerequisites in the deliberations involving the performance of any procedure on the upper femur that is designed to correct angular and/or rotational deformities. Clearly, a rotational osteotomy of the femur should not be done if there is greatly restricted rotational motion in one direction or another. Likewise, an angular osteotomy should not be accomplished if there is restriction of adduction or abduction, unless one is performing an osteotomy to compensate for such restriction. Furthermore, any procedure that rotates the acetabular fragment should not be done unless there is a satisfactory range of hip motion, especially flexion, abduction, and internal rotation.

Limb lengths should be accurately measured and recorded. Any variation must be taken into account when osteotomies on either side of the hip joint are being considered, simply because these procedures all have some significant potential effect on limb length (see Chapter 7). For example, a varus rotational osteotomy of the proximal femur usually produces some degree of temporary and possibly even permanent shortening in the lower limb. On the other hand either a pericapsular or innominate pelvic osteotomy almost always produces a measurable degree, although minor, of increased length of the limb. Thus in a limb that may already be shorter, a varus osteotomy of the proximal femur may further shorten the limb, whereas the reverse will ob-

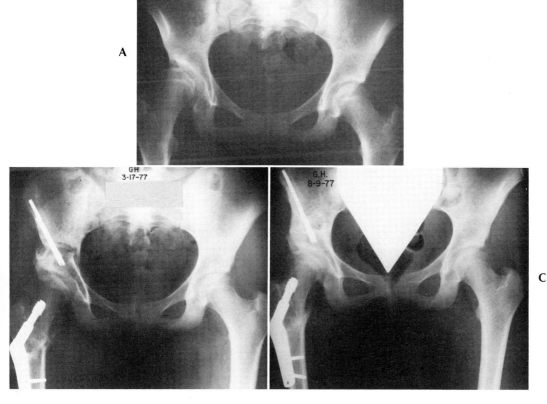

Fig. 6-4. A 13-year-old girl complained of a painful right hip, **A.** Earlier treatment for dislocation had consisted of an open reduction at age 2 years. The patient was 2.0 cm longer on the affected side. An innominate osteotomy was coupled with femoral shortening of 3.0 cm in order to equalize limb lengths, **B.** Five months later the patient walked with a normal gait and was asymptomatic. The valgus deformity of the femur should have been better corrected, **C.**

viously be true if a reconstructive pelvic osteotomy is accomplished. In most instances this will not be an influential issue, but occasionally it may necessitate surgery on both sides of the joint in order to avoid the need for subsequent treatment of the lower limb length inequality (Fig. 6-4).

SURGICAL PROCEDURES INVOLVED IN TREATMENT OF ACETABULAR DYSPLASIA

Once the roentgenographic and clinical data have been assembled, the problem has been accurately defined, and a decision has been reached justifying an operative approach, the surgeon must then select the surgical procedure or procedures that will best solve the entire problem. The available technical procedures include those either on the acetabular side, the femoral side, or a combination of both. Experience and thoughtful analysis are essential in order that the orthopedic surgeon may synthesize the most appropriate solution to the challenging problems that present themselves in the treatment of childhood hip dysplasia.

Operative procedures on the acetabular side

Correction of deformities of the acetabulum can be achieved in a variety of ways, largely depending on the age of the patient. In younger children whose acetabular-femoral relationships are congruent, and in whom the prerequisites have been met, an acetabular deformity can be corrected equally well by one or another of the reconstructive pelvic osteotomies. These procedures, appropriately executed, will correct the majority of instances of acetabular dysplasia in children under 15 years of age, in those cases where the demonstrable deformity is confined to the acetabular side of the joint. In children under 5 or 6 years of age I preferentially utilize the pericapsular osteotomy (Fig. 6-5); for children from 6 or 7 years of age through skeletal age 15 years, I prefer the innominate osteotomy of Salter (Figs. 6-6 and 6-7). However, it should be pointed out that, irrespective of the differences in the two osteotomies, the Salter osteotomy can be used effectively for all age groups through 15 years. The details of these procedures, includ-

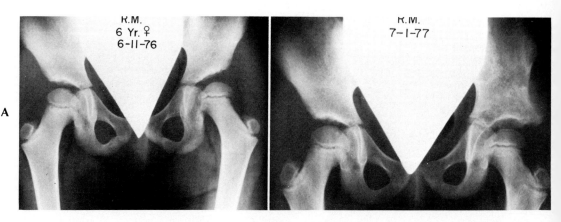

Fig. 6-5. This 6-year-old girl had been treated in early infancy for a dysplastic left hip. The preoperative pelvic x-ray film showed a sloping oblique acetabular roof, with upward displacement of the femur as evidenced by a broken Shenton line, **A.** One year after a pericapsular pelvic osteotomy, the acetabulum appeared much more normal, the femoral head was well covered, and the Shenton line had been restored to normal, **B.**

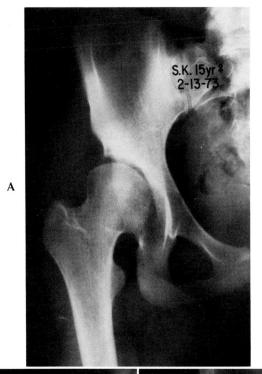
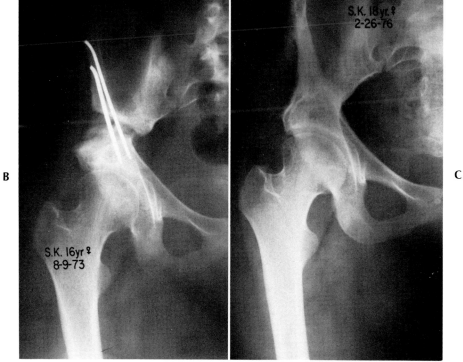

Fig. 6-6. This 15-year-old girl had a painful right hip following earlier treatment for congenital dislocation of the hip, **A.** Note early degenerative changes in the acetabulum. A redirectional (Salter) pelvic osteotomy was accomplished, **B,** and the result 2½ years later is seen in **C.** The patient had no pain and had a normal range of motion. Note improved, healthy appearance of rotated acetabular roof.

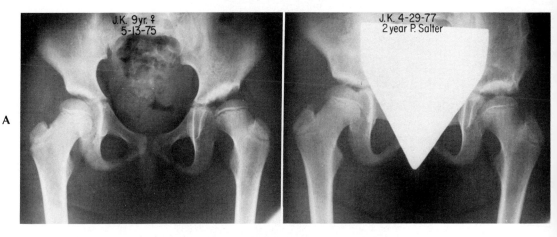

Fig. 6-7. This 9-year-old girl had a routine pelvic film made during a urologic evaluation. An abnormal left hip was encountered, **A,** for which a redirectional (Salter) pelvic osteotomy was accomplished, **B.**

ing their indications, prerequisites, complications, and so forth, have been described in Chapter 5.

In adolescents over age 15 years the problems of correcting acetabular dysplasia become greater because of increasing maturity of the skeleton and the reduced flexibility of the symphysis pubis and the other pelvic ligaments. In this situation an attempt to perform the Salter osteotomy amounts to a significant and sometimes overwhelming technical challenge. Furthermore, the partial pericapsular osteotomy of Pemberton cannot be done as he described it because the triradiate cartilage has long since become ossified. In these patients over age 15 years, therefore, a different surgical approach becomes necessary. If the femoral head can be seated well in the acetabulum in flexion, abduction, and internal rotation, and if there is a nearly normal range of hip motions, then I prefer the triple innominate osteotomy as described by Steel.[6] Based on a simple technical difference, however, Sutherland and Greenfield[8] have recommended that a "double" innominate osteotomy be done in these circumstances. Also, Wagner[10] and Eppright[2] have devised a very unique technique of producing acetabular rotation (dial osteotomy), which is similarly designed to provide a greater acetabular weight-bearing surface. Each of these is discussed in the following section.

Triple innominate osteotomy. As noted earlier, this procedure was developed by Steel[6] as a means of surgically rotating and redirecting the acetabulum after the age when the Salter osteotomy becomes difficult or impossible because of ligamentous rigidity about the symphysis pubis. By performing an osteotomy through the pubic and ischial rami, as well as through the ilium, a completely mobile inferior pelvic fragment is produced. which then can be rotated in any direction that covers the femoral head best.

Indications. I believe that the prime indication for the triple innominate osteotomy is a patient who has a deficient acetabulum and who is skeletally too old for the successful accomplishment of the innominate osteotomy of Salter. The definition of a "deficient acetabulum" requires some degree of quantitation and some degree of intuitive interpretation of the x-ray films in order to arrive at that determination. From the quantitative point of view the most commonly used method is that developed by Wiberg (p. 158). The actual configuration of the acetabular roof must also be taken into consideration in this determination. A sloping socket in which the major portion of weight-bearing stress is being exerted through the outer aspect of the acetabulum is just as likely to develop osteoarthritis as is a hip having a normal acetabular configuration, but with a C-E angle below 20 degrees. It is this interpretation of acetabular integrity that requires the intuition and judgment of experience. This, combined with a properly done C-E quantitation, can usually provide data that make it possible to determine whether or not some form of acetabular rotation is indicated.

Hip pain is a third indication, and because of the fact that painful symptoms may be the cause of restriction in a child's activities, pain can be even more pressing as an indication for surgery than the x-ray evaluation. Pain is rare in young children, but during adolescence intermittent painful hip symptoms following vigorous physical activities are not uncommon in instances of acetabular dysplasia. Once the pain begins, it usually becomes progressively worse with advancing years. Also, the development of a gluteus medius limp (Trendelenburg gait) resulting from acetabular insufficiency represents a positive indication, because this usually means that there is an unstable hip joint. This can be documented by weight-bearing roentgenograms. This examination may show that the femoral head tends to extrude when weight is borne on the hip. A painless limp developing in adolescence caused by hip instability will almost always become slowly more apparent, and the patient usually will develop hip pain resulting from osteoarthritis with the passage of time.

In summary, therefore, the three major indications for an acetabular rotation in adolescence consist of a deficient socket, as determined by the foregoing roentgenographic studies; hip pain; and a gluteus medius limp (Trendelenburg gait) caused by demonstrable hip joint instability.

Prerequisites. Even with good defensible indications, it is not appropriate to proceed with this operation unless all of the prerequisites are satisfied. Conceptually, the prerequisites are the same as for any reconstructive operation that rotates the acetabular roof over the femoral head. Thus they are essentially the same as for the innominate (Salter) or pericapsular (Pemberton) osteotomies. This means that the femoral head must be concentrically situated within the acetabulum; that there should be minimal deformity of the femoral head; that there must be a "reasonable" degree of congruency between the femoral head and acetabulum; and that there must be a good (not necessarily completely normal) range of hip motion, especially in the directions of flexion, abduction, and internal rotation. To what degree these prerequisites are critically adhered to will largely determine the success of the operation. Conversely, when adherence to these prerequisites is not enforced, the operation will likely fail or its result will be compromised.

Surgical technique. The patient is positioned supine on either a fracture table or a standard operating room table with the buttock on the affected side draped so that the ischial tuberosity can be exposed. The entire involved limb must be draped free so as to permit unrestricted motion of the hip.

With the hip and knee flexed to 90 degrees, a 3-inch transverse incision is made over the ischial ramus and tuberosity. The deep fascia is incised and the inferior border of the gluteus maximus

166 *Congenital dysplasia and dislocation of the hip*

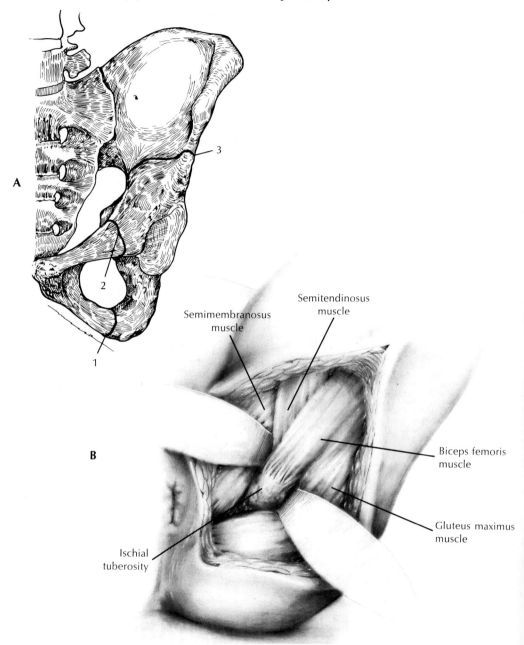

Fig. 6-8. All components of the innominate bone are sectioned in the triple innominate osteotomy, **A.** Two incisions are necessary in order to accomplish the procedure. The first is made transversely in the buttock directly over the prominence of the ischial tuberosity. With the hip flexed, this bony prominence is virtually subcutaneous, **B.** The ischium is exposed subperiosteally, and with a curved kidney pedicle clamp placed into the obturator foramen, the ischial ramus is osteotomized, **C.** Through an anterior-iliofemoral incision, the pubis is exposed subperiosteally and osteotomized just lateral to the iliopectoral eminence, **D.** Thereafter, the procedure of cutting the ilium is exactly as described in the redirectional osteotomy of Salter (Fig. 5-17). (Redrawn after Steel, H. H.: Triple osteotomy of the innominate bone, J. Bone Joint Surg. **55A:**343, 1973.)

muscle is identified and retracted laterally. The ischial ramus is then identified, and the entire circumference of the ramus is exposed subperiosteally just lateral to the origin of the hamstring muscles. The sciatic nerve is watched for, but it is not necessary to expose it. A curved kidney-pedicle clamp is placed behind the ischial ramus, and the ramus is osteotomized. This wound is then closed, gown and gloves are changed, and the instruments that have been used are discarded. This is deemed necessary because of the closed proximity of the perineum to the operative wound.[7]

The second incision consists of an anterior (iliofemoral) incision. It is the same as that employed in other innominate osteotomies. The superior ramus of the pubis must be exposed as far medially as the iliopectineal eminence; at this level the pubic ramus is subperiosteally exposed circumferentially as far as the obturator foramen. Care must be exercised so as not to injure the obturator nerve or vascular bundle. A curved clamp is then placed behind the pubic ramus, in the obuturator foramen, and the ramus is osteotomized.

Next the sciatic notch is exposed subperiosteally, just as in the innominate (Salter) osteotomy, and a Gigli saw is used to osteotomize the ilium in the same fashion. At this time the entire acetabulum can be freely moved into almost any position that most appropriately covers the femoral head. A full-thickness, wedge-shaped bone graft is taken from the crest of the ilium and is placed into the opening created between the acetabular and iliac fragments. These latter fragments and the graft are then trans-

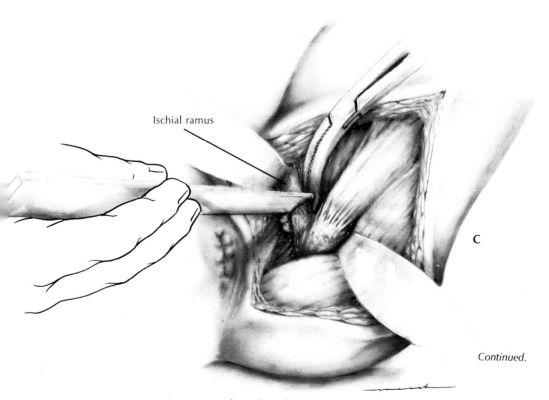

Continued.

Fig. 6-8, cont'd. For legend see opposite page.

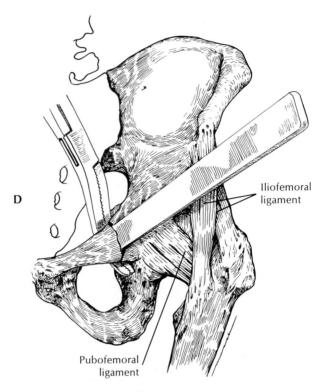

Fig. 6-8, cont'd. For legend see p. 166.

fixed with at least two large-sized Steinmann pins, preferably threaded (Fig. 6-8). Stability of the graft is tested and an x-ray film is taken in order to establish the position of the pins and to verify that they are not in the joint. The wound is closed and a one and one-half hip spica cast is applied.

Aftercare is identical with that employed in the Salter osteotomy, except that I prefer to use the cast for a minimum of 8 to 10 weeks because patients who are subjected to this operation are usually in an older skeletal age group (Fig. 6-9).

Contraindications and complications. The same contraindications apply in this procedure as were discussed in the case of the innominate (Salter) osteotomy. Essentially the same potential complications are inherent in the two procedures.

Double innominate osteotomy. In an effort to effect acetabular rotation and to avoid cutting all three segments of the innominate bone, Sutherland and Greenfield[8] have utilized a double osteotomy of the pelvis. Through a transverse suprapubic incision, the pelvic bone is cut just lateral to the symphysis pubis and medial to the point at which the bone branches into inferior and superior rami (Fig. 6-10). The ilium is then cut just as in the innominate or triple osteotomy, and the remainder of the operation is the same. Two incisions are required just as in the triple osteotomy, but it is not necessary to expose the gluteal area. One of the criticisms that has been voiced regarding Sutherland's procedure is that the distal (lateral) fragment can become very prominent in the pubic region if very much rotation of the acetabulum is accomplished. Sutherland believes that this

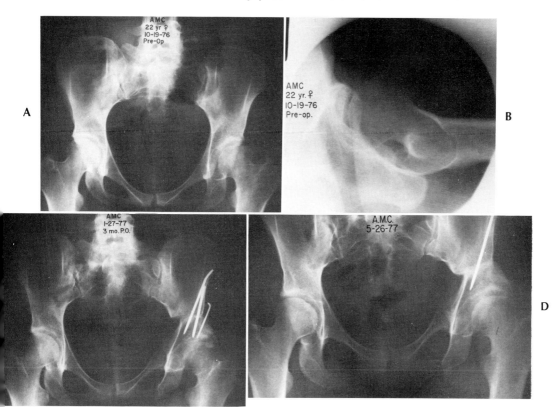

Fig. 6-9. The left hip of this 22-year-old woman was treated by open reduction at age 2 years. She was totally asymptomatic until age 20 years. Gradually increasing left hip pain prompted a pelvic roentgenogram. The anteroposterior view shows extrapelvic protrusion of the femoral head, **A**, and the groin lateral view demonstrates the defective acetabulum anteriorly, **B**. A triple innominate (Steel) osteotomy was accomplished, **C**, and the result following pin removal is seen in **D**. The remaining pin broke off during attempted removal. The patient has full weight bearing and is asymptomatic.

is not a significant problem. I have had no personal experience with this procedure and can, therefore, neither support nor criticize this objection or the operation itself.

Periacetabular "dial" osteotomy. Eppright,[2] Wagner,[10] and Kawamura[3] have utilized an osteotomy that rotates the acetabulum in a somewhat different way than in any of the innominate osteotomies previously described. Utilizing the same biologic concept that preservation of articular cartilage is essential to a long-lasting hip joint, the articular cartilage and subchondral bone of the acetabulum are rotated by means of a curved osteotomy that is made about the entire circumference of the hip socket (Fig. 6-11). It is a difficult and challenging procedure that requires specially made curved gouges resembling "spoons." In my current opinion this procedure exceeds the technical expertise of most surgeons. However, in the hands of a master surgeon, it appears to be an effective method of improving acetabular coverage of the femoral head in adolescents and young adults. The *indications* and *prerequisites* for this procedure conceptually are the same as for the innominate osteotomies previously discussed.

Surgical technique. Through an ante-

170 *Congenital dysplasia and dislocation of the hip*

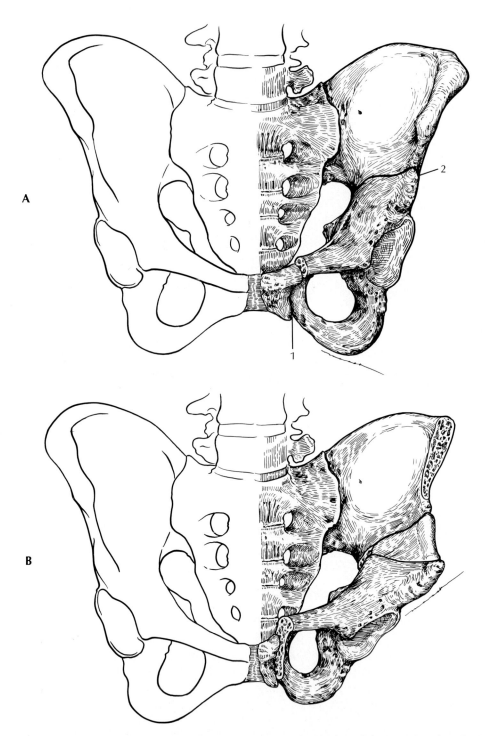

Fig. 6-10. A, The double innominate osteotomy consists of an osteotomy through the innominate bone just lateral to the symphysis pubis, *1*. The superior and inferior pubic rami are cut at this location. The second osteotomy is done through the iliac bone the same way as in the Salter or Steel osteotomy, *2*. Note the slight asymmetry of the superior pubic ramus created by rotation of the inferior pelvic fragment, **B,** as a result of the long lever arm. (Redrawn from unpublished work of Dr. D. H. Sutherland.)

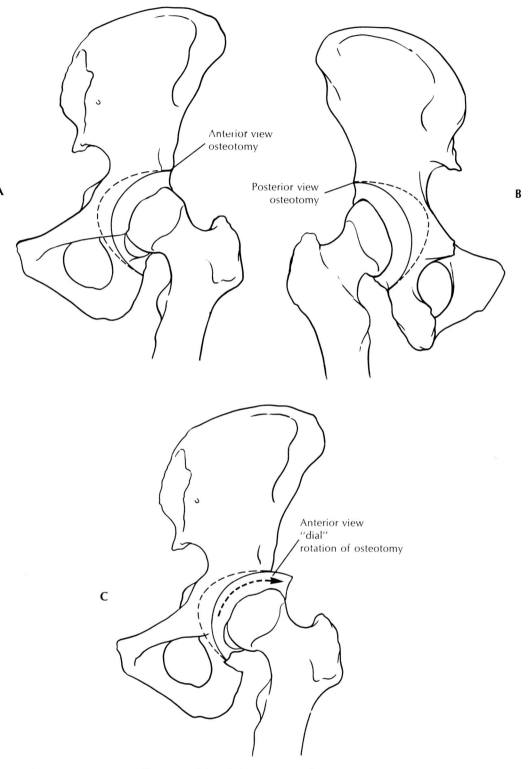

Fig. 6-11. Diagrammatic illustration of the "dial" osteotomy. The periarticular osteotomy is shown as it should be done anteriorly, **A**, and posteriorly, **B**. The entire fragment is then rotated outward in whatever direction best "covers" the femoral head, **C**.

rior (iliofemoral) incision, the hip joint and sciatic notch are exposed as in previous reconstructive procedures about the hip. The periacetabular portions of the innominate bone are exposed anteriorly, superiorly, and posteriorly. With protective retractors placed anteriorly between the capsule and the iliopsoas and pectineus muscles and posteriorly in the sciatic notch, an osteotomy is begun approximately ⅜ to ½ inch peripheral to the acetabular rim. The osteotomy is carried progressively deeper in a circumferential fashion about the acetabulum. As the posterior and inferior portions of the acetabulum are approached, the surgeon's index finger must be placed deeply behind the acetabulum in order to protect the sciatic nerve from the final cut into this portion of the pelvis.

Once the acetabulum has been completely osteotomized it can be rotated to cover the exposed femoral head. The fragment may or may not require transfixion by threaded Steinmann pins, depending on the degree of stability. A cast is applied just as in other innominate osteotomies.

Wagner[10] has devised at least three variations in performing this dial osteotomy. These technical variations are used according to the character of the pathology of the hip joint. These different procedures are highly sophisticated, and they require not only the expertise of a superb technical surgeon but also the specialized technical instruments essential for their effective accomplishment.

I have had no personal experience with any of the dial osteotomies, therefore, they cannot be recommended by me as standard treatment for the inadequate acetabulum in adolescents and adults. At the present time my preference for correction of this defect is the triple innominate osteotomy when a Salter osteotomy cannot be accomplished. It appears safer and technically simpler and has less potential complications than either the dial or the double innominate osteotomies.

Operative procedures on the femoral side

Proximal femoral osteotomy. It is uncommon to find a good indication for performing *exclusively* a proximal femoral osteotomy for dysplasia of the hip in older children and adolescents. Most often the *principal* identifiable deformity will be encountered on the acetabular side, and when corrective proximal femoral osteotomy is indicated, *usually* an acetabular rotation will be required in addition to the femoral procedure. Nevertheless, there are certain instances when the proximal femur is the exclusive and primary problem and when the femur is sufficiently deformed that it justifies the accomplishment of some form of corrective osteotomy at the intertrochanteric level. The goals of proximal femoral osteotomy are to correct deformity of the proximal femur, to enhance hip joint stability, and to improve femoral head coverage. In young children under 3 or 4 years of age and occasionally in older children, as demonstrated by Chuinard,[1] a substantial influence can be exerted on acetabular configuration and development by appropriately correcting established deformities in the proximal femur.

Indications. As suggested in the preceding paragraph, the indications for this operation consist of the following: (1) a demonstrable deformity of the proximal femur, which results in a poorly covered, relatively unstable hip, and (2) a hip having disturbed biomechanics as a result of an altered lever arm (usually coxa valga and excessive anteversion) (Fig. 6-2). As discussed previously in this section, the appropriate x-ray films must be available in order to establish the presence of these abnormalities.

Prerequisites It is essential that certain criteria be met prior to performing a proximal femoral osteotomy for dysplasia of the hip. These have already been dis cussed in Chapter 5, but they will be summarized here for emphasis. The head must be well seated in flexion, abduction, and internal rotation; the acetabular and femoral relationships must be congruent; there must be little deformity of the femoral head; and the ranges of hip motion must be essentially normal. Utilizing the earlier mentioned indications and adhering to these prerequisites, the results of proximal femoral osteotomy are likely to be very satisfactory. Failure to heed any of them will result in possible or probable failure.

Surgical technique. The technique of varus and/or rotational osteotomy of the femur has been discussed and illustrated thoroughly in Chapter 5, and the reader is referred to that section for details. In older adolescents and adults it is helpful to achieve some degree of extension of the osteotomy, thus creating what usually amounts to a triplane osteotomy; namely, varus rotation and extension. To what extent either of these corrections must be achieved is clearly an individual matter that can only be determined by accurate preoperative roentgenographic evaluation.

Wagner[9] has developed some very ingenious methods of correcting the many deformities of the proximal femur in adolescents and adults with sequelae of congenital dislocation of the hip. These deformities include varus and shortening of the neck-shaft angle of the femur, coxa valga, and relative overgrowth of the greater trochanter. Most of these deformities are the result of femoral head and physeal plate necrosis, and they therefore represent salvage procedures. These deformities and their treatment will be discussed in Chapter 8.

Combined acetabular rotation and proximal femoral osteotomy

It is not rare to encounter instances of dysplasia, not only in young children but also in adolescents who have sufficient deformities of both the acetabulum and the proximal femur to justify operations on both sides of the joint. These operations may be done either sequentially or simultaneously (Fig. 6-4). When it is anticipated that both sides need correction but the surgeon believes that they should be corrected at separate operations, then it is probably advisable to accomplish the acetabular correction first. This is because the improved fulcrum (socket) will render greater stability to the joint and make femoral osteotomy relatively easier to accomplish. In most instances correction will be done at separate operations, and in these cases it is better to do the acetabular rotation first, because the presence of an intact femur is essential for effective pelvic osteotomy.

In any case that requires both surgical procedures, it is clear that the same indications and prerequisites must be satisfied as for either operation done separately.

REFERENCES

1. Chuinard, E. G.: Femoral osteotomy in the treatment of congenital dysplasia of the hip, Orthop. Clin. North Am. **3:**157, 1972.
2. Eppright, R.: From motion picture presentation at AAOS annual meeting, Las Vegas, Nevada, Fall 1977.
3. Kawamura, B.: Dome osteotomy, C. D. H. Symposium, Royal Oak, Michigan, 1974.
4. Laage, H., Barnett, J. D., Brady, J. M., Dulligan, P. J., Jr., Fett, N. C., Jr., Gallegher, T. F., and Schneider, B. A.: Horizontal lateral roentgenography of the hip in children, J. Bone Joint Surg. **35A:**387, 1953.
5. Somerville, E. W.: Open reduction in congenital dislocation of the hip, J. Bone Joint Surg. **35B:**363, 1953.
6. Steel, H. H.: Triple osteotomy of the innominate bone, J. Bone Joint Surg. **55A:**343, 1973.
7. Steel, H. H.: Personal communication.
8. Sutherland, D. H., and Greenfield, R.: Medial pubic osteotomy in difficult Salter procedures, Proceedings of the Western Orthopaedic Association, J. Bone Joint Surg. **57A:**135, 1975.
9. Wagner, H.: Osteotomies for congenital hip dislocation. In The Hip Society: The hip, vol. IV, Proceedings of the fourth open scientific

meeting of The Hip Society, St. Louis, 1976, The C. V. Mosby Co., p. 45.
10. Wagner, H.: Presentation at 5th Annual International Symposium on Pediatric Orthopaedics, Chicago, Ill., June 1977.
11. Wiberg, G.: Relation between congenital subluxation of the hip and arthritis deformans (roentgenological study) Acta Orthop. Scand. **10:**351, 1939.

CHAPTER 7

Problems and complications in treatment

Problems in diagnosis
Problems in treatment
   Unusual pathology
   Problems caused by associated abnormalities
   Problems resulting from prior treatment
   Problems resulting from late diagnosis
Causes of complications during treatment
   Failure to define problem accurately
   Failure to achieve and maintain concentric reduction
   Failure to implement appropriate operative procedure
   Errors and technical failures in implementation
Complications during treatment
   Persistent subluxation
   Redislocation
   Osteonecrosis (epiphysitis)
   Chondrolysis and cartilage necrosis
   Restriction of hip joint motion
   Limb length inequality caused by stimulation following surgery

In the preceding chapters emphasis has been directed toward the recognition of the problem of congenital dislocation of the hip in its various manifestations and toward the treatment of the manifold expressions of this complex and capricious condition. If all instances of congenital dislocation of the hip were uniform in their behavior and pathology, and if they all responded in a consistent pattern to treatment, there would be little need for this section. However, since human disease is so variable and since there is such great diversification in the manifestations of congenital dislocation of the hip, it is only natural that occasional untoward results must inevitably occur, either in the diagnosis and definition of the problem, in the synthesis of the therapeutic program, or in the operative or nonoperative execution of such a program. Thus a very simple and logical classification of untoward circumstances would include: (1) *problems* in diagnosis and treatment and (2) *complications* of treatment in congenital dislocation of the hip.[13] These are philosophically different issues, and it is sometimes difficult to separate them from each other. However, for discussion purposes such a distinction seems reasonable.

PROBLEMS IN DIAGNOSIS

Problems in diagnosis have largely been covered in earlier sections. In order to emphasize these important issues, however, the following brief review is necessary. Such diagnostic pitfalls occur principally at two times—the neonatal period and late childhood. The most important is the period during the early days and months of infancy when the clinical and roentgenographic diagnostic parameters are so critically contingent on surgeons' expertise in newborn and neonatal physical examination and on their intelligent and knowledgeable interpretation of the newborn pelvic x-ray film. During this early period, as has been emphasized in Chapters 3 and 4, the challenges to the pediatrician, the family practitioner, and the orthopedic surgeon are ominously great, because of the subtle and capricious nature of the physical and roentgenographic determinations of hip dysplasia during this neonatal period. On the other hand, it is during this same neonatal period that the most attractive and valuable period for diagnosis presents itself, and if the diagnosis can be made at this time, the most rewarding results can be realized.

Realistically and practically, it is very important to emphasize the peculiarly vicarious nature of this neonatal condition. On the one hand, it is essential to establish and recognize that the diagnosis of dysplasia (or dislocation, if it exists) can *usually* be established during the newborn or neonatal period in the majority of instances. But, on the other hand, it is equally important to emphasize that *the diagnosis can be missed* in this neonatal period, even by an experienced and dedicated examiner. This possibility, therefore, mandates that repeated examinations be made during the early months of infancy and that a pelvic x-ray film be taken if suspicious findings exist.

Problems in diagnosis can also present themselves in older children with a dysplastic hip. The salient features supporting a diagnosis of dysplasia during this earlier period of childhood are almost exclusively radiographic, because physical findings are almost totally wanting at this time. As the child grows and becomes heavier, gait abnormalities slowly develop, either as a result of progressive hip joint weakness resulting from disturbed hip biomechanics or from the onset of hip pain. There is really no good solution to this diagnostic problem because of the consistent absence of any suggestive physical findings. Such problems are usually discovered incidentally (Fig. 7-1); the only alternative would be to require pelvic roentgenography in all children during the first year of life, prefer-

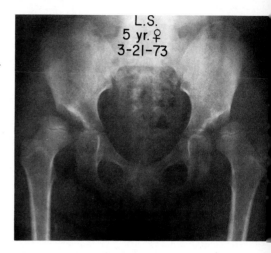

Fig. 7-1. This x-ray film was taken of a 5-year-old girl because of the recent onset of a limp bilaterally. She had no history of dislocated hips and was otherwise asymptomatic and healthy. Note dysplastic hips.

ably between 3 and 6 months of age. At present this does not seem to be practical, and, except for children in the high-risk group, its universal implementation seems untenable because of the low yield of positive diagnosis as compared to the number of pelvic x-ray films required. The important concepts to emphasize are that in the absence of x-ray evaluation the diagnosis is virtually impossible to make early in a child's life and that all children with lower limb abnormalities, those with gait abnormalities, and those in this high risk category should have pelvic x-ray films to rule out the possibility of hip dysplasia.

In instances of true dislocation problems of diagnosis are relatively insignificant. All that is required is an index of suspicion based on a thorough history, a competent physical examination, and a confirmatory pelvic x-ray examination. Failure to make the diagnosis of true *dislocation* after the age of 18 months should rarely occur in our sophisticated medical society if appropriate pediatric well-baby care is made available and is religiously implemented.

PROBLEMS IN TREATMENT

Problems in treatment of congenital dislocation of the hip can be grouped under the following categories: (1) problems caused by the unusual pathology of the dislocation; (2) problems caused by associated abnormalities; (3) problems resulting from prior treatment; and (4) problems resulting from late diagnosis. Although overlapping circumstances exist between each of these categories, they will be discussed separately.

Unusual pathology

Several problems in treatment can result from special or unusual characteristics of the dislocation. The fact that there is such a wide variation in the pathology of congenital dislocation of the hip from one patient to another makes this observation rather self-evident. For example, an *antenatal* dislocation will usually present greater problems than will a *postnatal* dislocation. A high-riding, relatively rigid dislocation must be dealt with somewhat differently than one that is more mobile and easily reducible. Other examples include instances where there is a shallow, poorly formed acetabulum as well as circumstances where there are significant angular or rotational deformities of the proximal femur. Such problems require careful analysis and definition so that an appropriate and effective treatment program can be synthesized.

Because of the increased length of duration of the dislocation (antenatal), there is a greater likelihood that adaptive changes will have taken place in the acetabulum and upper femur; as a result, the problems of reduction and maintenance of reduction are accentuated. Thus one must anticipate the need for a longer period of traction, a greater need for early muscle and soft tissue releases, and the greater possibility of the necessity for an open reduction in such instances. Furthermore, as mentioned in Chapter 3, I believe that if open reduction is required it should be done preferably from an anterior (iliofemoral) approach rather than from the medial (adductor) approach, in anticipation of the potential but unforeseen problems that might be encountered during the reduction. Under such circumstances the versatility of the anterior (iliofemoral) approach outweighs any advantages inherent in the greater simplicity of the medial (adductor) approach.

Similar difficulties may be encounterd in a high-riding, relatively rigid dislocation in older infants and young children. The height of the dislocation may make it impossible to achieve a significant degree of downward displacement in order to effect closed reduction. Even prolonged skeletal traction usually does not result in sufficient descent of the femoral head to obviate the need for open surgical intervention. Thus, one must be prepared, not only for the need of soft tissue releases, but also even for the need of femoral resection. In some *rare* instances, when proximal femoral deformities and acetabular deficiencies coexist, open reduction may have to be combined with femoral resection and simultaneous angular and rotational osteotomy of the proximal femur, along with pelvic osteotomy (Fig. 7-2). As mentioned in an earlier section, this decision often has to be made at the time of surgery; however, careful preoperative evaluation can increase the surgeon's index of suspicion for the need of such a complicated and technically difficult procedure.

Problems caused by associated abnormalities

Associated abnormalities that influence the therapeutic program in congenital dislocation of the hip include such unusual things as extension contracture of the knee (with or without congenital dislocation) and pelvic obliquity, resulting

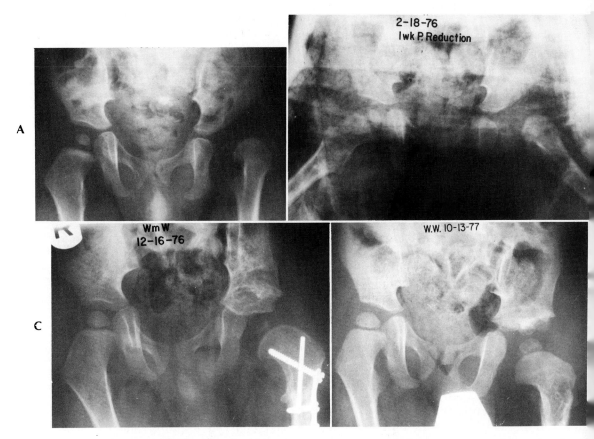

Fig. 7-2. At birth this 18-month-old boy was found to have a dislocated hip. Two previous efforts at closed reduction had been tried, **A.** After 2 weeks of skin traction, very little change in the level of the femoral head was accomplished, and an open reduction was attempted via the medial (adductor) approach. It was a difficult operative procedure, and a check film 1 week later revealed either redislocation or failure of the original reduction, **B.** As a result, an open reduction, femoral shortening, and pericapsular pelvic osteotomy were done and were successful, **C.** One year later satisfactory reduction is maintained and there is a normal range of movement, **D.**

either from lumbosacral congenital scoliosis or from an abduction contracture of the opposite hip. Muscular imbalance caused by some form of neurologic disease may also present a very significant problem in treatment, but these neuromuscular conditions involve considerations and deliberations that have been intentionally deleted from the scope of this text.

In those rare instances in which associated knee extension contractures or anterior dislocation of the tibia on the femur are present, a dislocated hip cannot and should not be reduced until the hamstring muscles can be relaxed by flexion of the knee and/or by reduction of the knee dislocation. Thus, as emphasized by Curtis,[2] no effort at hip reduction should ever be attempted until these knee problems have been corrected as well as possible (Fig. 7-3).

Occasionally, but rarely, pelvic obliquity can complicate efforts at hip reduction or stabilization. I have had no experience with problems in treatment o

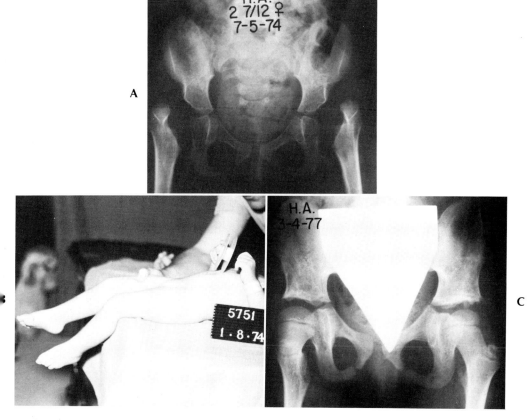

Fig. 7-3. Pelvic film of a bilateral dislocation of the hip in a 2½-year-old girl, **A.** These dislocations were antenatal and were associated with congenital bilateral knee extension contractures. Maximum flexion permitted was 30 degrees on the left, **B.** The quadriceps mechanism was lengthened so that greater than 90 degrees of flexion could be obtained before the hips were treated by open reduction and subsequent pericapsular pelvic osteotomy, **C.**

congenital dislocation of the hip stemming from pelvic obliquity caused by congenital lumbosacral scoliosis, but the observation that an abduction contracture of the opposite hip may contribute to the difficulties in treating a dysplastic or subluxated hip is well known. The treatment is correction of the abduction contracture by whatever means is necessary.

Problems resulting from prior treatment

The most common problems relating to prior treatment include muscle atrophy and weakness, osteoporosis of disuse, delayed ambulation, and restriction of hip joint motion, sometimes accompanied by contractures resulting from immobilization. All of these may exist in the face of a dislocation that was never reduced or in a situation where an effort at open reduction was made but the hip remained dislocated. In one consideration, therefore, these problems are the result of a complication, that is, either failure of initial effort at reduction or redislocation following reduction. These problems are discussed in greater detail on p. 188.

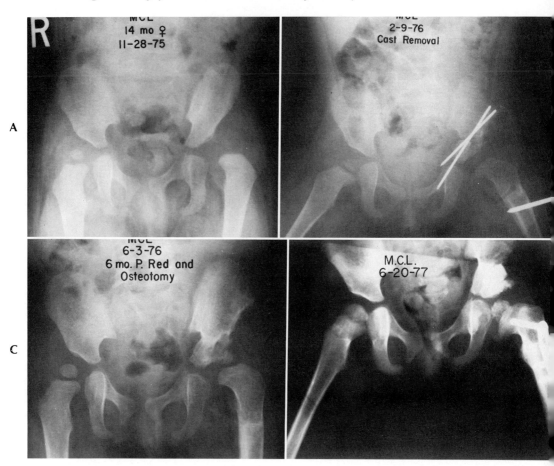

Fig. 7-4. This 14-month-old girl underwent attempted open reduction coupled with a redirectional pelvic osteotomy and a proximal femoral varus rotational osteotomy done simultaneously shortly after this film was taken, **A.** The result of the operative venture, which I do not condone at this age, is seen in **B.** At the time this patient was seen, 4 months after the cast and pin removal, the hip was stiff, the muscles were flabby, and there was poor tissue turgor, **C.** The patient was encouraged to ambulate without any encumbrances. Eight months later a very difficult repeat open reduction, femoral shortening, and modified pericapsular pelvic osteotomy were done simultaneously. The result 6 months later is seen in **D.**

When faced with a patient who has been previously treated but has a persisting dislocation, all of these potential problems must be thoroughly assessed and given appropriate consideration in the program of treatment. Thus prior to any efforts at gaining reduction by any means, muscle tone and bone strength must be regained, ranges of joint motion must be reestablished, and any hip joint contractures must be overcome. Usually this requires an extensive period of mobilization and ambulation (3 to 6 months) with special effort being made toward *ignoring* the fact that the hip is dislocated (Fig. 7-4). Not until the hip has regained its pretreatment mobility and the bone and muscle strengths have been restored should reduction of the hip again be attempted. The slate should be "wiped clean," so to speak, and the persisting hip dislocation should be approached with new and fresh therapeutic concept, utilizing the principles and techniques outlined in earlier chapters.

Problems resulting from late diagnosis

These problems result purely from the fact that greater adaptive changes will have taken place in either the acetabulum, the femur, or both, as a result of the delay in diagnosis. In the case of dysplasia, in early months this would not represent a serious issue unless dislocation takes place. In such instances where the hip is still in the socket (dysplasia or subluxation), usually simple abduction splinting is all that is required. At the other extreme, however, if the diagnosis is not made until after age 2 or 3 years, then operative correction will almost always be necessary, and in some instances the required surgery can be very complicated and difficult. In the most extreme situations involving children over age 10 years, currently very rare, the problem may be so great as to negate the advisability of any effort at reduction that is aimed at maintaining a mobile hip. Therefore, since delay in diagnosis does complicate treatment, the necessity for repeatedly emphasizing efforts at early diagnosis is evident.

CAUSES OF COMPLICATIONS DURING TREATMENT

Most complications are the result of one or more of the following circumstances: (1) failure to define the problem accurately; (2) failure to achieve a concentric reduction; (3) failure to implement the appropriate procedure; and (4) technical errors or failures in implementation of closed reduction, open reduction, or any reconstructive procedure. Rarely some complications occur that are unavoidable, irrespective of whether or not the errors mentioned above are assiduously avoided. But since complications are nearly always the result of treatment, it is essential that great care be exercised during treatment in order to avoid untoward results that so often lead to compromise of hip joint structure and function. Thus the following causes of these complications must be kept in view when undertaking the care of a child with congenital dislocation of the hip.

Failure to define problem accurately

It is axiomatic that the pathology of the hip be defined before appropriate treatment can be given. In the case of congenital dislocation of the hip this means that a thorough history be taken, that a thorough orthopedic physical examination be carefully done, that appropriate x-ray studies be carried out, and that all of the potential problems alluded to in the earlier section be considered. By this means one should be able to determine whether the hip is dislocated or not, whether it is a true congenital dislocation of the hip or the result of some form of muscle imbalance or other associated abnormalities, whether there is a significant deformity of the acetabulum or proximal femur, and whether or not conventional forms of treatment will likely be successful. Also it will help determine not only what procedures may be necessary but in what sequence they should be administered.

Failure to achieve and maintain concentric reduction

One of the most common and most significant complications in the treatment of congenital dislocation of the hip is the failure to achieve and maintain a concentric reduction of the femoral head in the acetabulum. Since this accomplishment is essential for there to be any reasonable chance for a normal hip, and since it is a *prerequisite* prior to performing *any* reconstructive procedure on the acetabulum or proximal femur, the magnitude of the problems created by failure to

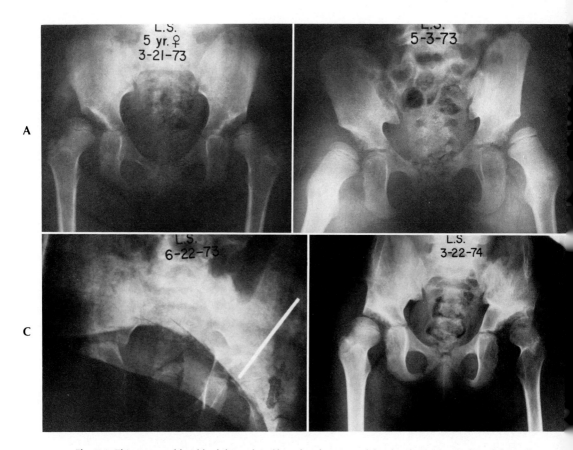

Fig. 7-5. This 5-year-old girl had this pelvic film taken because of the development of a limp bilaterally, **A.** A pelvic film with the thighs in abduction and internal rotation shows that the hips fail to seat well, which represents the major contraindication to any reconstructive pelvic osteotomy, **B.** Bilateral redirectional osteotomies were attempted, but the distal fragment on the left displaced medially, and the pin penetrated the joint, **C.** The end result 9 months later is bilaterally subluxated hips. The right hip is not improved over the preoperative status, and in the left hip the situation is worse, **D.** This patient illustrates the importance of having a concentric reduction prior to attempting any reconstructive procedure on the acetabulum or femur.

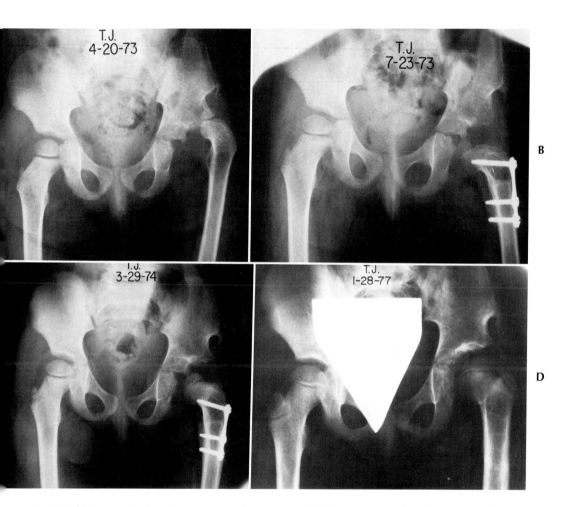

Fig. 7-6. This 5-year-old girl had a pelvic osteotomy accomplished 1 year previously in the presence of a dislocated hip. The result at the time I first saw her is seen in **A.** An open reduction aided by femoral shortening produced a very satisfactory and stable hip, **B.** The character of the acetabulum even in this age group was surprisingly good. Eight months later the hip remained stable, **C,** and 2 years later the acetabulum showed continued improvement, **D.** This case illustrates that a pelvic osteotomy is *not* designed to gain reduction, and it also demonstrates the great remodeling power of the acetabulum even at age 5 years; *if* the femoral head becomes concentrically reduced.

achieve and maintain concentric reduction is clear (Fig. 7-5).

The causes of failure to achieve a concentric reduction usually consist of one or more of the following: (1) failure to institute traction in children under age 2 or 3 years; (2) failure to explore and inspect the joint at time of open reduction; (3) failure to remove any interposed soft tissue, including hypertrophic fat pad and/or infolded limbus when encountered at open reduction; (4) failure to perform adequate soft tissue releases during reduction (specifically the iliopsoas tendon, the transverse acetabular ligament, and the anterior-inferior joint capsule); (5) failure to perform necessary femoral resection *and* soft tissue releases in children over age 3 years; and (6) difficulty in determining adequacy of reduction by available clinical and radiographic evaluation.

These errors in technique, or in judgment, are for the most part avoidable; it should only be rarely that a concentric reduction cannot be achieved and verified by radiography in a child age 4 years or younger on the initial surgical effort. X-ray films at the time of either open or closed reduction are very valuable, and arthrography must occasionally be employed as an aid to making the all-important determination of whether a concentric reduction has been accomplished. Once achieved, of course, the reduction must be maintained by appropriate immobilization in a position that avoids any extremes of abduction or rotation. This reduction must be retained until the hip becomes stable, either as a result of normal growth and remodeling in infants and young children or as the result or reconstructive procedures in older children.

Failure to implement appropriate operative procedure

If efforts at conscientious closed reduction are unsuccessful, then some form of operative intervention becomes necessary in order to achieve a satisfactory reduction. The selection of the proper procedure and careful adherence to the indications and prerequisites for the operation are critical to achieving a successful surgical venture. If one selects the wrong approach or the wrong technical procedure or if too many variables are added to the operation, failure will very likely ensue. These considerations relate to the very important issue involving definition of the problem. They also are a reflection of one's understanding of the purpose and goals of the operation. For example, a medial (adductor) approach should not be employed in instances of high-riding, rigid dislocations in any infant or child, and it is largely contraindicated in all children over 30 months of age. A pelvic osteotomy should *never* be used as a means of *obtaining* reduction; such osteotomies are designed as reconstructive procedures to improve femoral head coverage and enhance stability, not to gain reduction (Fig. 7-6). A proximal femoral osteotomy should only be used to correct a deformity of the proximal femur and thereby enhance hip joint stability never as a means of *gaining* reduction or

Fig. 7-7. This patient illustrates four major disasters—failure to gain reduction prior to performing a reconstructive pelvic osteotomy, failure to rotate the inferior fragment, failure to transfix the fragments with the pin, and penetration of the joint by the pin. Any one of these can result in complete failure of the operation. The initial dislocation was encountered in a 2-year-old girl, **A.** The result of the four technical errors is seen in **B.** After appropriate unencumbered ambulation, an open reduction of each hip through the anterior approach was accomplished 1 week apart, **C.** Six months later a pericapsular pelvic osteotomy was done on the left hip, **D,** and 7 years later a redirectional osteotomy was attempted on the right hip, **E.**

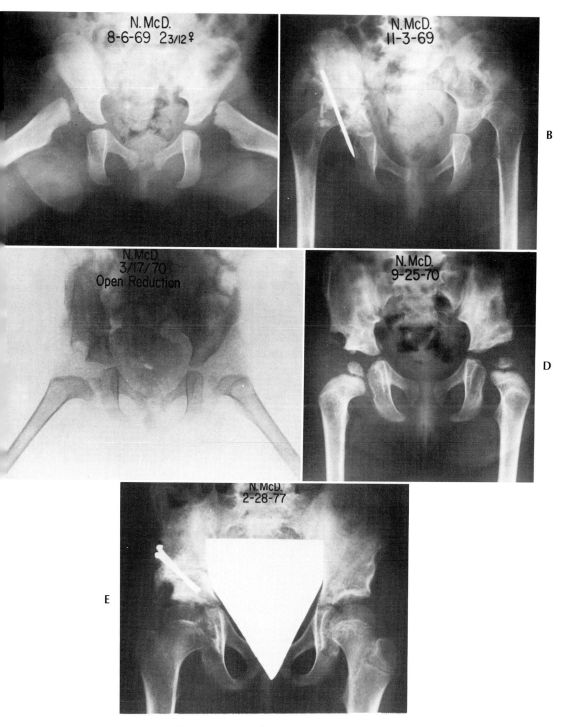

Fig. 7-7. For legend see opposite page.

necessarily solving any problems or deformity in the acetabulum, especially in older children. Furthermore, a pelvic osteotomy or a proximal femoral osteotomy done *prior* to achieving concentric reduction will invariably fail to accomplish its intended purpose and therefore will only complicate any future therapeutic efforts.

Errors and technical failures in implementation

These causes of complications are usually a result of any one or all of several possible situations. One of these is failure to adhere to the need for gentleness of reduction and maintenance of reduction of the hip and thighs in a position that does *not* compromise femoral head circulation. Forcible, manipulative reductions are contraindicated because of the high probability of producing excessive pressure on the femoral head. Also, forced positions of reduction and maintenance are likewise contraindicated. Another error is injudicious trauma to the articular cartilage of the femoral head and to the femoral head vasculature at the time of open reduction. If one recalls that the articular cartilage of the femoral head is a sensitive growth center and that the viability of the head rests largely with the capsular vasculature, the need for meticulous care in the handling of these structures is self-evident.

Technical failure in accomplishment of a concentric reduction has been discussed earlier. Other technical errors include failure to rotate the inferior fragment properly in the innominate (Salter) osteotomy (Fig. 7-7); failure to transfix the innominate osteotomy properly, thus allowing posteromedial displacement of the distal fragment (Fig. 7-5); penetration of the hip joint by transfixion devices (Fig. 7-4); improper accomplishment and fixation of the fragments of a proximal femoral osteotomy, which then results in an unattractive and complicating deformity (Fig. 7-8); and, finally, failure to release the iliopsoas tendon when performing an innominate osteotomy, thus resulting in increased pressure on the femoral head. In general these causes of complications of treatment are all avoidable and should not occur except in extremely unusual circumstances.

COMPLICATIONS DURING TREATMENT

Complications that occur as a result of the technical errors in the preceding paragraph include the following: (1) persistent subluxation; (2) redislocation; (3) osteonecrosis (epiphysitis) and its sequelae; (4) chondrolysis and cartilage necrosis; (5) restriction of hip joint motion; and (6) limb length inequality. Because most of these complications result in some degree of compromise of hip joint function, extreme care and precaution must be exercised in prevention or avoidance of such untoward results. Following are a further definition of each of these complications and a discussion of their treatment.

Persistent subluxation

This complication is almost always the direct result of failure to obtain or maintain concentric reduction. Once such instances are recognized, all efforts must be made toward reducing the hip concentrically. Above all, absolutely no consideration should be given to any reconstructive procedures, on either the acetabulum or the proximal femur, until this complete reduction is accomplished (Fig. 7-5).

In most cases of subluxation or incomplete dislocation, the slate must again be "wiped clean" and a totally fresh program developed. The principles and therapeutic approach outlined in earlier chapters must be reinstituted. Thus in children in the younger age group (under 2 years) who have not previously

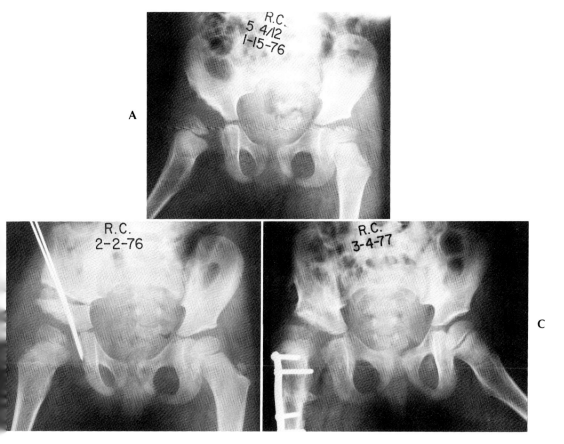

Fig. 7-8. This 5-year-old girl had a history of closed reduction of a dislocated hip on the right at age 2½ years. A limp persisted and a pelvic film revealed subluxation of the hip, a dysplastic acetabulum, and possible increased femoral anteversion, **A.** A redirectional pelvic osteotomy was attempted, but there was inadequate rotation of the inferior fragment and the pins penetrated the joint, **B.** Despite an inadequately reduced and unstable hip, a proximal femoral rotational osteotomy was done; however, it was a failure because the prerequisites for femoral osteotomy were not heeded, **C.**

been subjected to surgery, skin traction is utilized for an arbitrary period of 2 weeks, followed by an effort at accomplishing gentle, closed reduction. If there have been previous surgical efforts at open reduction, I have found traction to be futile because of scarring about the hip joint. At the time the closed reduction is attempted, appropriate arrangements should be made in anticipation of the possible need for an open reduction. At this time an arthrogram *may* be helpful in defining the acetabular femoral relationships, but in most instances I have relied on the plain films to determine whether a concentric reduction has been achieved. If doubt persists about the adequacy of reduction, either with or without arthrography, it is then appropriate to proceed with immediate open reduction, because almost surely there will be some obstruction to reduction that must be removed. If the patient is under 2 years of age, has not been operated on before, and has no other factors that would contraindicate a medial (adductor) surgical approach, then this may be the best procedure. If the child is over 2 years of age, has been previously operated on, or has unusual features of the dislocation that would argue against the medial (adductor) technique, then the best surgical solution is executed through the anterior (iliofemoral) approach because of its greater versatility. In those *rare* instances where arthrography (when employed) shows an infolded limbus to be the obstruction to complete reduction, then the anterior (iliofemoral) approach is preferable because the limbus cannot be adequately dealt with by the medial (adductor) approach.

In nearly all cases institution of this therapeutic program will achieve a concentric reduction. Subsequent follow-up care should be the same as described on earlier pages. It should again be emphasized that if prior treatment has resulted in any stiffness, muscle atrophy, scarring, or osteoporosis caused by immobilization, these factors should be remedied by an appropriate period of mobilization prior to instituting this program.

Redislocation

In most so-called redislocations the actual situation probably reflects either failure of concentric reduction or failure of reduction at all. Nevertheless, some are caused by failure of adequate, postreduction immobilization or by failure to *enhance* stability by appropriate reconstructive procedures such as iliac osteotomy, proximal femoral osteotomy, or both. The issues dealing with failure to obtain concentric reduction and failure to gain reduction at all have been covered in the preceding sections. The complication of true redislocation requires first of all

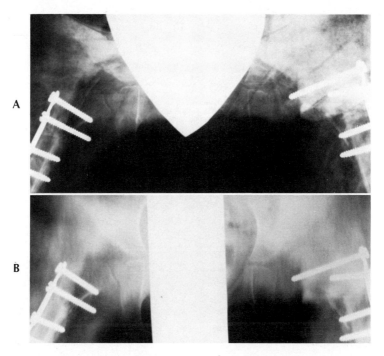

Fig. 7-9. The presence of overlying plaster made interpretation of this pelvic x-ray film difficult, **A.** Tomography gave much better detail and verified that the right hip was reduced but that there was distinct subluxation on the left, **B.** (Courtesy Dr. K. M. Samuelson.)

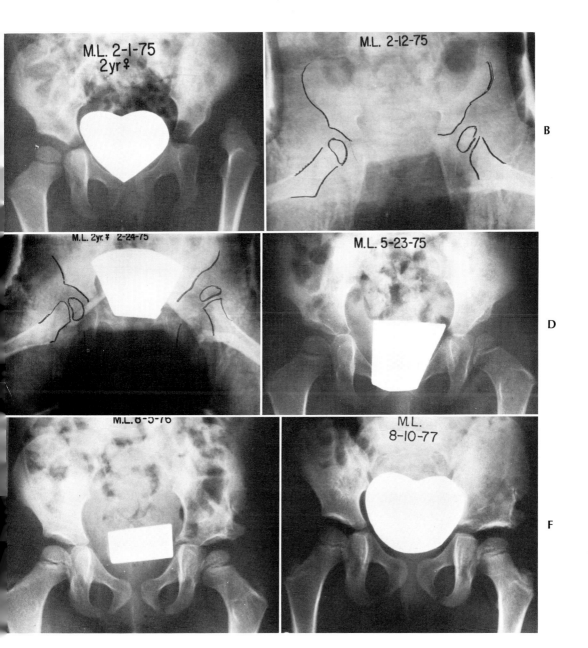

Fig. 7-10. A 2-year-old girl with dislocation of the left hip, **A.** After 2 weeks of traction a closed reduction was attempted, with a reduction that appeared satisfactory, **B.** Twelve days later a check film revealed an obvious redislocation, **C.** As a result an open reduction was accomplished via the medial (adductor) approach, **D.** One year later, because of failure of the acetabulum to improve in its configuration, a pericapsular osteotomy was accomplished. Three months postoperatively the femoral head was well covered, **E,** and 1 year later the hip was even better developed with a viable femoral head, **F.**

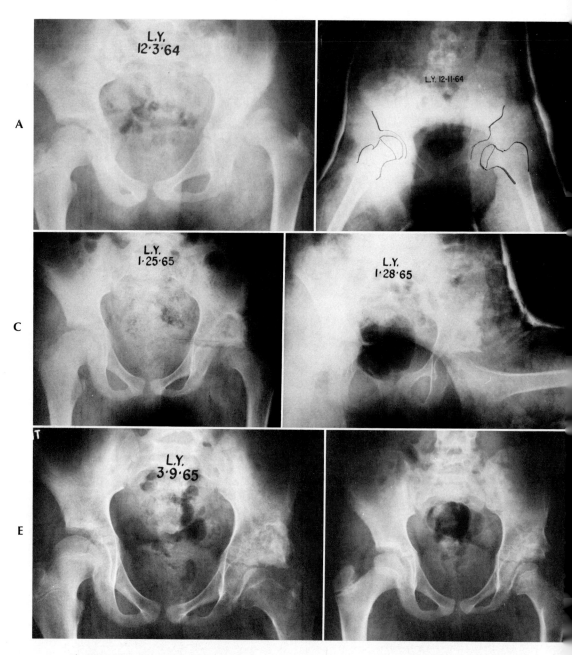

Fig. 7-11. This 9-year-old Navajo girl had an untreated dislocation of the left hip, **A.** An open reduction accompanied by a pericapsular pelvic osteotomy was accomplished after 3 weeks of skeletal traction, **B.** When the cast was removed 6 weeks later, a redislocation was evident, **C.** Three days later an effort at closed reduction was successful, **D** and **E.** This hip joint shows a satisfactory appearance 1 year later, **F,** and 5½ years later when the patient was last seen, **G.** The mistake in this instance was removing the cast too soon in an older patient, but it also shows that an effort at closed reduction under such circumstances may be effective.

that it be recognized. The sooner one can identify this complication, the simpler and more effective will be its treatment. X-ray examination at appropriate intervals following reduction is mandatory. If there is doubt about the reduction or if the x-ray film is unsatisfactory because of overlying plaster, either the plaster must be cut out or one must resort to more sophisticated measures such as tomography of the pelvis[12] (Fig. 7-9) or even computerized tomography scans.

Once the diagnosis of redislocation is established, the cast should be removed immediately and a program instituted toward regaining reduction. Depending on how soon after the original reduction that redislocation is discovered, the decision is made whether or not *immediate* efforts at reduction should be carried out. If a *closed* reduction was accomplished originally and the redislocation is picked up early in the postreduction period, then another effort at closed reduction is appropriate. If unsuccessful, an open procedure is indicated (Fig. 7-10). Likewise, in the instances when initial *open* reduction has been carried out, if redislocation is discovered early, a similar effort at *closed* reduction is justified (Fig. 7-11). In all circumstances an analysis of the factors that might explain the redislocation should obviously be made and appropriate corrective measures taken (Fig. 7-12).

If, on the other hand, redislocation occurs or is not identified until several weeks following the initial reduction, then a totally different therapeutic approach must be instituted. By this time adaptive shortening of the soft tissues will have occurred and, in the case of open reduction, there will be some induration and scarring of the soft tissues in addition to their adaptive shortening. Efforts at closed reduction will almost always be ineffective, and an open reduction should not be done until the skin and soft tissues have softened up and hip motions have returned to prereduction ranges (Fig. 7-4). This means that a delay of several weeks or 2 or 3 months should be utilized in order to prepare the hip for another effort at reduction. During this time the patient should be totally unencumbered by splints, braces, or casts, and ambulation should be encouraged. In the case of a younger child under age 2 or 3 years, if a repeat *closed* reduction is planned, prereduction traction should again be implemented. If a repeat *open* reduction is planned, it has been my experience that traction is *not* helpful because of the scarring from previous surgery. Also, as a result of the additional length of immobilization imposed, traction may even be deleterious, because of the possible increased atrophy and osteoporosis that it may produce.

Clearly, if redislocation does occur, the causes must be identified, if possible, and each must be analyzed in order to avoid subsequent redislocation. In some instances correction of these problems may require some sort of stabilizing procedure such as innominate osteotomy or proximal femoral osteotomy, but, of course, *never* until a concentric reduction has

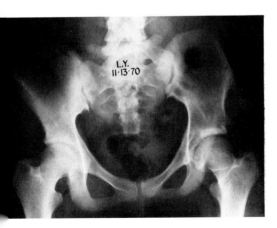

Fig. 7-11, cont'd. For legend see opposite page.

192 Congenital dysplasia and dislocation of the hip

again been achieved. It may be that femoral shortening should also be done, in the event that it was not done at the time of the initial open reduction. In older children (over age 6 years) it is possible that a salvage procedure such as a Colonna arthroplasty (see Chapter 8) may be required. Considerable experience is required in order to synthesize a proper solution to the problems involved in redislocation of the hip, and each case must obviously be solved on an individual basis.

Osteonecrosis (epiphysitis)

The causes and implications of osteonecrosis of the femoral head during and following treatment of congenital hip dislocation have been discussed earlier. The manifold problems presented by this complication reflect the need for early identification of necrosis and the development of an appropriate program of treatment when it occurs. The roentgenographic diagnostic features of femoral head necrosis are rather easily recognized (Fig. 7-13). Initially it is evidenced

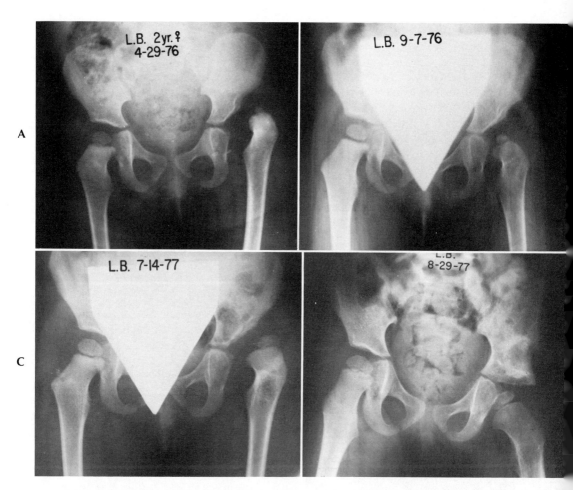

Fig. 7-12. Pelvic film, **A,** of a 2-year-old Navajo girl who underwent successful closed reduction following preliminary skin traction, **B.** Postoperative splinting was discontinued voluntarily by the mother, with resulting redislocation 10 months later, **C.** Open reduction and pelvic osteotomy were then done, **D.**

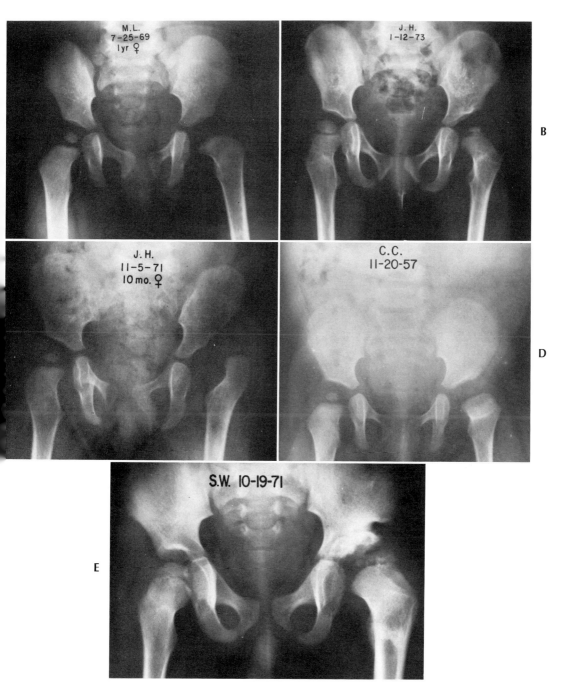

Fig. 7-13. Roentgenographic changes that are diagnostic of osteonecrosis include delay in appearance of the femoral head, **A;** failure of the femoral head ossification center to grow commensurate with its companion center, **B,** even though it was present prior to reduction, **C;** shortening and widening of the femoral neck, **D;** and flattening and fragmented ossification, **E.**

194 *Congenital dysplasia and dislocation of the hip*

by significant and otherwise unexplainable delay in ossification of the femoral head if it were not ossified prior to treatment. If the head had ossified prior to treatment, necrosis may be manifested by failure of the femoral head to grow at the normal rate, increased density of the ossification center, widening and shortening of the femoral neck, and irregularity in femoral head ossification. Ultimately deformities of the head, neck, and proximal femur may be evident, all governed by the degree and location of the necrosis (Fig. 7-14).

Once femoral head necrosis is identified, there are several different courses it may follow. In fortunate circumstances the necrosis is minimal and essentially complete healing takes place. In other circumstances complete necrosis may occur and the femoral head may subsequently become deformed. It may extrude from the socket and lose its spherical contour. Various degrees of physeal plate growth retardation may occur, resulting in shortening of the neck, and either a varus or valgus attitude of the head may develop along with eventual relative "overgrowth" of the greater trochanter (Fig. 7-14). Anticipation of these possible deformities resulting from necrosis is obviously essential to their proper treatment.

Early in the course of treatment of

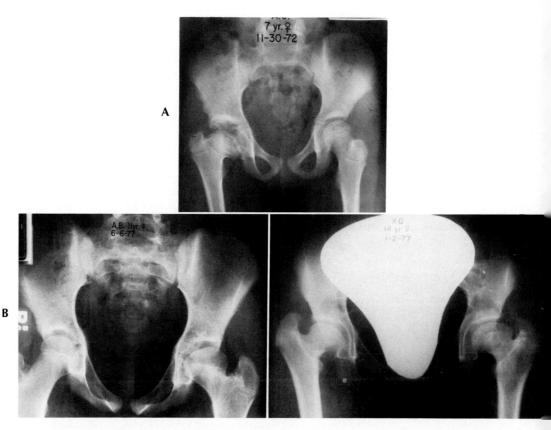

Fig. 7-14. The deformities of the proximal femur secondary to osseous necrosis include shortening and varus of the neck, **A**, shortening and valgus of the neck, **B**, and "overgrowth" of the greater trochanter, **C**.

femoral head necrosis, the primary goal is to maintain reduction and containment of the femoral head in the acetabulum. The concept is the same as that currently utilized in the treatment of the Perthes disease. In femoral head necrosis following treatment of congenital dislocation of the hip, "healing" or ossification of the necrotic head takes place much faster than in the Perthes disease and containment is usually easier to achieve and maintain.

The subsequent deformities of the femoral head, however, represent a significant therapeutic challenge and mandate that routine periodic pelvic x-ray films be taken in order to establish the presence of a treatable deformity.

The most distressing deformity and the most difficult to treat is that in which the femoral head loses its sphericity. This is often followed by reciprocal adaptive changes in the acetabulum, occasionally

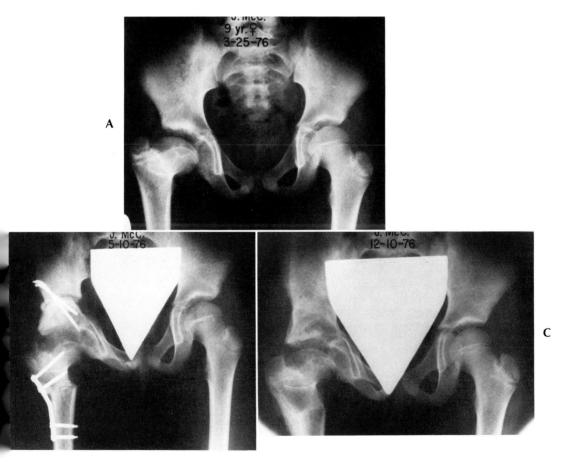

Fig. 7-15. This 9-year-old girl developed coxa plana, coxa vara, and relative overgrowth of the greater trochanter, **A,** as sequelae of earlier treatment of a dislocated hip. Combined valgus osteotomy, redirectional pelvic osteotomy, and greater trochanteric arrest were accomplished at the same operation, **B.** The pelvic osteotomy was considered necessary despite lack of femoral head sphericity, because the valgus osteotomy of the femur would tend to produce extrapelvic protrusion and because there was need for lengthening of the limb. The result 8 months after surgery shows a well-covered femoral head and 1 full inch (2.5 cm) of correction of limb lengths, **C.**

resulting in obliquity of the acetabular roof. Sometimes the acetabular change is sufficiently great to justify pelvic osteotomy (Fig. 7-15), but, unfortunately, the femoral head deformation cannot be treated as well.

Angular deformities of the neck-shaft angle, resulting from asymmetric epiphyseal arrest, may require varus or valgus intertrochanteric osteotomy. Care must be exercised that the valgus osteotomy does not uncover the femoral head too much, and varus osteotomy must be done cautiously, because of the possible altered growth potential in the physeal plate. It is possible that a permanent varus deformity of the neck-shaft angle may result if the normal growth characteristics of the proximal femur are compromised. This concern is especially appropriate in children over age 6 or 7 years because of the reduced capacity of the proximal femur for remodeling.

Relative overgrowth of the greater trochanter, as the result of the discrepancy between the normal growth of the trochanter and retarded growth of the femoral head, eventuates in progressive

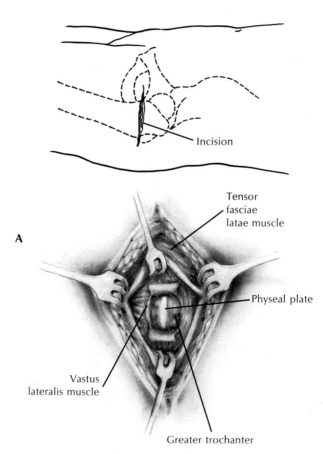

Fig. 7-16. My technique of performing apophyseal arrest of the greater trochanter. A transverse incision is made over the prominence of the greater trochanter. A vertical incision is made in the tensor faciae latae muscle, and the periosteum and perichondrium over the greater trochanteric apophysis are elevated, **A.** A ¾-inch square plug of bone is removed, and the physis is thoroughly curetted, **B.** The bone plug is then rotated 90 degrees and impacted into its original site, **C.**

Problems and complications in treatment 197

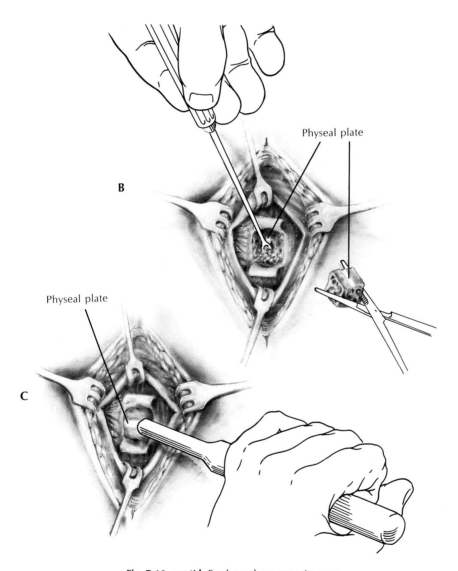

Fig. 7-16, cont'd. For legend see opposite page.

reduction in the strength of the abductor mechanism. Compere and associates[1] were able to reproduce this deformity in lower animals by arresting the growth of the capital epiphysis. Later, Hoyt and associates[6] accomplished the same thing in dogs. In Hoyt's study it was observed that patients who had previously had a normal gait gradually developed a positive Trendelenburg gait because the effective strength of the abductor muscles progressively deteriorated as they were effectively lengthened. This occurred because the distance between the origin (iliac crest) and the insertion (trochanter) became progressively closer together. The important thing is to recognize *early* the development of this proximal femoral deformity. If this complication can be diagnosed before the Trendelenburg test becomes positive, and preferably before the trochanter has exceeded the height of the superior portion of the femoral head (a positive articulotrochanteric [ATD] distance as shown in Fig. 7-17), simple correction can be achieved by fusion of the greater trochanteric apophyseal plate as has been so beautifully demonstrated by Langeskiöld and Salenius[8] (Fig. 7-16). Postoperative healing is rapid, and full unrestricted weight bearing can be exercised within 4 weeks. No cast is required. If a deformity (usually varus) of the neck-shaft angle also exists, then intertrochanteric valgus osteotomy can be combined with the apophyseal arrest (Fig. 7-17). In some cases when an accompanying acetabular deficiency is present, innominate osteotomy may be combined with valgus intertrochanteric osteotomy and apophyseal arrest (Fig. 7-15). On the other hand if the diagnosis is made late, after fusion of the apophysis, or long after the development of a positive Trendelenburg gait, then the only operative treatment is downward transplantation of the greater trochanter onto the proximal femoral shaft (Fig. 7-18). This is a much greater operative procedure than simple apophyseal arrest, because postoperative cast immobilization in abduction is necessary until strong osseous union of the trans-

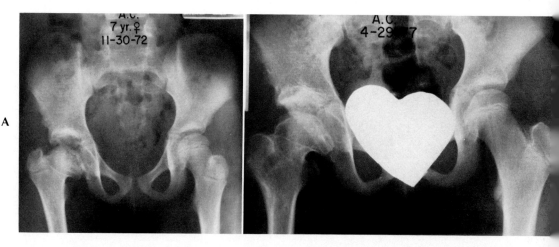

Fig. 7-17. An example of varus deformity of the femoral neck and relative overgrowth of the greater trochanter following femoral head necrosis, **A.** An open reduction and subsequent pericapsular pelvic osteotomy had been done earlier. An x-ray film showing the results of valgus osteotomy accompanied by greater trochanteric apophyseal growth arrest is seen in **B.** The valgus osteotomy resulted in a gain of ½ inch.

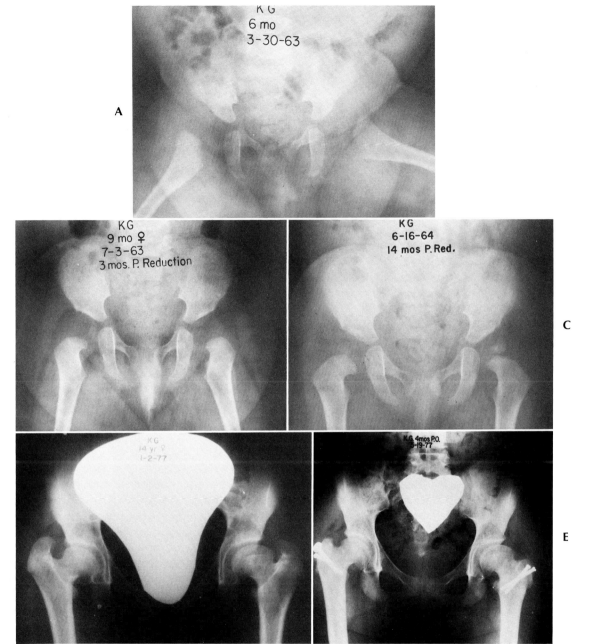

Fig. 7-18. Pelvic film of a 6-month-old girl with bilateral dislocation of the hip, **A.** After closed reduction and maintenance in the "frog-leg" position for 3 months, the hips appear reduced, although they are slightly more laterally displaced than desirable, **B.** One year later the hips remain reduced, but evidence of femoral head necrosis is seen bilaterally, more so on the right than on the left, **C.** Twelve years later the hips are reduced, but the femoral necks are somewhat short (not in varus) and the greater trochanters have shown considerable "overgrowth," **D.** This patient had slowly developed a Trendelenburg gait that she described as "walking like a duck." The greater trochanters were transplanted distally, **E.** Ideally, the trochanter on the right should have been transplanted more distally. In this instance there was no need for valgus osteotomy, and she was skeletally too old for simple trochanteric apophyseal arrest. Her positive Trendelenburg gait was reversed by the operation.

planted trochanter to the upper femoral shaft has taken place. The convalescence is likewise much delayed.

Femoral head and physeal plate necrosis not only produced the obvious deformities of the proximal femur mentioned in the preceding paragraph, but they also result in varying degrees of shortening of the involved lower limb. The amount of limb length discrepancy will differ considerably, depending on the degree of necrosis and the skeletal age at which it occurs. In general the approach to the limb length inequality is much the same as for progressive limb length discrepancies resulting from other physeal plate arrests. However, the discrepancies are not usually great and rarely exceed 2 or 3 cm unless total necrosis occurs early in infancy or childhood.

In instances where innominate osteotomy may be indicated, this discrepancy can largely be corrected by the osteotomy. In other patients whose hip joints do not require such reconstructive surgery, contralateral distal femoral epiphysiodesis at the appropriate skeletal age may be indicated. However, since many of these discrepancies are accompanied by significantly abnormal hip joints on the same side, some of which will almost surely require subsequent hip arthroplasty, the question of whether equalization by growth arrest of the opposite limb should be accomplished could well be challenged in some cases. For example, at least 3 cm of length can often be gained at the time of a total hip arthroplasty. If the patient can tolerate this amount of lower limb length inequality until arthroplasty needs to be performed, then this concept will obviate the need for growth arrest and will permit one to preserve the length and cosmetic integrity of the opposite normal limb. Obviously no rigid approach to this problem appears defensible, for each case must be evaluated individually.

Chondrolysis and cartilage necrosis

The condition known as chondrolysis is primarily a clinical and radiologic manifestation, and its etiology, pathology, and pathogenesis are poorly understood. The term has frequently been used synonymously with "cartilage necrosis," but it is uncertain whether the two conditions are the same, or even similar, in etiology, pathogenesis, and pathology.[10] Because I consider these to be separate and distinct entities, each will be discussed separately.

Chondrolysis

Etiology. Though more frequently associated with slipped capital femoral epiphysis, chondrolysis is occasionally seen following treatment of congenital dislocation of the hip. The proposed theories of etiology are numerous, reflecting the enigmatic nature of this particular entity. Some authors have incriminated surgical or nonsurgical trauma, ischemia, infection, prolonged immobilization, and endocrine and metabolic disorders. There are distinct racial tendencies in the cases of chondrolysis[7,9] associated with slipped capital femoral epiphysis, suggesting a genetic factor; however, in most instances of chondrolysis in congenital dislocation of the hip, such racial influences do not seem to be evident. The most plausible etiology suggests an autoimmune mechanism. Eisenstein and Rothschild[3] have proposed that a proteoglycan may act as an antigen that releases enzymes that interfere with the process of synthesizing articular cartilage. This is an attractive hypothesis, but irrefutable proof is yet lacking.

Pathology. The gross and histologic findings in chondrolysis have shown a thickened, edematous, and hyperemic synovial membrane, with perivascular lymphocyte and plasma cell infiltrates. The articular cartilage is diffusely thinned and fibrillated with a lusterless and pitted surface. Changes of advanced chondromalacia may be evident, although the subchondral bone shows some degree of atrophy along with some degree of marrow fibrosis.[9]

Clinical manifestations. The clinical manifestations of chondrolysis of the hip are heralded by the gradual onset of pain and progressive loss of range of joint motion, often with hip flexion contractures. There is a radiographic reduction in width of the cartilage (clear) space and an accompanying reduced osseous density of the femoral head and neck as well as the acetabulum (Fig. 7-19). Subchondral irregularities on both sides of the joint may be evident. Chondrolysis may or may not be associated with radiographic evidence of osteonecrosis of the femoral head. Some increase in size of the femoral head and neck may be observed, very likely the result of prolonged hyperemia. Early physeal plate closure may also occur.

Except for stiffness and limp, other symptoms such as pain at rest are usually missing, and the patient is also afebrile

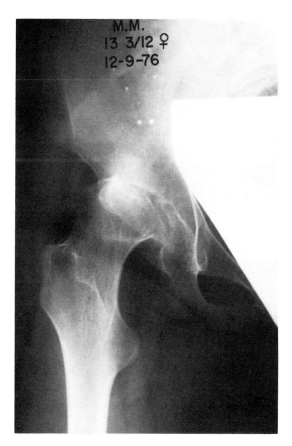

Fig. 7-19. An example of chondrolysis is seen in the hip roentgenogram of this 13-year-old girl. Loss of cartilage space, bone atrophy, and subchondral irregularity are clearly demonstrated. For complete case history see Fig. 7-21.

and lacking constitutional symptoms. Laboratory studies are nearly always within normal limits. The sedimentation rate, white blood count, RA factor, antistreptolysin O (ASO) titer, lupus erythematosus (LE) preparation, and levels of febrile agglutinins, enzymes, and serum electrolytes are practically never significantly altered. However, in some instances, increases in serum immunoglobulins and C-3 compliment have been noted.[3]

Treatment. Since the etiology of the problem is not known, specific therapy directed toward treating its cause is clearly not available. Consequently the manifestations of the disease rather than its primary etiology must be treated. This may explain why the results of treatment are so highly variable.

There are four major therapeutic modalities that have provided the best therapeutic results in my experience. These consist of (1) prolonged traction, either skin or skeletal, depending on the patient's age; (2) daily physical therapy; (3) aspirin to therapeutic dosages; and (4) prolonged nonweight-bearing activities on crutches.

Traction is empirically designed to relieve any muscle spasm, to correct any deformities or contractures, and to reduce the intra-articular pressure on the articular cartilage. Traction is exerted 24 hours a day, and the amount of weight used is in proportion to body weight. Generally speaking, the same amount of weight used is the same as that employed for treatment of a femoral shaft fracture in comparable age/weight groups. Also the same supervision of the traction must be exercised as for fracture treatment. It is essential that the hip be kept in some degree of flexion during the period of traction in order to avoid any increased intra-articular pressure imposed by traction placed with full extension of the hip, wherein the capsule will become taut.

During the periods of daily therapy the traction, of course, must be discontinued.

The *physical therapy* is designed to maintain some degree of physiologic muscle tone by means of simple isometric contractions of the muscle while the traction is still being exerted. More importantly, however, the therapy is directed toward increasing the ranges of motion of the hip and toward maintaining the ranges of motion of the knee and ankle.

The concept that motion is salubrious to the health and nutrition of the joint is the major justification for this aspect of therapy. It is preferably administered by a qualified physical therapist in the hospital, but under appropriate circumstances a parent may conduct the program just as well at home. The ranges of joint motion must be encouraged by simple active assistive exercises, *never* by passive stretching, and never to the point of pain. During this period of therapy the traction is usually discontinued. The duration of traction will vary from patient to patient, and the patient's clinical response largely determines the requisite length of time. It usually is necessary to maintain traction continuously for a minimum of 6 weeks and then gradually to reduce the duration of daytime traction as the range of motion improves. Nighttime skin traction is continued until the maximum range of motion has been achieved or until detectable improvement stops. This may be as long as 2 years (Fig. 7-20). In some situations the problem cannot be solved conservatively, and fusion or arthroplasty in unilateral instances and arthroplasty in bilateral cases must be accomplished (Fig. 7-21).

Aspirin has long been known to have a beneficial effect on articular cartilage, even though the exact mechanism by which it exerts this effect is not well understood. It is prescribed in the amount that will produce a therapeutic blood level of 20 to 30 mg/100 ml. Ordinarily

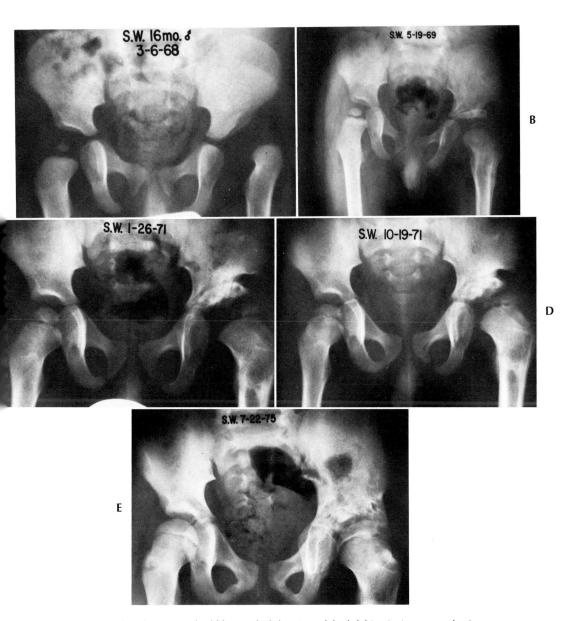

Fig. 7-20. Pelvic film of a 16-month-old boy with dislocation of the left hip, **A.** An open reduction was followed by a pericapsular pelvic osteotomy, at which time the hip joint was apparently entered through the posterior cut in the ilium, **B.** Postoperatively ankylosis of the hip was present and the roentgenogram showed bone necrosis, subchondral irregularities, and bony atrophy, **C.** The patient was placed in skin traction at night, and gradual improvement in the appearance of the hip can be seen, **D.** Ranges of motion slowly improved. After 2 years of nighttime skin traction and 4 years later, the ranges of hip motion approached normal, and there was considerable improvement in the hip x-ray film, **E.** Note the distortion of the ischial and pubic segments of the pelvis secondary to prolonged hyperemia. (Courtesy Dr. W. E. Hess.)

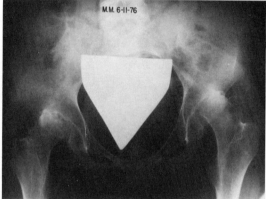
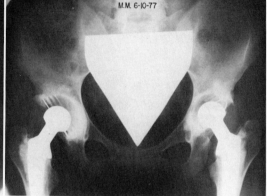

Fig. 7-21. This 12-year-old girl was treated at age 2 years for bilateral dislocation of the hip. Ten years later she developed gradual onset of pain and limp in both hips. The x-ray film of the pelvis showed abnormalities in configuration of the proximal femur as well as a reduced cartilage space and bone atrophy, **A.** One year later the cartilage space is completely gone, there are gross changes in the subchondral bone, and there is severe bony atrophy, **B.** "Bilabiation" of the femoral head is evident, resulting from the extrapelvic protrusion and collapse. All routine laboratory studies, including rheumatoid arthritis (RA) factor, lupus erythematosus (LE) preparation, and sedimentation rate were normal. Because of failure to respond to prolonged traction, nonweight-bearing, and oral medications, bilateral total hip arthroplasty was done, **C.**

this requires 100 mg/kg/day of aspirin. The usual care involved in aspirin therapy must be observed, specifically relating to any audiologic or gastrointestinal symptoms, and to any possible bleeding diathesis.

Ambulation is not allowed until the hip has lost its irritability and any significant contractures have been overcome. Then the skeletal traction pin (if it were used) is removed, and skin traction is instituted both day and night. Nonweight-bearing crutch ambulation is permitted, and daily therapy is continued. The duration of nonweight-bearing activities is governed by the same concepts as that utilized following surgical osteotomies or arthroplasties such as cup and femoral head replacement; that is, full weight bearing is not permitted until approximately 6 months from the onset of initial treatment. This gives the articular cartilage in the growing patient an opportunity to repair itself, to hypertrophy, and to mature sufficiently so that gradual resumption of weight bearing may be instituted. The patient gradually progresses to full weight bearing depending on the maintenance of a painless, satisfactory range of motion. Unrestricted activities are resumed at a highly individualized rate.

The foregoing therapeutic program is best instituted in a hospital setting; however, it undoubtedly can be implemented in an appropriate home situation. Though the program is rather long, tedious, and sometimes tiring, my results continue to justify its use.

Cartilage necrosis. Salter and Field[11] have shown that prolonged, uninterrupted immobilization of a joint or excessive pressure on the joint surfaces leads to necrosis of the articular cartilage. The degree of necrosis seems to be governed by the duration of the immobilization and/or the degree of pressure exerted. It has been shown that continued motion of the diarthrodial joint is essential to its normal nutrition; thus any time the hip joint undergoes prolonged immobilization, some degree of articular cartilage necrosis may occur. Also if greater than normal intra-articular pressure is exerted after reduction of a dislocated hip or if asymmetry of pressure resulting from a nonconcentric reduction (subluxation) is imposed on the femoral head articular cartilage, there is a greater likelihood that cartilage necrosis will occur.

Pathology. Experimentally, Salter and Field[11] have shown that necrosis of cartilage may be caused by continuous compression. Early changes in the cartilage consist simply of loss of normal luster and translucency, associated with loss of staining power of the nuclei in the superficial and transitional zones. These changes progress to partial loss of cartilage, with loss of nuclear staining power in all layers, and ultimately a full-thickness loss of articular cartilage can be seen at points of maximum compression, exposing the subchondral bone, which becomes hypertrophic. In all advanced cases there are intra-articular adhesions at the edges of areas of pressure necrosis.

Clinical manifestations. The physical and roentgenographic findings in cartilage necrosis are much the same as those encountered in chondrolysis, thus explaining the frequent association of the two conditions. Whether or not they are the same pathologic process becomes largely academic from a therapeutic standpoint, because once either is established, the treatment available is the same for both.

Treatment of cartilage necrosis is best done by prevention. This means strict avoidance of these etiologic factors that were outlined above. Once necrosis develops, however, the treatment program that I prefer is essentially the same as that outlined in the therapy of chondrolysis.

In nearly all cases of chondrolysis and cartilage necrosis there will eventually develop some degree of lost motion of the hip and some degree of permanent compromise of hip joint wear, leading eventually to the need for further reconstructive procedures in adult life. It is difficult to know the long-term beneficial effects of the treatment program discussed in this section, but the greater range of motion gained and the improved appearance of the joint, roentgenographically, appear to justify the efforts.

Not all instances of chondrolysis or necrosis will respond effectively to this therapy program, and some cases that appear at early ages to be chondrolysis may actually be some other condition such as juvenile rheumatoid arthritis, femoral head osteonecrosis, or pauciarticular rheumatoid arthritis, as described by Griffin and associates.[5] In these particular patients the response to any form of treatment will be highly unpredictable.

Restriction of hip joint motion

The two major causes of restricted hip joint motion are intra-articular scarring

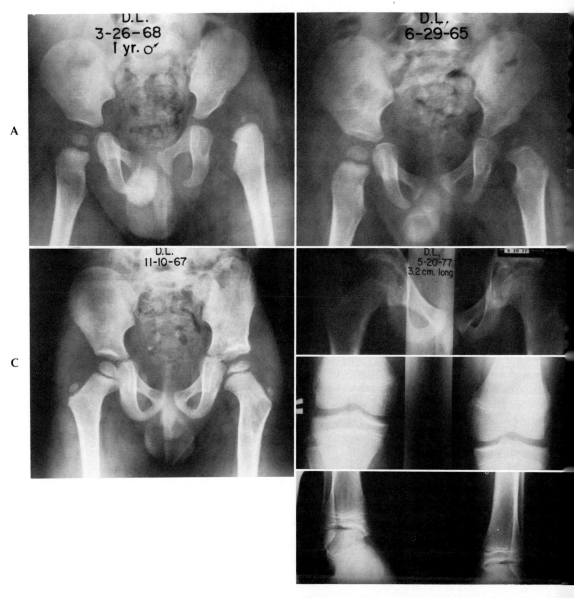

Fig. 7-22. Limb length inequality caused by treatment of hip dislocation is seen in this 1-year-old boy with dislocation of the left hip, **A.** A closed reduction was easily accomplished, **B.** The appearance of the hip after combined pelvic and proximal femoral osteotomy is seen in **C.** At age 13 years the affected lower limb is 3.2 cm longer than the other leg, undoubtedly the result of surgical stimulation of skeletal growth, **D.**

(cartilage necrosis, chondrolysis, and arthrofibrosis) and incongruity of joint surface. The latter is the result of deformation of the femoral head as a result of the sequelae of osteonecrosis along with associated acetabular deformities. In the absence of both of these complications, a growing child, simply by pursuing everyday activities, usually will regain a relatively normal range of motion following treatment of congenital dislocation of the hip.

Treatment of the intra-articular problems has already been discussed in the preceding section. The difficulties produced by joint incongruity are difficult to approach, because of the bony deformity that exists. The usual deformity in the femur will be a flattened, enlarged femoral head very similar to that seen in the Perthes disease. Treatment, therefore, parallels that utilized in the Perthes disease. Thus in younger children who yet have considerable remodeling capacity of the femoral head, an effort at gaining and maintaining concentric reduction of the deformed head must be exercised. This usually requires a period of traction in which the femoral head is gradually reduced into the socket and then held there by some form of bracing or casting until some degree of remodeling of the femoral head can occur. In young adolescents, when the femoral head has largely attained its adult shape, it may be necessary to exise the portion of the femoral head extruding laterally from the acetabulum. This procedure is known as "cheilectomy." Popularized by Garceau,[4] it can be used to obtain improved abduction of the hip; occasionally some improved rotation can also be realized.

A femoral head deformity of the degree seen in the Perthes disease is rather uncommon in congenital hip dislocation, and just as often the incongruity will be the result of a deformity both in the acetabulum and in the femoral head. In these instances there is very little that can be done surgically to regain motion of the hip. Judgment must be exercised in making the decision as to whether any effort at improving motion by this means is worthwhile. In such patients the employment of arthrography may have some value in providing a picture of the true configuration of either the acetabulum, the femoral head, or both. This is essential prior to making such a decision.

Limb length inequality caused by stimulation following surgery

A little-known and poorly emphasized complication following surgical treatment of congenital dislocation of the hip is limb length inequality resulting from stimulation of growth of the operated side. This discrepancy can sometimes be sufficiently great to require a surgical equalization procedure (Fig. 7-22).

The reasons for the increased length of the limb are multiple and have considerable relationship to the age at which various surgical procedures are carried out. Either a pericapsular or innominate osteotomy can produce increased length up to 1 or 2 cm. Osteotomy of the femur, especially in the proximal subtrochanteric and intertrochanteric areas, can stimulate growth to a similar degree, just as fractures of the proximal femur stimulate growth in growing children. The result of growth stimulation of combined operations on the proximal femur and acetabulum can sometimes produce a discrepancy in excess of 3.0 cm, which then justifies growth arrest if the inequality is recognized in time to correct it by that simple measure.

This complication can be recognized only by long-term and conscientious follow-up examinations, and it requires careful periodic documentation of limb lengths on any child having had operative treatment of congenital dislocation of the hip. It thus further reinforces the need for systematic follow-up examinations in all children who have been treated for congenital dislocation of the hip until they have reached skeletal maturity.

REFERENCES

1. Compere, E. L., Garrison, M., and Fahey, J. J.: Deformities of femur resulting from arrestment of growth of capital and greater trochanteric epiphyses, J. Bone Joint Surg. **22**:909, 1940.
2. Curtis, B.: Unpublished data.
3. Eisenstein, A., and Rothschild, S.: Biochemical abnormalities in patients with slipped capital femoral epiphysis and chondrolysis, J. Bone Joint Surg. **58A**:459, 1976.
4. Garceau, G.: Unpublished data.
5. Griffin, P. P., Tachdjian, M. O., and Green, W. J.: Pauciarticular arthritis in children, J.A.M.A. **184**:145, 1963.
6. Hoyt, W. A., Troyer, M. L., Reef, T., and Sheik, S.: The proximal femoral epiphyses; experimental and correlated clinical observations of their potential, Proceedings of the AAOS, January 1966, J. Bone Joint Surg. **48A**:1026, 1966.
7. Jones, B. S.: Adolescent chondrolysis of the hip joint, S. Afr. Med. J., p. 196, February 1971.
8. Langenskiöld, A., and Salenius, P.: Epiphysiodesis of the greater trochanter, Acta Orthop. Scand. **38**:199, 1967.
9. Moule, N. J., and Golding, J. S. R.: Idiopathic chondrolysis of the hip, Clin. Radiol. **25**:247, 1974.
10. Salter, R. B.: Personal communication.
11. Salter, R. B., and Field, P.: The effects of continuous compression on living articular cartilage, J. Bone Joint Surg. **42A**:31, 1960.
12. Samuelson, K. M., Nixon, G. W., and Morrow, R. E.: Tomography for evaluation of congenital dislocation of the hip while in a spica cast, J. Bone Joint Surg. **56A**:844, 1974.
13. Wagner, H.: Personal communication.

CHAPTER 8

Salvage procedures

Introduction, purposes, and goals
Problems requiring salvage procedures
Colonna arthroplasty
    Indications
    Prerequisites and contraindications
    Surgical technique
    Postoperative care
    Special complications
Chiari osteotomy
    Indications
    Prerequisites
    Surgical technique
    Postoperative care
    Complications and unique characteristics
Shelf procedures
    Indications
    Surgical technique
Reconstructive proximal femoral osteotomies
Trochanteric arthroplasty ("stick femur" procedure)
    Surgical technique
Arthrodesis
    Indications
    Prerequisites
    Surgical technique

INTRODUCTION, PURPOSES, AND GOALS

The primary emphasis of the preceding chapters has been on recognizing the various problems associated with congenital dysplasia and dislocation of the hip. Therapeutic efforts have been conceived and developed with the idea that a reasonably normal hip having lasting qualities will result if the diagnosis is made early and if the treatment program is executed properly. In most circumstances a satisfactory result can therefore be expected, but for a variety of reasons there will be a certain number of patients whose problems are such that a salvage procedure is all that can be used in an effort to retrieve former untoward results and to improve the functional capacity of the hip. To some extent these salvage operations are also designed to prepare the hip for a more successful and more easily performed secondary operation such as a total hip arthroplasty at a later time. This chapter, therefore, will deal with the problems for which there is not a good long-range solution and for which the only form of treatment is a compromise procedure that is designed either to arthrodese the hip joint or to prolong and improve the function of the hip until a more definitive procedure becomes necessary in adult life. The operations that fall into this category include Colonna arthroplasty, Chiari osteotomy, shelf procedures, reconstructive proximal femoral osteotomies, trochanteric arthroplasty ("stick femur" procedure), and arthrodesis. Except for arthrodesis and the osteotomies, these salvage operations have one thing in common—each, in a different way, utilizes an interposed fibrocartilaginous capsule as a weight-bearing tissue. It is for this reason that such operations cannot be put in the same category as the innominate osteotomies, wherein normal hyaline articular carti-

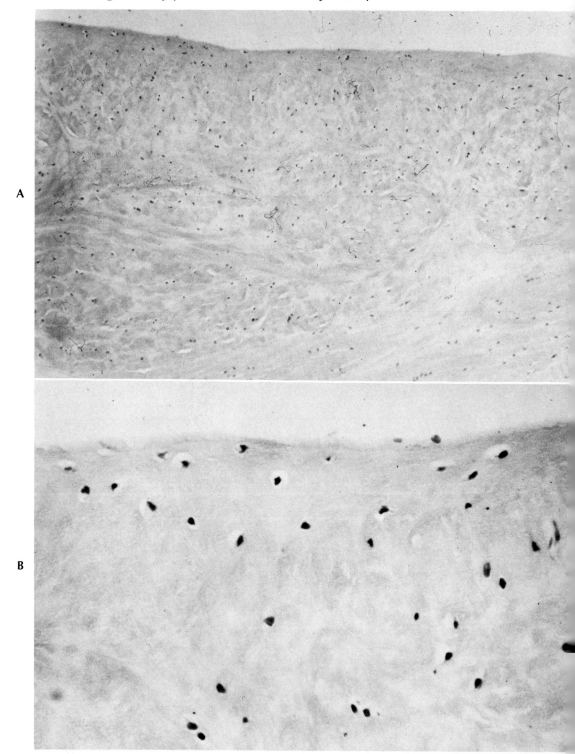

Fig. 8-1. For legend see opposite page.

lage serves as the weight-bearing structure. I consider operations such as pelvic support osteotomy[18] ineffective and outmoded, and they will therefore be discussed purely for historical value.

PROBLEMS REQUIRING SALVAGE PROCEDURES

The most common problems that necessitate the use of a salvage operation are the following: (1) late diagnosis of a dislocated hip (in children over 5 or 6 years of skeletal age); (2) persistent subluxation with incongruity of femoral head and acetabulum; (3) persistent dislocation following repeated attempts at reduction; (4) deformities of the acetabulum caused by failures of prior surgery; and (5) fibrous or bony ankylosis of the hip in a poor functional position. The causes of these problems are discussed in considerable detail in Chapter 6. With greater and better understanding of the behavior of congenital dislocation of the hip and with improved technical expertise in the solution of the many problems presented by this condition, the need for such a chapter as this should probably gradually disappear.

COLONNA ARTHROPLASTY

In 1936 Colonna[6] developed a procedure that was designed to gain stable reduction in older children in whom simpler procedures had either failed or were ineffective. The acetabulum was reamed and deepened, and the redundant capsule was sewn over the femoral head in order to serve as an interposed membrane. It thus qualifies as a fascial arthroplasty. The Colonna arthroplasty was developed in response to the following fundamental concepts: (1) In some instances the acetabulum will not accept the dislocated femoral head, or if it does there will be a gross incongruity. As a result excessive pressure will be exerted on various areas on the articular cartilage, leading to cartilage necrosis. (2) The superior portion of the joint capsule has become adapted to weight bearing and has undergone some degree of metaplasia into fibrocartilage or even possibly immature hyaline cartilage (Fig. 8-1), and therefore may well serve as a long-term weight-bearing structure. (3) It is better that a unilateral dislocation be reduced into its original modified acetabulum than to leave it persistently dislocated. Based on these concepts, I have performed a large number of Colonna arthroplasties during the past 20 years and find it one of the most rewarding operative procedures in the salvage treatment of congenital dislocation of the hip, *provided* that the indications and prerequisites are given proper consideration and that the surgical technique is meticulously and rigidly followed.[1,4,17]

Indications

The prime indication for this operation is a virginal unilateral hip dislocation in a child over 6 or 7 years of age[1] (Fig. 8-2). Another indication is a child in a similar age group with a persistently dislocated hip that has been subjected to previous efforts at operative reduction along with other reconstructive procedures (Fig. 8-3). In these latter instances the anatomy will usually be so disturbed or the scarring so great that any other reconstructive

Fig. 8-1. Histologic section of the capsule directly overlying the femoral head in a complete dislocation of the hip in a 6-year-old white girl. Most of the tissue is composed of hyalinized dense white fibrous tissue containing healthy cellular elements, **A.** In the areas closer to the surface, utilizing polarized light, evidence of fibrocartilage can be identified (× 120), **B.** It is this tissue that serves as the weight-bearing support on the surface of the newly created acetabulum.

212 *Congenital dysplasia and dislocation of the hip*

procedure will be contraindicated. A final but more controversial indication is a *bilateral* virginal hip dislocation in a child over the age of 6 years. Fortunately this circumstance will rarely ever be encountered in this country except in our more remote areas where treatment may have been either unavailable or refused.

It is very important to emphasize that for satisfactory results from the Colonna procedure the hip must be *completely dislocated* in order that sufficient weight-bearing capsule will be available for interposition between the femoral head and the newly created bony acetabulum. Rarely a subluxated hip may be considered for this operation, but, as will be discussed subsequently, these conditions are better suited for the Chiari osteotomy.

Prerequisites and contraindications

The most important criteria to be met prior to undertaking this very challenging operation are as follows: (1) child over 6

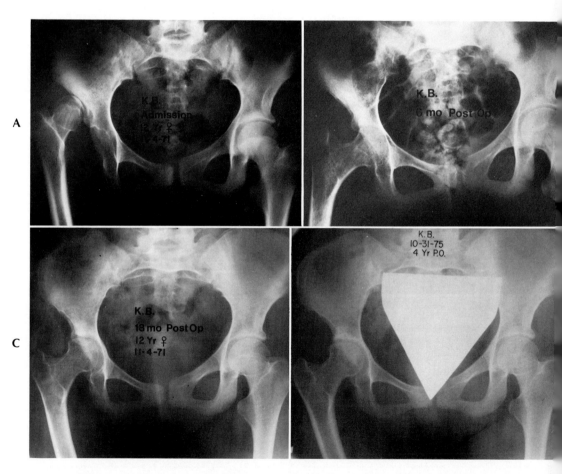

Fig. 8-2. An example of a good candidate for a Colonna arthroplasty is this 12-year-old girl with a unilateral dislocation of the right hip, **A.** Pelvic film 6 months postoperatively shows a well-seated, viable femoral head. She lacks only 10 degrees of inward rotation in an otherwise normal range of motion, **B.** A roentgenogram taken 18 months postoperatively shows increase in the cartilage space, **C.** Four years postoperatively the patient has a normal range of motion, no limp, and no pain, **D.** Undoubtedly total hip arthroplasty will eventually be necessary, but the goals of a salvage procedure have been realized.

or 7 years of age; (2) complete dislocation, having adequate capsule to cover the femoral head; (3) remote likelihood that any lesser or different procedure will be effective; (4) absence of any recent infection in the involved joint region; and (5) absence of any sign of central nervous system disease. These prerequisites are discussed in greater detail below.

The procedure preferably should *not* be done in young children under age 6 years, primarily because the articular cartilage of the acetabulum must be completely reamed out. Since this is one of the major growth centers of the acetabulum, it is likely that some degree of reduction in ultimate size of the socket may eventuate. The older the child, the less likely this is to occur. This observation is more conceptual than proved, but because of this possibility I have restricted the performance of Colonna arthroplasty to children over 6 or 7 years of age.

In order to perform the arthroplasty as

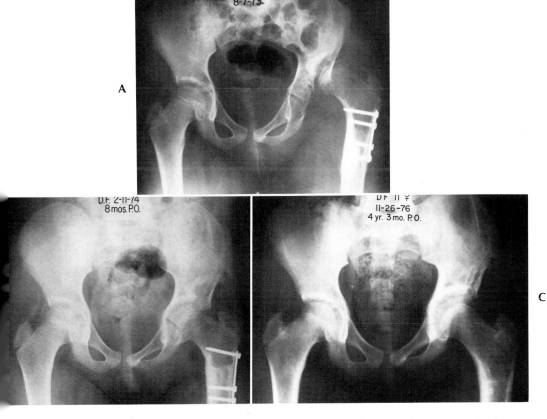

Fig. 8-3. This 7-year-old girl had undergone two attempts at open reduction and a varus rotational osteotomy as treatment for congenital dislocation. Unfortunately the hip remained dislocated in a false acetabulum, **A.** A Colonna arthroplasty aided by a femoral shortening resulted in a satisfactory reduction, **B.** Three years later the femur was well reduced, **C.** There is a normal range of motion and she has no limp or pain.

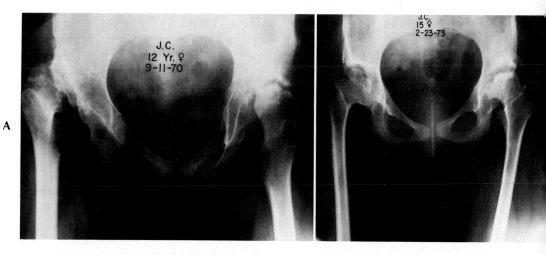

Fig. 8-4. This 12-year-old girl had undergone multiple previous surgical procedures for bilateral congenital dislocation of the hip. At the time that I saw her both hips were severely restricted in their motions, which were painful. She had a very grotesque gait, almost impossible to describe, **A.** On each hip a modified Colonna arthroplasty was accomplished, utilizing the horizontal split capsular technique. Two and one half years later she had a substantial increase in range of hip motion, and her hips were painless, **B.** The ranges of motion, however, were less than desirable. Clearly, these were salvage procedures designed to "buy time" until total hip arthroplasties could be done.

described by Colonna, the femoral head should be completely dislocated from the socket, otherwise there will not be enough joint capsule to cover the femoral head with the smooth and glistening capsule that is so essential to a good result. In rare instances in which there has been no alternative, I have done a modified Colonna arthroplasty in hips not completely dislocated. It is necessary to split the capsule horizontally and spread the capsule out around the femoral head. Although improvement in motion and better reduction are achieved (Fig. 8-4), the functional result is far below those instances of dislocation in which the capsule is large and redundant.

Since this is a salvage procedure, it obviously should not be done if a less extensive, simpler operation will accomplish the necessary goal. This determination can largely be reached by making a thorough analysis of the problem and by then comparing the conclusions reached with the indications and prerequisites of other procedures discussed earlier. To repeat, a Colonna arthroplasty is only justified when no other operation will accomplish the goals intended.

The need for absence of any recent infection is self-evident in any operation on the hip, but this concern is especially important when performing such an extensive procedure as the Colonna arthroplasty. Because of the major instrumentation in the joint, the wide dissection of the capsule, and the exposure of large areas of cancellous bone, the potential devastating effects of infection are obvious.

Absence of any sign of central nervous system disease is essential because of the great tendency for these patients to form heterotopic bone in and about joints. In a few children with cerebral palsy and myelodysplasia on whom I have performed the Colonna arthroplasty, the tendency to develop myositis ossificans

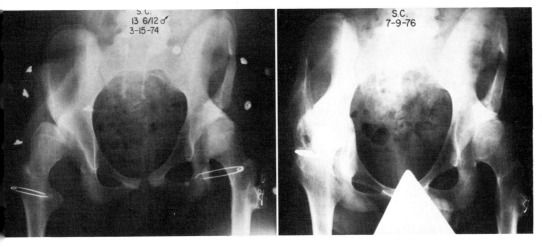

Fig. 8-5. An example of the unfavorable response of neurologically impaired patients to Colonna arthroplasty is shown in this 13-year-old boy with myelodysplasia and paralytic dislocation of the right hip, **A.** A Colonna arthroplasty coupled with iliopsoas transfer to the greater trochanter was accomplished. The hip developed ankylosis resulting from periarticular ossification, **B.**

and heterotopic bone about the joint capsule has been a major factor resulting in compromise of subsequent hip motion (Fig. 8-5). As a consequence I consider any suggestion of central nervous system disease a relative contraindication to performing this operation.

Surgical technique

Some significant modifications have been made in the technique of this operation as originally described by Colonna, but the essentials of the procedure are unchanged because they are critical to achieving its purpose. Thus the two basic concepts of creating an enlarged and deepened socket at the level of the original acetabulum and covering the femoral head with the capsule of the hip joint are the most significant technical aspects of the procedure.

With the patient lying supine on the operating table, a sandbag is placed under the affected buttock and the lower limb is draped free. A generous anterior (iliofemoral) incision is made and extended downward over the lateral aspect of the proximal thigh in the same manner as for open reduction and femoral resection illustrated in Fig. 5-5.

Once the capsule has been exposed, it must be stripped off the ilium and freed from the overlying soft tissues throughout its entire attachment over the anterior, superior, and posterior aspects of the acetabulum (Fig. 8-6). In this process the abductor muscles are stripped extensively from their origin on the iliac crest in order that they may be recessed distally if necessary. Also, the iliopsoas muscle is sectioned at or near its insertion. The capsule is then incised in a direction paralleling its fibers, and the capsule is severed at its attachments to the anterior and superior aspects of the acetabular margin. The joint can then be explored, but the femoral head can rarely be reduced into the socket without extreme force, and this should *never* be used.

Next the distal lateral extension of the incision is deepened and the fascia lata is cut transversely. The femur is exposed

Text continued on p. 222.

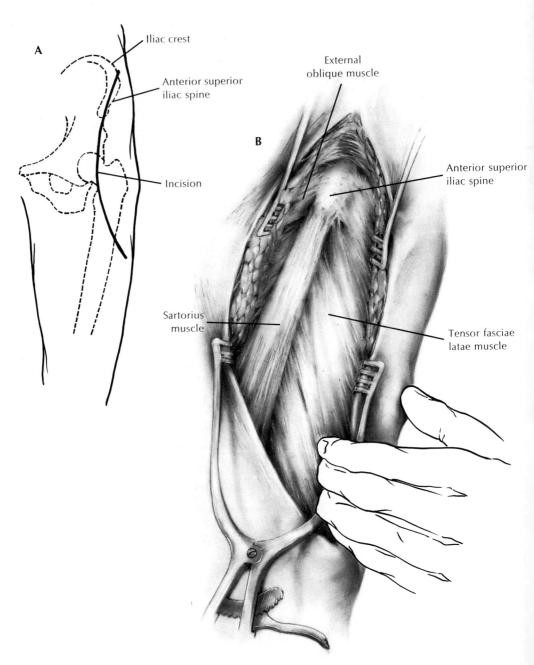

Fig. 8-6. For legend see opposite page.

Salvage procedures 217

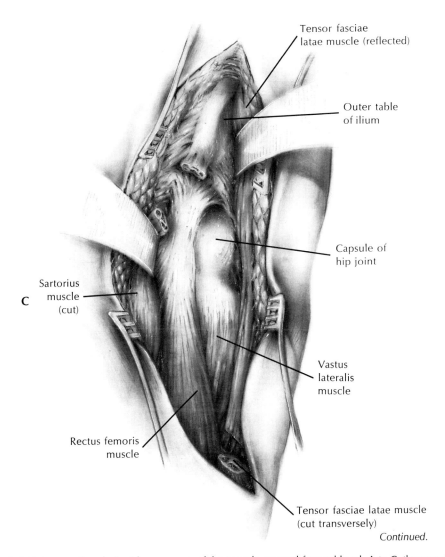

Fig. 8-6. Colonna arthroplasty. After exposure of the capsule-covered femoral head, **A** to **C,** the capsule is completely and circumferentially incised at its attachment to the acetabular rim, **D.** Then, after appropriate extension of the operative incision, the femur is osteotomized and the fragments are allowed to overlap, **E.** (Note: a longitudinal "score" on the femur is designed to maintain rotational orientation.) The proximal fragment, consisting of the head and neck of the femur, is gently retracted posteriorly by means of a retractor placed in the sciatic notch, **F.** The acetabulum is then cleared of soft tissue and cartilage and is reamed deeply into the inner table of the ilium, **G.** The redundant capsule is then trimmed and the free edges of the capsule are sutured over the femoral head, **H.** The capsule-covered femoral head is then reduced into the newly created bony acetabulum and an appropriate internal fixation device is applied to the femur, **I.**

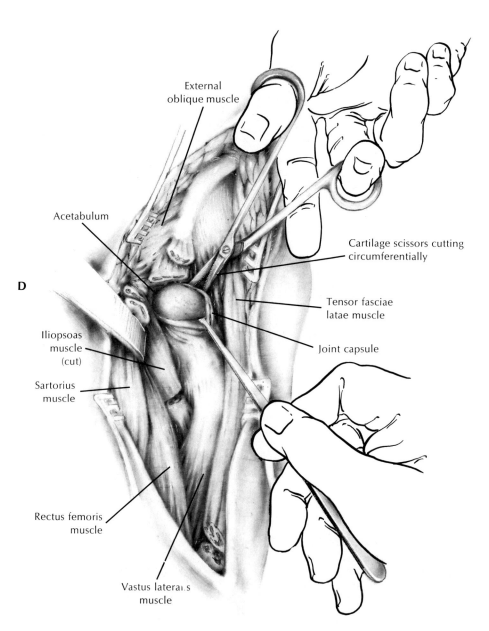

Fig. 8-6, cont'd. For legend see p. 217.

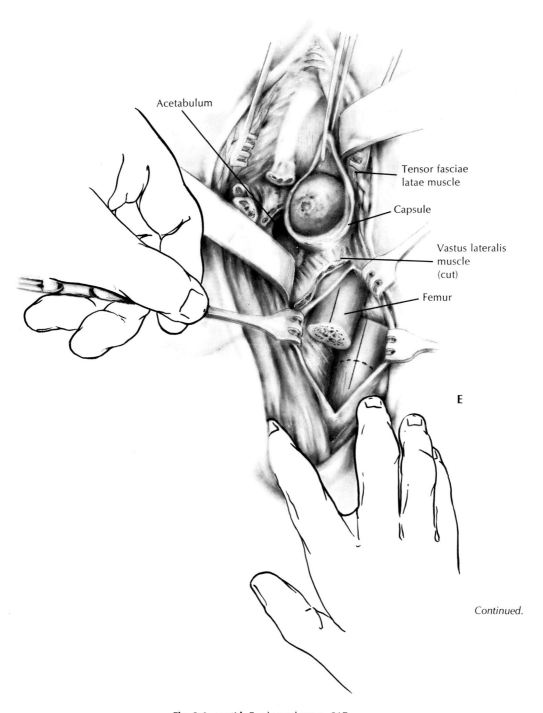

Fig. 8-6, cont'd. For legend see p. 217.

220 Congenital dysplasia and dislocation of the hip

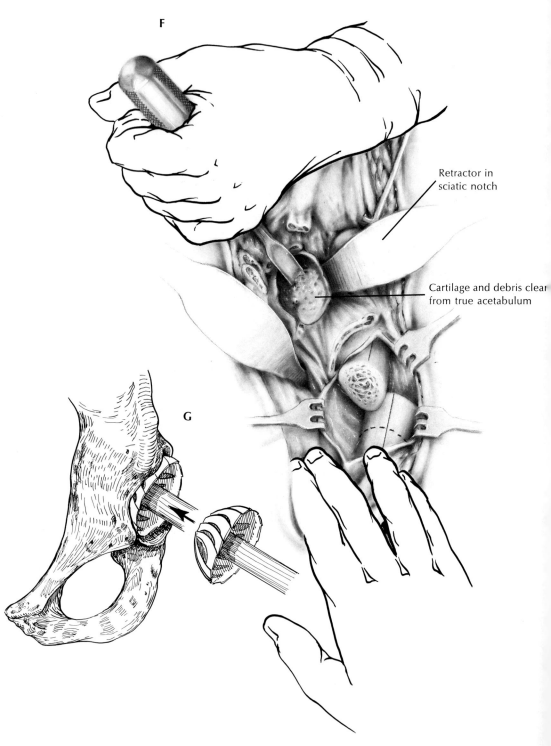

Fig. 8-6, cont'd. For legend see p. 217.

Salvage procedures 221

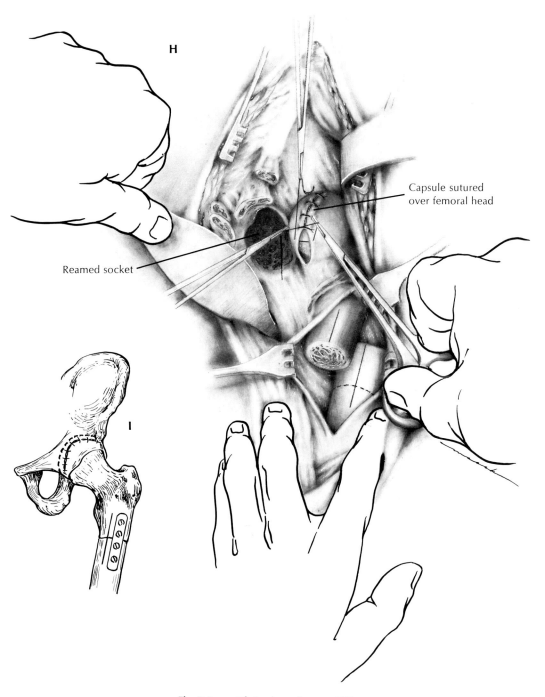

Fig. 8-6, cont'd. For legend see p. 217.

over its proximal 3 inches in order to perform a femoral resection. The femur is cut at the level of the lesser trochanter and the distal fragment is allowed to overlap the proximal. At this juncture the proximal fragment will be surprisingly free, and the femoral head can easily be brought down to the level of the acetabulum. The remainder of the capsule is then separated from the acetabular margin, except for the most posterior and inferior portions. In the posterior dissection care must be exercised so as not to cut or damage the external rotator muscles, because much of the blood supply to the capsule is located in these structures.

The proximal fragment with its attached capsule is then reflected posteriorly, and this provides adequate exposure of the acetabulum. The articular cartilage of the socket and all other soft tissues, including the ligamentum teres, are removed with a curved gouge and rongeur in preparation for the acetabular reamers, which then deepen and enlarge the socket symmetrically to the appropriate size and depth. In order to provide maximum depth, which ensures adequate femoral head coverage, it is essential to ream the socket to the inner table of the ilium. In rare instances it may be necessary to create a stellate osteotomy of the inner table in order to gain increased depth.

The capsule is then trimmed and fashioned so that it can be sewn over the femoral head, with care being taken to see that the thickened portion of the capsule previously situated over the weight-bearing portion of the femoral head is maintained in this position. It is carefully trimmed so that there is no redundancy but so that the capsule can move freely over the head. When adhesions exist between the head and the capsule as a result of previous surgical intervention, these must by lysed. However, invariably under these circumstances the ultimate range of motion will be compromised, because many of the adhesions probably will re-form. The capsule-covered head is then gently placed into the enlarged and deepened acetabulum. If appropriate releases have been done, it will be possible to displace the femoral head downward a short distance from the acetabulum with gentle distraction in order to assure that there is not any excessive pressure on the head.

The distal fragment of the femur is then allowed to overlap the proximal fragment in its newly reduced position, and the amount of overlapping femur is resected from the distal fragment just as described and illustrated in Fig. 5-5. Any previously existing rotational or angular deformity of the femur is corrected, and a plate or nail-plate combination is applied for internal fixation. The hip is then carried through a range of motion to test stability. Usually it will be stable through 90 degrees of flexion, through full abduction, and with acceptable degrees of rotation. An x-ray film is taken on the table to determine the adequacy and concentricity of reduction as well as to verify the position of the internal fixation devices.

The wound is closed and a one and one-half hip spica cast is applied with the hip and knee in about 30 degrees of flexion, about 20 degrees of hip abduction, and neutral rotation. An x-ray film is again taken after application of the cast to ascertain maintenance of reduction.

Postoperative care

One week after surgery another x-ray film should be taken in order to evaluate the status of the reduction. If the femoral head appears well reduced, the cast remains on for 6 weeks, after which time the anterior half of the cast is removed and the posterior shell is maintained for night splinting. An x-ray film should again be taken to determine whether the reduction has been maintained and whether the osteotomy has healed sufficiently for permanent removal of the cast. Usually this will be the case. Physical therapy is then begun, consisting of active assistive range of motion exercises in the hip, knee, and ankle and muscle-strengthening exercises. The posterior shell of the cast is used at night and is gradually removed during the daytime as the stability of the reduction is demonstrated. The posterior shell is then removed permanently 3 months after surgery. Crutch ambulation with no weight bearing on the involved limb is begun at about 12 weeks postoperatively. Graduated weight bearing is then begun at 4 months after surgery; full weight bearing is not permitted until 6 months postoperatively. Range-of-motion and muscle-strengthening exercises are continued throughout the convalescent period. The reason why weight bearing should be discouraged is based on the same principle as for the nonweight-bearing requirement following prosthetic and cup arthroplasties. That is, it is hoped that the interposed capsule can undergo maturation and can adapt to the new weight bearing function imposed on it. An arbitrary period of 4 to 6 months has been selected for this to take place.

Long-term follow-up evaluation of Colonna arthroplasty shows that many of these hip joints eventually develop loss of cartilage space and that they ultimately become painful and more stiff,[21] requiring a more formal and more definitive procedure in later adult life. However, this arthroplasty does fulfill the two major purposes of a salvage procedure, that is, it prolongs the functional use of a movable hip until an age when implants can be confidently placed in the hip, and it results in an improvement of the bone stock of the hip joint so that subsequent total hip joint replacements or other adult procedures can be more easily and safely accomplished.[8]

Special complications

Although the entire subject of complications has been covered in Chapter 7, there are certain complications that are unusually unique to the Colonna arthroplasty because of the very nature of the operation. These consist of cartilage

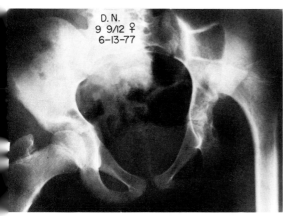
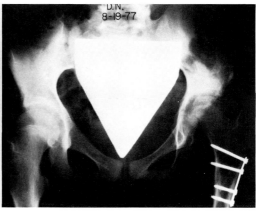

Fig. 8-7. Preoperative pelvic roentgenograms in a 10-year-old girl with unilateral congenital dislocation of the left hip, **A.** A Colonna arthroplasty was done, assisted by a femoral shortening. She did very well for 2 years and then developed pain in the hip, accompanied by a decrease in range of hip motions. X-ray films, **B,** suggest that chondrolysis occurred, even as late as 2 years after the definitive surgery.

necrosis, chondrolysis, and osteonecrosis of the femoral head. Any one of these complications, in turn, may lead to stiffness, which is occasionally painful and which on occasion may reach the point of fibrous ankylosis. This complication was very frequent prior to the development of femoral resection, as mentioned earlier; some have even labeled the Colonna arthroplasty "Italian for fusion."[14] There is no question that there is a greater potential for cartilage and osseous necrosis in this operation than in any other salvage procedure and, as illustrated in Fig. 8-7, that this complication can occur even as long as 18 months after surgery. This operation and its complications underscore the need for great attention to the technical details when the operation is being performed, and it also emphasizes the point made earlier, that is, the operation should not be done if a less extensive procedure can achieve the necessary goals.

CHIARI OSTEOTOMY

In 1955 Chiari[3] developed an ingenious osteotomy of the ilium, which, when properly done, can provide a very satisfactory weight-bearing superior roof of the acetabulum in hips having a previously deficient socket. The procedure was originally designed to be a definitive reconstructive procedure, and, prior to the development of the innominate osteotomies of Pemberton and Salter, it was done for almost all types of dislocated and subluxated hips. Over the years it has gradually assumed its more appropriate position of a salvage procedure that is appropriately suited for the subluxated hip having femoral head and acetabular incongruities, in which the femoral head cannot be seated concentrically in the acetabulum (Fig. 8-8). There may be extensions of this rather confined indication, but the best results will be obtained utilizing this rigid indication.

The fundamental concept in this operation is illustrated in the diagrams seen in Fig. 8-9. The iliac osteotomy is made as close to the osteochondral juncture of the roof of the acetabulum as possible, just between the capsule (below) and the reflected head of the rectus femoris muscle (above). The distal fragment of the transected ilium is displaced medially, taking the capsule inward to cover the raw bone surface of the superior fragment. Thus the capsule serves as an interposed fibrous

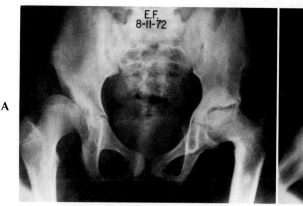
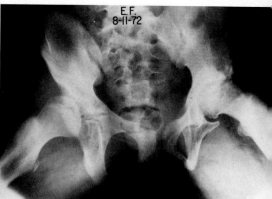

Fig. 8-8. An indication for the Chiari osteotomy is seen in this 11-year-old girl with a subluxated right hip following failure of previous treatment, **A.** A pelvic film with the thighs in abduction and internal rotation shows lack of concentric reduction, **B.**

membrane over the weight-bearing area, somewhat similar to that situation created in the Colonna arthroplasty. However, there is one very significant difference between the two procedures, that is, the Chiari osteotomy is basically an extra-articular operation. This is a rather simple concept that has far-reaching implications, as is discussed on p. 229.

Indications

Although the most appropriate indication for this osteotomy is a child over age 3 or 4 years who has a subluxated hip with incongruity of the femoral head and acetabulum, other indications do exist that I consider marginal. Some employ the Chiari osteotomy in cases of complete dislocation, and others have performed the procedure in patients whose femoral heads can be concentrically situated in the acetabulum (good candidates for any one of the reconstructive pelvic rotational osteotomies such as Pemberton, Salter, and Steel). In two separate studies done by surgeons in the Shriners Hospitals[2,7] on the Chiari osteotomy, it was found that the poorest results were achieved in in-

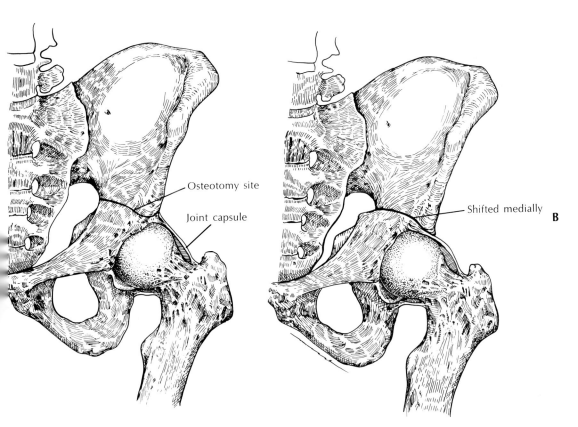

Fig. 8-9. This diagrammatic representation of the Chiari osteotomy attempts to illustrate the principles of the procedure. The osteotomy must be made precisely at the osteochondral juncture of the acetabular rim, directly on top of the superior joint capsule as it attaches to the acetabular rim, **A.** The osteotomy, which is made in an arcuate (pericapsular) direction over the roof of the acetabulum, is directed upward between 20 and 30 degrees. The distal fragment is then displaced medially so that the capsule-covered head comes to lie under the osteotomized surface of the superior fragment, **B.** It thus represents a modified capsular arthroplasty.

stances of complete dislocation of the hip, cases that I believe are good candidates for the Colonna arthroplasty.

I currently believe that the indications for the Chiari osteotomy as a salvage procedure in congenital dislocation of the hip are as follows: (1) an unstable dysplastic or subluxated hip with positive Trendelenburg gait; (2) painful subluxation of the hip (nonconcentric reduction), especially as demonstrated on weight-bearing films; (3) incongruity of the acetabulofemoral relationships; and (4) the presence of a contraindication for any *reconstructive* pelvic osteotomy.

Prerequisites

Consistent with the somewhat restricted indications for the operation, the prerequisites are likewise rather limited. They are, however, extremely important. The age group should range from 3 years through early adult life, that is, prior to the age for total hip arthroplasty. There should be a satisfactory range of motion, especially in flexion, and there should be no significant contractures of the hip.

There should be a reasonably satisfactory cartilage space, and the outer rim of the true acetabular rim must not be too high. Finally, just as in the instance of Colonna arthroplasty, the likelihood should be remote that any other less extensive and substantially more lasting procedure can accomplish the same necessary goals. When neither the indications nor the prerequisites are met, the operation is contraindicated. It is important that when the acetabulum is too high the osteotomy may not permit displacement of the distal fragment (Fig. 8-10). This is a rare circumstance, but it is a most distressing pitfall and must be watched for.

Surgical technique

With the patient lying supine on a standard operating room table, a sandbag is placed under the buttock of the affected side and the hip is draped free. An anterior (iliofemoral) incision is made, the same as for either of the reconstructive iliac osteotomies. Though not commonly necessary, one should be prepared to do femoral osteotomy and shortening if

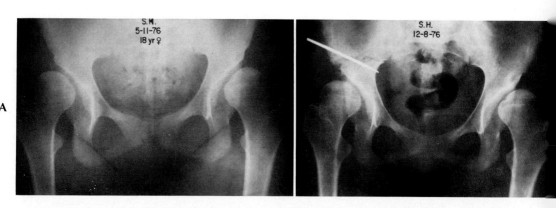

Fig. 8-10. When the acetabular rim of a severely dysplastic hip is too high, a properly done Chiari osteotomy cannot be accomplished. This 18-year-old girl complained of increasing pain and limp on the right, and a pelvic x-ray film was taken, **A,** which showed significant upward displacement of both acetabula and femoral heads. The osteotomy had to be placed so high that medial displacement of the distal fragment was impossible, **B.** This instance would probably call for a modification of the Chiari osteotomy in which the cut is "dome-shaped" rather than directed obliquely upward. (Courtesy Dr. Rae J. Johnston.)

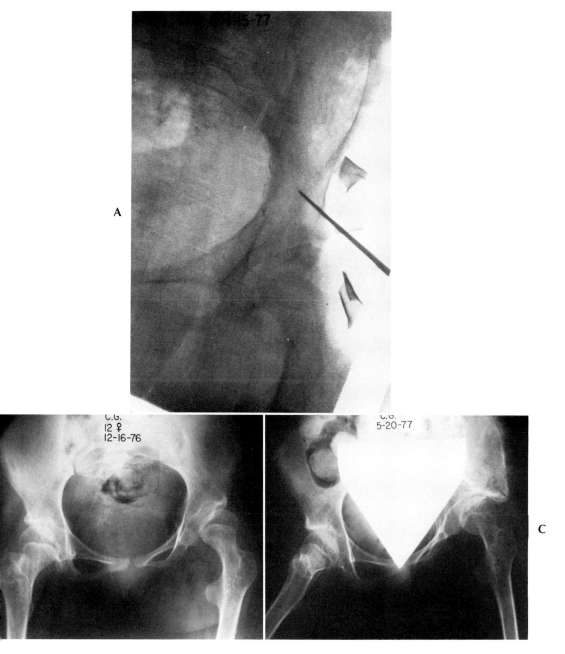

Fig. 8-11. The pelvic osteotomy must be made precisely at the rim of the acetabulum, and an intraoperative localizing x-ray film is essential in order to make that determination. In this patient the osteotomy was made about 1.0 cm lower than the level of the osteotome, **A.** The results of a well-done Chiari osteotomy on this same patient are seen preoperatively in **B** and 5 months later in **C.**

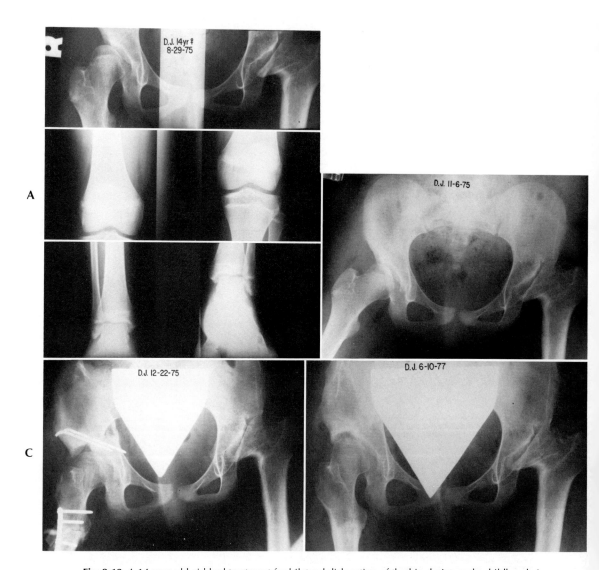

Fig. 8-12. A 14-year-old girl had treatment for bilateral dislocation of the hip during early childhood. An orthoroentgenogram showed significant (5.0 cm) limb length inequality, **A.** An abduction internal rotation film showed failure of the femoral head to seat concentrically in the acetabulum, **B.** There was pain in the right hip but no pain in the severely deformed left hip. A Chiari osteotomy coupled with a femoral shortening of 5.0 cm was accomplished, **C.** Eighteen months later the limb lengths were essentially equal and she had a painless gait, **D.** Some varus at the intertrochanteric level would have been appropriate.

necessary, but the incision need not be extended laterally until that determination is made. The ilium is exposed subperiosteally on both inner and outer tables, and retractors are placed in the sciatic notch. The outer table of the ilium is stripped subperiosteally down to the capsule of the hip joint, and the reflected head of the rectus femoris muscle is exposed and excised. This then exposes the attachment of the capsule to the acetabular rim. An osteotome is driven into the ilium at the osteochondral juncture, just at the upper level of the capsule, and a localizing pelvic x-ray film is taken (Fig. 8-11). This roentgenographic localization is extremely *important* because if the osteotomy is not made at the exact position desired, the procedure will fail and the resulting situation will be worse than if no operation had been done at all. If the x-ray localization of the placement of the osteotomy is appropriate, a curved osteotomy is made in a pericapsular fashion, with the angle of the osteotomy being directed upward about 20 to 30 degrees. The osteotomy is completed through the sciatic notch by means of a Gigli saw. Any irregularities in the osteotomized fragments should be smoothed off with a rongeur. In some instances one may want to combine the Chiari osteotomy with femoral shortening (Fig. 8-12).

The lower limb is placed in abduction, and the distal fragment is displaced medially for nearly the full width of the ilium at the osteotomy site. The capsule-covered head will be seen to disappear under the proximal fragment, which then serves as the future roof of the acetabulum (Fig. 8-9). Two threaded Steinmann pins are used to transfix the osteotomy site, and an x-ray film is taken to verify the position of the osteotomy, the coverage of the femoral head, and the location of the pins. The wound is closed and a one and one-half hip spica cast is applied.

Postoperative care

One week after surgery a pelvic x-ray film is taken to verify maintenance of the position of the osteotomy and the femoral head; at 6 or 8 weeks, depending on the age of the patient, the anterior half of the cast is removed, leaving the posterior shell for use as a day and night splint. Physical therapy is begun just as with the Colonna arthroplasty. Because of the similarity of principle in the two operations—a capsular arthroplasty—I impose the same weight-bearing restrictions in the Chiari osteotomy during convalescence as in the Colonna arthroplasty.

Complications and unique characteristics

There are certain technical features of this operation that are extremely critical to its success, and there is such little margin for error that it becomes one of the most technically demanding operations in hip surgery. If the osteotomy is made too high, a step-off will result in the weight-bearing portion of the acetabulum, and this may even disturb the stability of the hip joint sufficiently to result in a redislocation (Fig. 8-13). On the other hand if the osteotomy is made too low, into the articular cartilage, considerable stiffness and arthrofibrosis may result (Fig. 8-14). If the distal fragment is displaced too far medially, the configuration of the acetabulum will be altered, resulting in incongruity of the femoral head and acetabulum (Fig. 8-15). Also, if transfixion pins are not used, then the osteotomy can easily slip in one direction or another.

The osteotomy creates certain biomechanical changes in the hip that are not associated with any of the other iliac osteotomies. These have been summarized by Noel[15] and can be listed as follows:
1. The center of gravity is displaced medially, thus potentially enhancing the strength of the abductor muscles.

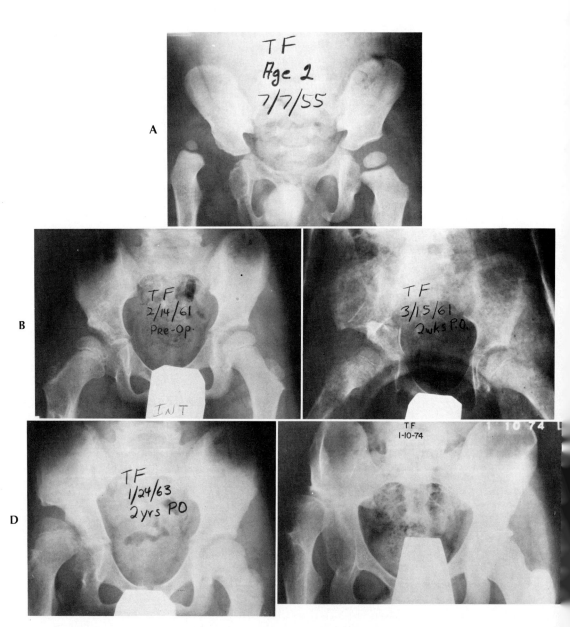

Fig. 8-13. An example of a Chiari osteotomy having been made too high is illustrated in this male patient, whose initial pelvic film is seen at 2 years of age, **A.** Six years later the hip is reduced, but the acetabulum is deficient, **B.** A Chiari osteotomy was attempted, but the osteotomy was made too high, **C.** Two years postoperatively the femoral head was subluxating upward because of the fact that the true acetabulum is actually made more oblique by the Chiari osteotomy and because there is no superior buttress to prevent subluxation, **D.** Eleven years later, at age 19 years, the femoral head has dislocated into the false acetabulum created by the osteotomy, **E.** (Courtesy Dr. Loren Larsen.)

2. The limb is shortened slightly; consequently, there is no tendency to increase the pressure on the femoral head.
3. The acetabulum is enlarged; therefore, the surface area of weight-bearing is increased.
4. It is an extra-articular procedure, which reduces the likelihood of joint stiffness.

On the other hand there are certain characteristics that are potential disadvantages. These include:

1. An increased obliquity of the true acetabulum
2. Slight shortening of the limb
3. Alteration of the pelvic ring

Since the distal fragment is displaced medially, there has to be a variable degree of reduction in the pelvic diameter, and the question of its influence on subsequent childbearing has often been raised. Gilbert[9] made a study of Chiari osteotomies several years postoperatively and concluded that any compromise of pelvic inlet or outlet that might have been

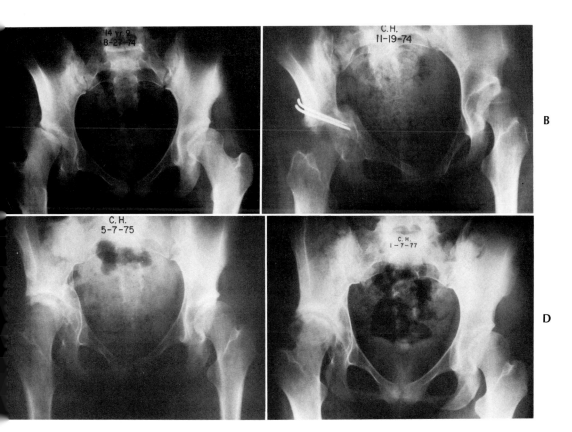

Fig. 8-14. An example of joint stiffness and arthrofibrosis is demonstrated by this 14-year-old girl who was complaining of a painful limp on the right hip, **A.** Note the coxa valga, extrapelvic protrusion, obliquity of the acetabulum, and early degenerative change. The osteotomy was made very slightly low, but satisfactory displacement was accomplished, **B.** The pins are anteriorly and posteriorly placed and are not in the joint. Following cast and pin removal the patient's hip was very stiff, but the femoral head remained well covered by an acetabulum with good configuration, **C.** Despite the appearance of the joint, 2 years later the motion had returned almost completely to normal and the patient was pain-free, **D.** A varus osteotomy, with or without femoral shortening, could have been done at the same operation.

232 Congenital dysplasia and dislocation of the hip

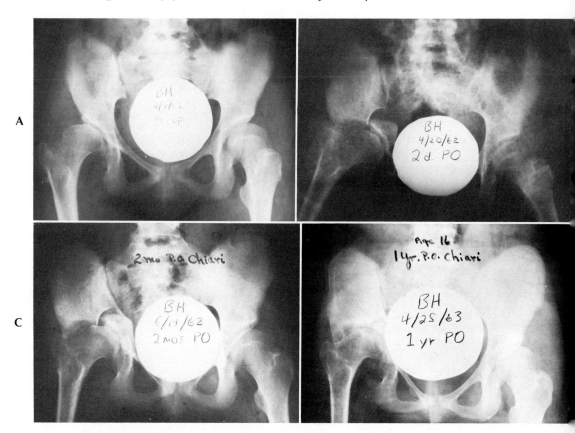

Fig. 8-15. The distal fragment of a Chiari osteotomy can become displaced too far medially, as shown in this 15-year-old girl who had persistent extrapelvic protrusion of the femoral head and an inadequate acetabulum following treatment for "dislocated hip in childhood," **A.** A Chiari osteotomy was accomplished, but the displacement of the distal fragment was too far medially, **B.** When the cast was removed 2 months later, there was a "step-off" in the acetabular roof and the femoral head was too far medial, **C.** Despite this offset, the acetabulum remodeled considerably, leaving a pain-free hip 1 year later, **D.** (Courtesy Dr. Loren Larsen.)

created at the time of the osteotomy ostensibly was subsequently compensated for. At skeletal maturity there was no demonstrable change in the configuration of the true pelvis attributable to the osteotomy. He explained that the proximal fragment often displaces laterally; thus the pelvis was actually altered less than was originally believed.

It has been my observation that the depth of the newly created acetabulum resulting from the Chiari osteotomy gradually diminishes over the subsequent years of growth, if it is done during the growing years. What appeared to be excellent coverage shortly after removal of the operative cast resulted in gradual extrusion of the head of the femur in many instances (Fig. 8-16). My explanation for this is as follows: The entire circumference of the acetabulum is displaced medially, which carries with it the articular cartilage and triradiate cartilage, the two major growth centers of the acetabulum. These cartilage centers continue to grow and gradually tend to remodel the

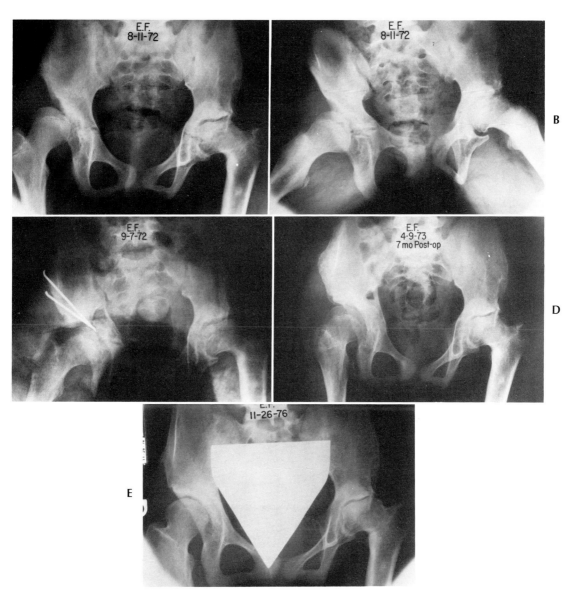

Fig. 8-16. In this patient it can be seen that when a Chiari osteotomy is done at an age when there is remaining skeletal growth there will be a tendency for the femur to extrude with growth, despite early good coverage. A 10-year-old Oriental girl had as a child, multiple surgical procedures on both hips for bilateral congenital dislocation. The residuals showed an ankylosed but painless hip on the left and a subluxated severely dysplastic and painful hip on the right, **A.** The abduction internal rotation film shows poor congruity between femoral head and acetabulum, **B.** A Chiari osteotomy was accomplished, with satisfactory displacement of the distal fragment, **C.** Seven months postoperatively the osteotomy was well healed and the femoral head well covered, **D.** Three and one-half years later at skeletal maturity there is a slight degree of increased lateral displacement of the femoral head, **E.** Note remodeling of inner wall of pelvis. The patient has a pain-free gait with a normal range of motion.

acetabulum. In the process the femoral head is slowly displaced laterally.

Long-term follow-up studies of the Chiari osteotomy continue to support its value as a salvage procedure, which accomplishes in a slightly different way what the Colonna arthroplasty does. It enhances function and reduces pain (when present) in the hip joint and improves the basic bone stock as a preparation for future reconstructive procedures in later adult life.

SHELF PROCEDURES

Prior to the development of the innominate osteotomy concept, several different techniques were utilized that attempted to provide a bony buttress or fulcrum in those instances of inadequate acetabula. Because these operations added onto or extended outward the bony roof of the acetabulum, they were called "shelves." These procedures have experienced cycles of enthusiasm, but in the majority of instances the recently developed and expanded techniques of innominate osteotomy and acetabular rotation have largely eliminated the need for shelf operations. Nevertheless, because there may be an occasional instance when this operation will be indicated and because it has served some individuals very well,[11,23] it deserves discussion. I however, have had no personal experience with shelf procedures.

The basic concept for shelf techniques emphasizes the use of bone grafts placed onto the roof of the acetabulum, either within or directly over the capsule of the exposed femoral head. The result, therefore, is a capsule-covered buttress, designed to stabilize the hip and increase the weight-bearing area of the femoral head and acetabulum. The acetabulum is unchanged and there is no alteration in the location of the center of gravity, which thus remains somewhat more lateral than desired. It therefore differs significantly from the Salter or Steel procedures, because the acetabulum is not rotated or altered in its position, and it differs from the Chiari osteotomy because there is no medial displacement of the acetabulum.

Indications

The same indications apply for this operation as apply for the pelvic osteotomy, that is, a deficient acetabulum in an older child or adolescent who exhibits pain, limp, or both. According to Wilson,[23] the procedure should not be done unless the hip is symptomatic. Others have believed that the simple presence of an asymptomatic but clearly deficient socket is justification for its accomplishment. Conceptually, the *prerequisites* are the same as for any one of the reconstructive iliac osteotomies described in Chapter 5.

Surgical technique

The shelf operation that appeals most to me is that described and illustrated by Wilson.[23] For the satisfactory accomplishment of this or any bone shelf procedure it is essential that the surgeon pay meticulous attention to the technical details of the procedure. In order for the shelf to perform its weight-bearing function, it must obviously be placed precisely at the weight-bearing level of the acetabulum. Failure to recognize or to adhere to this critical detail has resulted in many past failures of the procedure; for, deprived of any weight-bearing function, the shelf will slowly undergo atrophy and will eventually disappear. The procedure described by Wilson utilizes a partial-thickness capsulectomy and placement of an iliac bone shelf on the remaining capsule under direct vision (Fig. 8-17).

The patient is operated on in a supine position with a sandbag placed under the operated buttock. Through an anterior

Text continued on p. 240.

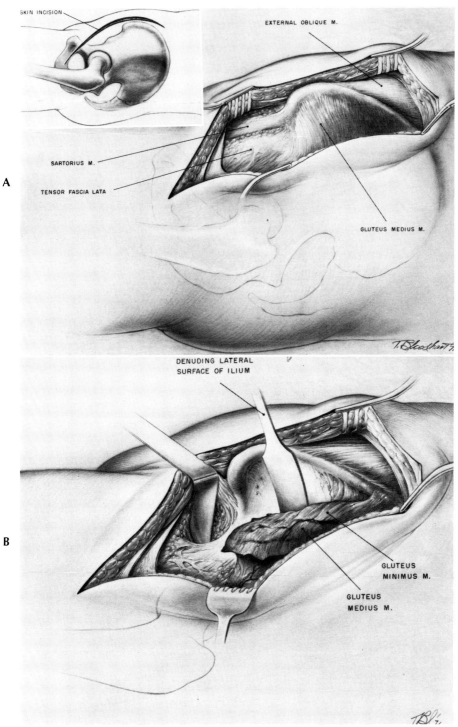

Fig. 8-17. For legend see p. 239.

Continued.

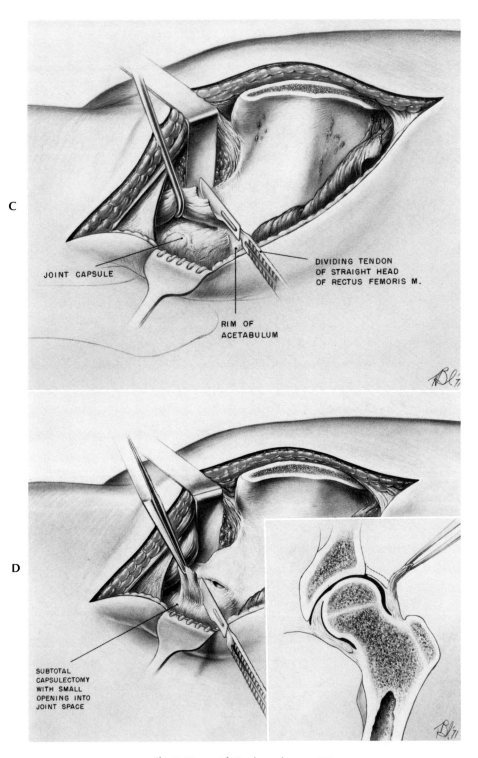

Fig. 8-17, cont'd. For legend see p. 239.

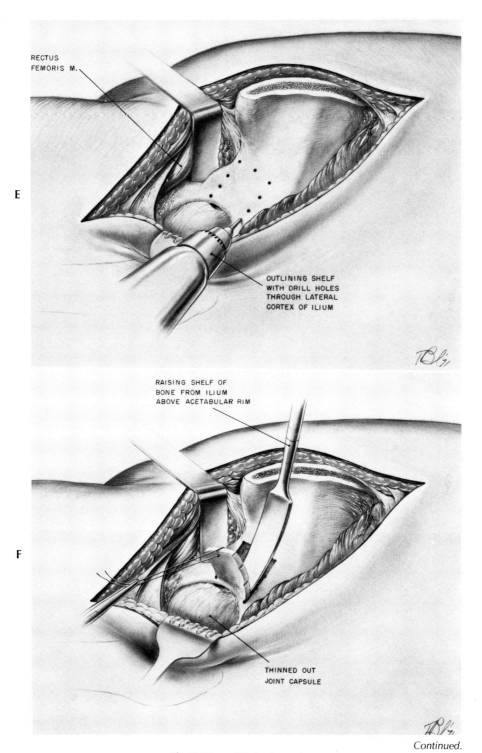

Fig. 8-17, cont'd. For legend see p. 239.

Continued.

238 *Congenital dysplasia and dislocation of the hip*

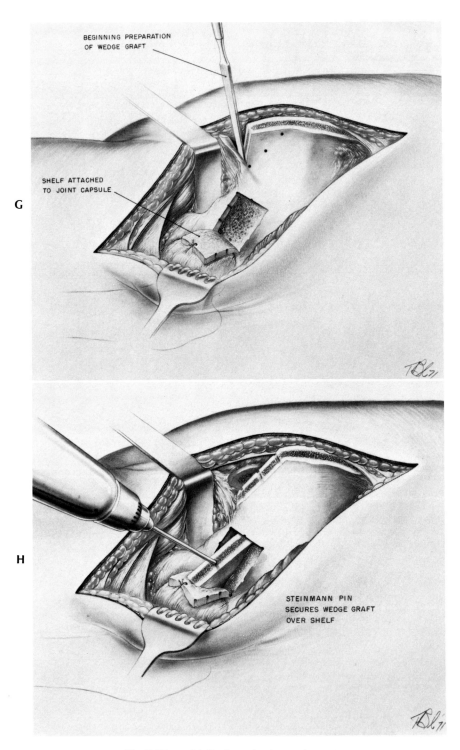

Fig. 8-17, cont'd. For legend see opposite page.

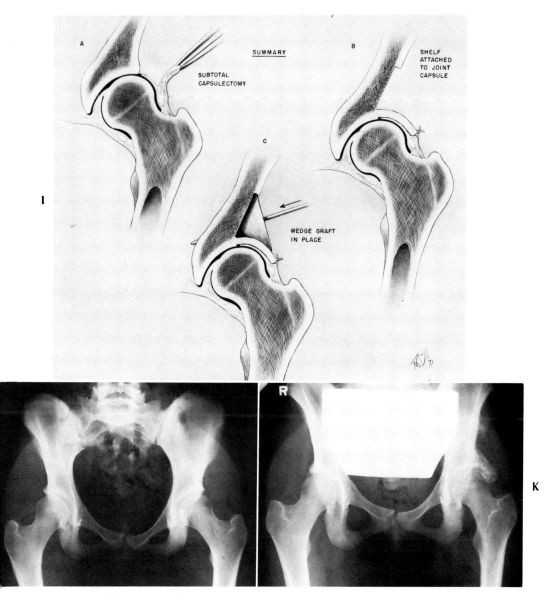

Fig. 8-17. The technique of accomplishing the Wilson acetabular "shelf." **A,** The incision and surgical exposure of the ilium. **B,** Subperiosteal exposure of the iliac wing. **C,** Further exposure of the hip joint capsule, accompanied by tenotomy of the rectus femoris muscle. Partial capsulectomy is then made over the superior aspect of the residual joint capsule, **D,** in order to create an interposed capsular membrane as a weight-bearing structure. Utilizing drill holes in the outer cortex, **E,** a flap of bone is created that can be reflected directly over the superior portion of the femoral head and joint capsule, **F.** A generous-sized, full-thickness iliac graft is obtained from the anterior superior iliac spine, **G,** and the graft is placed in the defect created by the flap. It is transfixed by a smooth (or threaded) fixation pin, **H.** A diagrammatic summary of the procedure is seen in **I.** Preoperative and immediate postoperative roentgenograms of an illustrative case are seen in **J** and **K.** (J and K from Wilson, J. C.: Surgical treatment of the dysplastic acetabulum in adolescence, Clin. Orthop. **98:**137, 1974.)

(iliofemoral) incision the entire anterior half of both tables of the ilium is exposed subperiosteally. The iliac apophysis is reflected in the process, and the sartorius muscle and straight heads of the rectus femoris muscle are sectioned. The capsule is then exposed widely and a small aperture is made in the capsule to identify the exact location of the lateral acetabular margin. A meticulous partial capsulectomy is accomplished over the superior aspect of the femoral head, leaving about ⅛ inch thickness of capsule intact over the femoral head. A 2.5 to 3.0 cm area of the outer ilium is outlined with drill holes directly above the area of capsulectomy. These drill holes are then connected with an osteotome, and this flap of bone is reflected downward onto the remaining capsule and accurately aligned with the lateral acetabular margin. This is the most critical part of the operation. Next a triangular, full-thickness graft is removed from the anterior iliac crest and is impacted into the defect created by the reflected flap of bone. This fimly holds and supports the flap against the capsule-covered head. The graft is secured by a threaded Steinmann pin in order to assure maintenance of proper position of the flap and the graft. This position is verified by a roentgenogram taken on the operating table. Additional cancellous iliac grafts can then be added as desired. Closure is followed by a one and one-half hip spica cast, which remains on for 8 weeks. Alternately, as preferred by Wilson, the patient may be placed in balanced suspension utilizing a proximal tibial pin for 4 weeks, followed

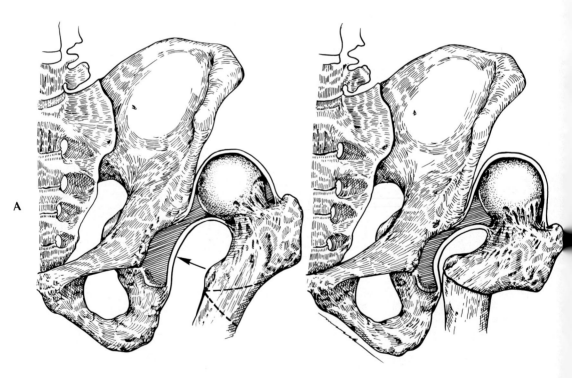

Fig. 8-18. The Schanz "pelvic-support" osteotomy leaves the femoral head and neck in their dislocated position, **A.** The lesser trochanter is placed into the capsule-covered acetabulum by means of a closing wedge osteotomy of the proximal femur, **B.**

by plaster immobilization. An example of a patient operated on by Wilson's technique is seen in Fig. 8-17.

RECONSTRUCTIVE PROXIMAL FEMORAL OSTEOTOMIES

Various types of proximal femoral osteotomies have been used over the years in the salvage treatment of congenital dislocation of the hip. The early osteotomies were usually performed in older patients with painful lurching gaits. The osteotomies described by Lorenz,[13] Schanz,[18] and Hass[10] were based on the concept of surgically shifting the femur closer to the center of gravity so that the body weight is transferred more directly along the axis of the femoral shaft.

The "pelvic-support" osteotomy of Schanz[18] was designed to produce stability in a dislocated hip by a valgus angulation osteotomy, which usually placed the lesser trochanter into the acetabulum, leaving the dislocation unreduced (Fig. 8-18). Two primary goals—enhancement of stability and displacement of the center of gravity medially—were achieved. The accomplishments in many cases were improvement in gait and relief of pain, when present. The Lorenz "bifurcation"[13] osteotomy was designed to accomplish similar goals in a technically slightly different way (Fig. 8-19). The current objections to these operations are twofold: (1) a grossly abnormal hip joint mechanism is created, and (2) future efforts at reconstruction are compromised because of the deformity produced (Fig. 10-10).

I have not accomplished either of these

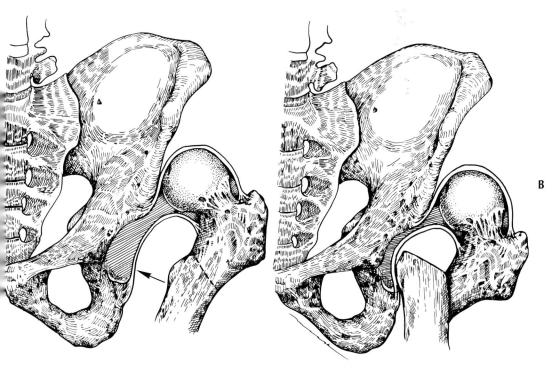

Fig. 8-19. The Lorenz "bifurcation" osteotomy leaves the femoral head and neck in their dislocated positions, **A.** After osteotomy the proximal end of the distal fragment is placed into the acetabulum, with the capsule serving as an interposed membrane, **B.** (After Lorenz, A.: Über die Behandlung der irreponiblen angeborenen Hüftluxation und der Schenkelhals pseudoarthrosen mittels Gabelung [Bifurkation des oberen Femurendes], Wien. Klin. Wochenschr. **32:**997, 1919.)

operations for congenital dislocation of the hip in over 20 years. It is now generally held that these procedures are no longer appropriate in salvaging hip joint function in adult congenital dislocation of the hip. They have been superseded by the other salvage procedures previously discussed. However, even though they have been appropriately relegated to the category of "historical operations," they justify the foregoing brief discussion in order to explain why they are no longer acceptable.

On the other hand there are certain reconstructive procedures on the proximal femur that can salvage and improve hip joint function in a deformed proximal femur of congenital dislocation of the hip. These osteotomies are technically very demanding and have been beautifully described and illustrated by Wagner.[19] Their basic goal is to reconstruct the proximal femur so as to provide the following: (1) improved hip function, (2) reduced pain, and (3) bone stock for any future resurfacing or implant procedure.

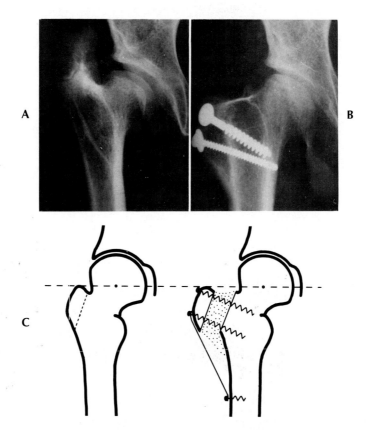

Fig. 8-20. Reshaping of proximal end of femur in 12-year-old girl by displacement of major trochanter only. **A,** Before surgery. **B,** Two years after surgery. **C,** Lateral displacement of major trochanter for elongation of lever arm of abductor muscles. Distance between fragment of trochanter and femur is maintained by two position screws, and traction force of abductor muscles is neutralized by tension band wire. Bone cleft must be filled with cancellous bone grafts. (From Wagner, H.: Osteotomies for congenital hip dislocation. In The Hip Society: The hip, vol. IV, Proceedings of the fourth open scientific meeting of The Hip Society, St. Louis, 1976, The C. V. Mosby Co., p. 45.)

Most of them are applicable only to subluxated and dysplastic hips rather than to completely dislocated hips. Some of the methods by which the hip can be salvaged by proximal femoral osteotomy are illustrated in Figs. 8-20 and 8-21 as described by Wagner.[19]

TROCHANTERIC ARTHROPLASTY ("STICK FEMUR" PROCEDURE)

In rare instances of congenital dislocation of the hip, the entire femoral head becomes destroyed from necrosis, resulting from either aseptic or septic causes. In young children it is inappropriate to use implants, and, since there is no femoral head and there is insufficient neck to gain any stability, one is forced either to leave the hip out of the socket or to perform a trochanteric arthroplasty as a salvage procedure.

The trochanteric arthroplasty basically and originally described by Colonna[5] has been popularized by Westin,[22] Larsen,[12]

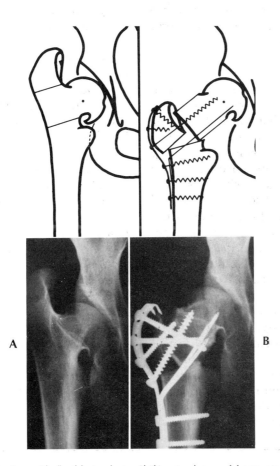

Fig. 8-21. Internal fixation with flexible implants. Shifting tendency of fragments on medial aspect is controlled by three Kirschner wires inserted diagonally. Tension forces on lateral aspect and varization tendency of femoral neck as well are neutralized by semitubular plate attached to lateral surface of bone that acts as a tension band. **A,** Sixteen-year-old girl with dysplastic hip. **B,** Eight weeks after intertrochanteric double osteotomy. (From Wagner, H.: Osteotomies for congenital hip dislocation. In The Hip Society: The hip, vol. IV, Proceedings of the fourth open scientific meeting of The Hip Society, St. Louis, 1976, The C. V. Mosby Co., p. 45.)

and Weissman.[20] Because of the straightness of the femur that results, Westin[22] has labeled it the "stick femur" operation. The concept is based on the following two unique characteristics of the problem: (1) the greater trochanter is viable and therefore retains its growth potential; and (2) when the hyaline cartilage–covered trochanter is placed inside the influence of the acetabulum, the trochanter tends to assume a globular shape, similar to a femoral head. The detached abductor muscles must then be transferred downward in order to provide hip stability and some degree of abductor function (Fig. 8-22).

Surgical technique

The hip is approached either through an anterior (iliofemoral) or a lateral incision over the trochanter with an extension upward on the iliac crest. The abductor muscles are removed by sharp dissection from their insertion onto the greater trochanter, which is then smoothed and shaped so as to be placed into the acetabulum. In the process the remnants of the femoral neck are removed, thus creating a perfectly straight proximal femur. The acetabulum is then cleared of all debris, exposing whatever is left of its articular cartilage, with care being exercised so as not to damage the cartilage unnecessarily. The trochanter is placed inside the acetabulum and is usually found to be stable in abduction. The hip abductor muscles are then inserted into the proximal femur under mild tension. The femur can at this point be osteotomized just below the new insertion of the abductor muscles, in order to create a new "neck-shaft" angle (Fig. 8-22). I, however, prefer to do this osteotomy 6 weeks later in order to reduce the number of variables at the time of the initial procedure. A pelvic x-ray film is taken to verify appropriate position of the greater trochanter in the acetabulum. The wound is then closed.

After wound closure a one and one-half hip spica cast is applied with the femur in as much abduction as necessary to provide stability of the reduction. Another x-ray film should be taken after the cast is applied and again 1 week later.

Four to 6 weeks after surgery the cast is removed and the subtrochanteric osteotomy is done, if it was not done previously. In some situations it may be better to wait until some degree of hip motion has been achieved before the osteotomy is done, but this is an individual matter. Abductor muscle–strengthening exercises are part of a very aggressive therapy program that must be carried out faithfully until maximum improvement in range of motion and muscle strength has been achieved. Graduated weight bearing is begun as soon as the osteotomy has healed, but weight bearing must be resumed slowly in order to protect the transferred abductor muscles as well as the osteotomy.

As one would expect, with growth the angulation osteotomy gradually straightens out. If the procedure is done during the early years of childhood, the femur will once more become completely straight, or nearly so, at the end of skeletal growth. Nevertheless, the basic effectiveness of the operation is not vitiated.

Fig. 8-22. The "stick femur" procedure requires that the remnants of the head and neck be removed in order to create a straight upper femur, **A.** The abductor muscles are then removed from their insertion on the greater trochanter and are reattached to the femur, just distal to the greater trochanteric physis. The greater trochanter is then placed into the acetabulum with the femur in wide abduction, **B.** After stability of the reduction has been established, varus osteotomy is accomplished just below the attached abductor muscles, **C.** This is best accomplished at a second stage 6 to 8 weeks after the initial procedure.

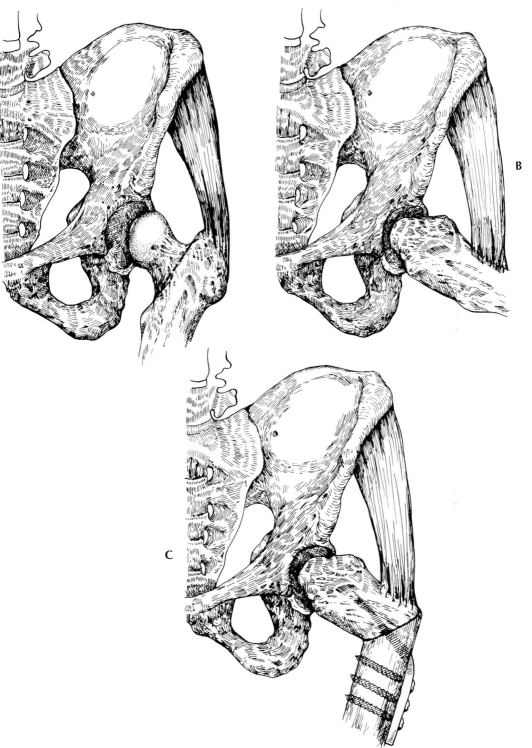

Fig. 8-22. For legend see opposite page.

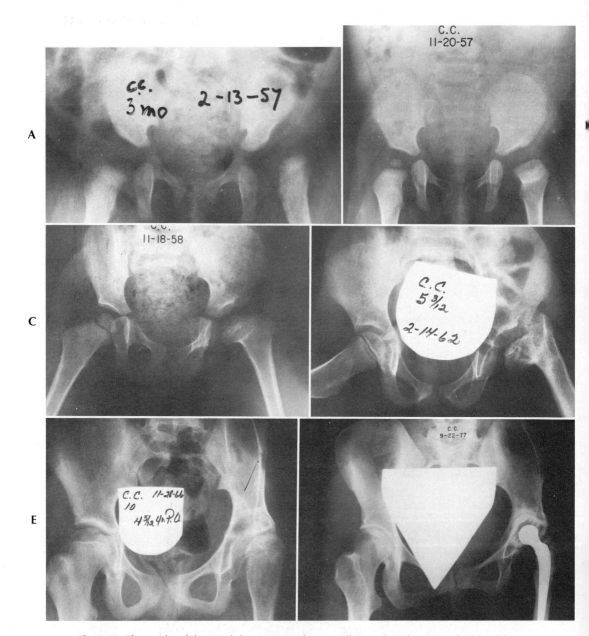

Fig. 8-23. The results of the "stick-femur" procedure are illustrated in this 3-month-old girl having a dislocation of the left hip, **A.** Nine months later, following closed reduction, there is obvious evidence of femoral head necrosis. The femoral neck is shortened and widened, and the ossification center has not appeared, **B.** One year later there is further evidence of severe femoral head necrosis, with varus deformity of the neck-shaft angle, continued delay in the femoral head ossification, and beginning relative "overgrowth" of the greater trochanter, **C.** Reciprocal defective acetabular development is also evident. At 5 years of age the femoral head is grossly deformed and the greater trochanter has "overgrown" even further, now abutting against the ilium on abduction, **D.** Excision of the deformed, rudimentary head and neck of the femur was accomplished, the greater trochanter was placed into the acetabulum, and the abductor muscles were transferred to the proximal shaft. Shortly thereafter a pelvic osteotomy was done, and the result 4½ years postoperatively is seen in **E.** Seven years later, because of increasing pain and decreasing motion, a total hip arthroplasty was done, utilizing custom-made implants. Three years after total hip replacement she is pain-free, has a satisfactory range of motion, but has a severe gluteal "lurch," **F.**

Femoral length, although compromised initially, is usually maintained at acceptable levels, a variable degree of pain-free motion results, and reasonable stock for future reconstructive procedures is preserved (Fig. 8-23).

ARTHRODESIS

Arthrodesis is the ultimate operation performed when the hip cannot be salvaged as a functional, moving joint. Fortunately, the need for this operation is becoming increasingly rare, but when there is no other operation that can be effectively employed to salvage a movable hip, and when sufficient pain or significant deformity is present, arthrodesis may be a very effective solution (Fig. 8-24). Price and Lovell[16] have shown that this is a very satisfactory means of salvaging a destroyed hip in select cases.

Currently, hip fusion does not need to be considered permanent, because in adult life a fusion can be taken down and a total hip arthroplasty effectively performed. Thus, in a sense, arthrodesis represents a salvage procedure because it does prolong function (not movable) and provides stock for a possible future reconstructive operation.

Indications

It is difficult to develop specific indications for arthrodesis, because the need for doing the operation usually surfaces as a "last resort." There are three circumstances in which arthrodesis can be justified: (1) disabling pain caused by a destroyed hip, (2) a handicapping deformity, and (3) a completely dislocated hip in an adolescent whose opposite hip is essentially normal. A combination of indications may present themselves, but the ultimate decision to do this particular procedure is made only after all factors have been given full consideration and after all of the possible alternatives have been excluded as not feasible.

Prerequisites

The major prerequisite for fusion is the presence of adequate bone stock to accomplish the procedure. However, it is also very important that the opposite hip have a satisfactory range of motion, that the ipsolateral knee have a good range of

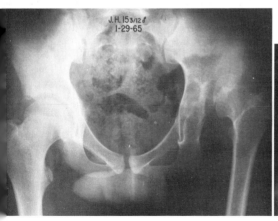 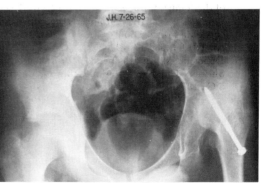

Fig. 8-24. The ultimate salvage procedure is hip fusion. A 15-year-old boy had a complete untreated dislocation of the left hip, present since infancy, **A.** He wanted to be a farm worker, and, therefore, arthrodesis was accomplished, **B.** It would have been desirable to gain more length. The patient has been lost to follow-up.

motion, that there is no fixed pelvic obliquity, and that no significant congenital or acquired problems in the lumbosacral spine are present. The reason for this latter prerequisite is the fact that a fused hip transfers greater stress to the lower spine during ambulation, standing, and sitting.

Surgical technique

The technical aspects of accomplishing a fusion of the hip are well described and illustrated in standard operative texts. Because of this and because of the rarity of ever having to perform this operation in patients with congenital dislocation of the hip, no further discussion here is considered necessary.

REFERENCES

1. Buehler, C. E., and Coleman, S. S.: Colonna arthroplasty for dislocation of the hip in the older child, J. Bone Joint Surg. **54A**:1799, 1972.
2. Campbell, P.: Presentation at Chief Surgeons' Meeting, Greenville, S.C., 1974.
3. Chiari, K.: Ergebnisse mit der Beckenosteotomie als Pfannendachplastik, Z. Orthop. **87**:14, 1955.
4. Chung, S. M., Scholl, H. W., Ralston, E. L., and Pendergrass, E.: The Colonna capsular arthroplasty: a long-term follow up study of 56 patients, J. Bone Joint Surg. **53A**:1511, 1971.
5. Colonna, P. C.: A new type of reconstruction operation for old ununited fracture of the neck of the femur, J. Bone Joint Surg. **17**:110, 1935.
6. Colonna, P. C.: An arthroplastic operation for congenital dislocation of the hip, Surg. Gynecol. Obstet. **63**:777, 1936.
7. Donovan, M., and associates: Presentation at Shriners' Chief Surgeons' Meeting, Greenville, S.C., 1974.
8. Dunn, H. K., and Hess, W. E.: Total hip reconstruction in chronically dislocated hips, J. Bone Joint Surg. **58A**:838, 1976.
9. Gilbert, R. J.: The Chiari procedure for acetabular insufficiency, J. Bone Joint Surg. **56A**:1538, 1974.
10. Hass, J.: A subtrochanteric osteotomy for pelvic support, J. Bone Joint Surg. **25**:281, 1943.
11. Heyman, C.: Long-term results following a bone-shelf operation for congenital and some other dislocations of the hip in children, J. Bone Joint Surg. **45A**:1113, 1963.
12. Larsen, I. J.: Discussion of "The stick femur," J. Bone Joint Surg. **52B**:779, 1970.
13. Lorenz, A.: Über die Behandlung der irreponiblen angeborenen Hüftluxation und der Schenkelhals pseudoarthrosen mittels Gabelung (Bifurkation des oberen Femurendes), Wien. Klin. Wochenschr. **32**:997, 1919.
14. Milligan, P. R.: Personal communication.
15. Noel, S.: Personal communication; unpublished data.
16. Price, C. T., and Lovell, W. W.: Arthrodesis of the hip in children, read at annual meeting, A.O.A., Boca Raton, Florida, June 1977.
17. Ritter, M. A., and Wilson, P. D.: Colonna capsular arthroplasty, a long-term follow-up of forty hips, J. Bone Joint Surg. **50A**:1305, 1968.
18. Schanz, A.: Zur Behandlung der veralteten angeborenen Hüftverrenkung, Münch. Med. Wochenschr. **69**:930, 1922.
19. Wagner, H.: Osteotomies for congenital hip dislocation. In The Hip Society: The hip, vol. IV, Proceedings of the fourth open scientific meeting of The Hip Society, St. Louis, 1976, The C. V. Mosby Co., p. 45.
20. Weissman, S. L.: Transplantation of the trochanteric epiphysis into the acetabulum after septic arthritis of the hip, J. Bone Joint Surg. **49A**:1647, 1967.
21. Westin, G. W.: Personal communication.
22. Westin, G. W.: The stick femur, J. Bone Joint Surg. **52B**:778, 1970.
23. Wilson, J. C.: Surgical treatment of the dysplastic acetabulum in adolescence, Clin. Orthop. **98**:137, 1974.

CHAPTER 9

"Teratologic" congenital dislocation

Pathology
Treatment in arthrogryposis
  Unilateral or bilateral dislocation
  Anterior vs posterior dislocation
  Ambulation potential and associated abnormalities
  Ranges of hip and knee motion
  Character of acetabulum
  Age of patient
  Operative approach
  Summary

Because of the unusual problems inherent in certain hip dislocations, a separate section is justified in order to emphasize the difference in philosophy and concepts that surround their treatment. It is not intended to discuss the dislocations associated with myelomeningocele and myelodysplasia, which, because of the paralysis of the lower limbs, represent a totally different set of problems. Rather this section will deal with treatment of teratologic congenital hip dislocations, not only in those cases associated with multiple other congenital abnormalities, but also in the interesting condition known as arthrogryposis multiplex congenita.

According to Middleton[4] the condition now commonly known as arthrogryposis multiplex congenita was described as early as 1841 by Otto. However, the term itself was introduced by Stern in 1923.[7] A simple term to describe the same condition was proposed by Sheldon in 1932.[5]

He preferred the name "amyoplasia congenita" because he believed that the condition was a primary deficiency of muscles or muscle fibers. Adams and associates[1] believe that there are two distinct clinical syndromes and pathologic processes—"neuropathic" and "myopathic" forms of the disease. Irrespective of the etiology, the treatment of hip disorders in this condition is identical. The problem in either instance is the stiffness and rigidity of the joints, which may be responsible for many intrauterine anatomic deformities and even fractures of long bones, especially the femur, during parturition (Fig. 9-1).

The absence of normal muscle function compromises efforts at maintaining reduction of a hip dislocation; in addition there is a striking tendency for arthrogrypotic joints to develop even further stiffness following open surgery (Fig. 9-2). Some of these patients become gainful contributing citizens in adult life, whereas others become totally disabled as a result of the devastating disability imposed by the lack of effective muscle and joint function. Many just "disappear" in adult life, leaving no trace of their whereabouts. In a search of all patients seen at the Intermountain Unit of the Shriners Hospital in Salt Lake City, only two patients over age 21 years were able to be located, although no record of the deaths of the remaining patients was uncovered.[3]

PATHOLOGY

A teratologic or atypical dislocation usually shows very marked and advanced changes in the hip joint at the time of birth. It is also frequently accompanied by other congenital abnormalities, both skeletal and visceral. Hass[2] reviewed forty-seven cases of atypical dislocations of the hip and concluded that many of these patients showed evidence of intrauterine postural influences. At least thirty-five of these patients had other accompanying congenital deformities. Hass further believed that the pathologic changes in the hip observed in the patient with early intrauterine dislocation paralleled those of a typical dislocation at 3 or 4 years of age. However, most authors have believed that a teratologic dislocation is quite a separate and distinct entity from the typical dislocation, and it further seems generally agreed that the deformity must occur early in utero and that it may be a primary germ plasm defect.

The acetabulum usually is small, and the roof is somewhat oblique or flattened. The acetabular cavity is filled with fibrofatty tissue, and the ligamentum teres is usually thickened. The femoral head may vary considerable in size and is often somewhat flattened on its medial side. Soft tissue planes may be poorly developed and difficult to define. The angle of anteversion of the femoral head may vary considerably and may even be in retroversion, in contrast to the typical dislocation in which the angle of anteversion is almost invariably increased.

Stanisavljevic and Mitchell[6] proposed that many of the anatomic findings in a teratologic dislocation are probably caused by lack of normal contact between the femoral head and acetabulum during the early development of the hip joint. This supports the concept mentioned earlier that in teratologic dislocation

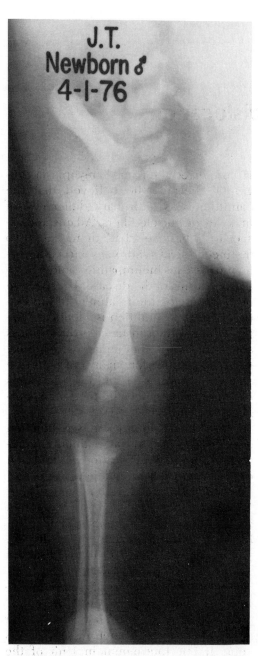

Fig. 9-1. X-ray film of right lower limb on a newborn boy with typical arthrogryposis of all four limbs. The right hip was dislocated, the feet were clubbed, and the hands were deformed. In addition, there was a fracture of the proximal femur on the side of the dislocated hip, which was present and probably was incurred on delivery.

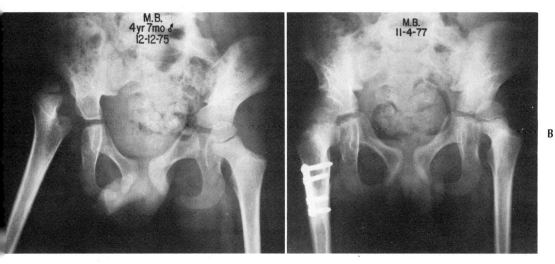

Fig. 9-2. Pelvic x-ray film of a 4½-year-old boy with severe arthrogryposis of all four lower limbs. The left hip is in its normal position relative to the acetabulum but is subluxated anteriorly. The right hip is clearly dislocated, producing a limb length inequality and pelvic obliquity, **A**. Two years after open reduction, aided by femoral shortening, the hip is well reduced and the limb length inequality and pelvic obliquity have been corrected, but the motion of the hip is substantially less than prior to surgery, **B**.

the pathology is the result of a very early intrauterine dislocation. Thus some authors were able to show that in four of five instances of teratologic dislocation the limbus in the superoposterior portion of the acetabulum was absent; in the fifth case it was deformed.

TREATMENT IN ARTHROGRYPOSIS

It is apparent from the preceding discussion that there are many complicating factors with which one has to contend in developing a sound solution to the problem of the dislocated hip in arthrogryposis. The major issues for consideration are these: (1) Is the dislocation unilateral or bilateral? (2) Is the dislocation anterior or posterior? (3) Is there good ambulation potential and what are the associated abnormalities? (4) What are the ranges of hip and knee motion? (5) What is the character of the acetabulum? and (6) What is the age of the patient? All of these factors must be taken into account in the deliberations involving treatment.

Unilateral or bilateral dislocation

A bilateral complete dislocation of the hips in patients with arthrogryposis is not very disabling when one considers the extremely low demand usually placed on such hips. Furthermore, left untreated, the dislocated hips usually have very acceptable ranges of motion. Because the true arthrogrypotic hip dislocation almost invariably requires open reduction in order to gain reduction, and because the hip tends to lose some degree of motion following such surgery in these patients, one is forced to make the decision in bilateral dislocations as to whether to leave the hips dislocated with the good ranges of motion or to take a chance on losing motion as a result of treatment. There is no rigid guideline to follow, and often the factors mentioned earlier will have a strong influence on that decision.

If there is a unilateral dislocation, on the other hand, there are several reasons for attempting reduction. In arthrogryposis the unilateral dislocation may lead to

252 Congenital dysplasia and dislocation of the hip

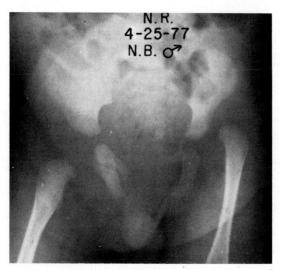

Fig. 9-3. Pelvic x-ray of a newborn boy who had an obvious irreducible dislocation of the left hip at birth. There were other visceral and skeletal abnormalities, including absence of the left radius with so-called radial club hand. The reduced size of the pelvis and proximal femur are consistent with an antenatal dislocation. I believe that this patient is not a candidate for open reduction via the medial (adductor) approach.

the development of a fixed pelvic obliquity, which can compromise sitting balance (Fig. 9-3); a short limb will persist that makes ambulation and bracing more difficult; and the parents will usually want the hip reduced if it is at all reasonable. I therefore, usually prefer to attempt reductions on unilateral dislocations in arthrogryposis, *provided that* the other factors support that decision and if it is *not* an anterior dislocation (see below).

Anterior vs posterior dislocation

A significant number of congenital dislocations of the hip in arthrogryposis will be anterior (Fig. 9-4), and the characteristics of this dislocation deserve special mention. There is usually very little shortening, and there is a greatly reduced tendency toward an adduction contracture on the involved side. Thus neither pelvic obliquity nor limb length inequality are so likely to be present in the anterior dislocation. Furthermore, the ranges of motion will usually be satisfactory. In these anteriorly displaced femoral heads, therefore, I tend to leave the hip dislocated, unless other factors mitigate strongly against so doing.

Ambulation potential and associated abnormalities

Clearly, any efforts at achieving reduction of the dislocated hips in these children must be directly related to the likelihood for effective ambulation. When there is extensive compromise of upper limb function, gross restriction of knee motion, and severely deformed feet, one's enthusiasm for doing major surgery on dislocated hips must be significantly lessened. The major consideration may be directed toward making the patient a better wheelchair sitter rather than to giving serious thought to ambulation.

Ranges of hip and knee motion

In a patient who is ambulatory or potentially so, the ranges of hip and knee motion play a significant role in deter-

Fig. 9-4. Pelvic x-ray film of a patient with arthrogryposis multiplex congenita, **A.** The right hip is dislocated posterosuperiorly, and the left hip is subluxated anteriorly (note poor acetabular development). Other physical abnormalities include severe club feet and mild, diffuse amyoplasia. At 18 months of age the patient still did not walk. His feet had been reasonably well corrected. The hip remained unreduced, having resisted all conservative efforts, **B.** When he began to ambulate at age 3 years, an open reduction through the medial (adductor) approach was accomplished, **C.** One year later because of poor acetabular development a pelvic osteotomy was done, **D.** Three and one-half years later the hip remained stable, although retaining the "windswept" appearance, **E.** The left hip remained subluxated anteriorly but was very functional with a satisfactory range of motion. I would ordinarily not favor the medial approach, but in this instance it succeeded, probably because the hip was not too high riding.

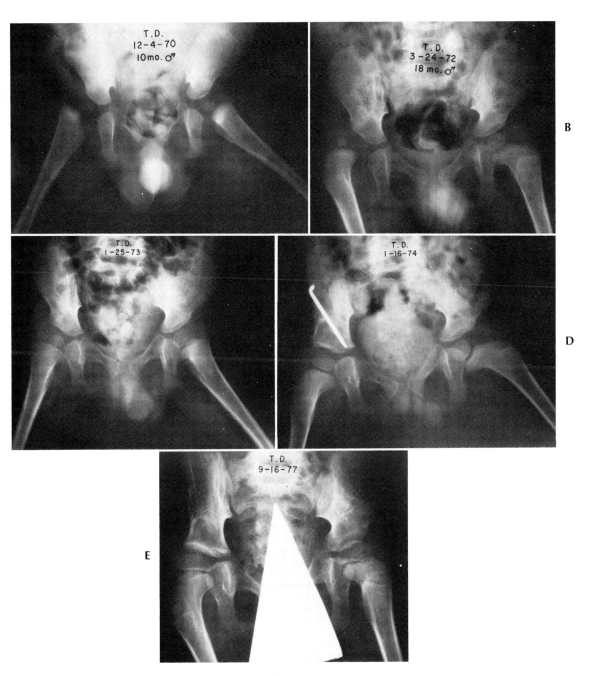

Fig. 9-4. For legend see opposite page.

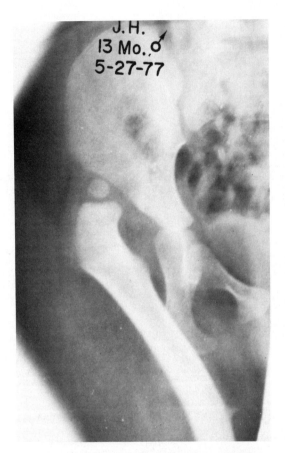

Fig. 9-5. The severe degree of acetabular dysplasia encountered in teratologic hip dislocation is suggested by this pelvic x-ray film of a 13-month-old boy having all of the clinical features of severe arthrogryposis, in addition to an antenatal hip dislocation.

mining the desirability of reducing the hip. For example, if the opposite hip or the ipsilateral knee has grossly restricted ranges of motion, then all efforts should be expended toward maintaining the motion in the involved hip. These factors may argue against surgical efforts at reduction that may substantially further compromise the previously existing motion in these particular patients.

Character of acetabulum

Since all arthrogrypotic hip dislocations are antenatal, and because the femoral head has been out of the acetabulum for a variable and unknown period of time, the degree of acetabular dysplasia may in some instances be very severe (Fig. 9-5). This determination may be difficult to make, because of the fact that only the ossification center can be seen on plain x-ray films. Arthrography may be helpful in these instances, but even this modality may not provide enough information in severe or doubtful cases. In any event the severity of the dysplastic changes must be identified as well as possible before undertaking surgical correction.

Age of patient

The older the child before reduction is attempted, the more difficult the challenge will be, even in otherwise normal children. However, in children with arthrogryposis the problems are even greater, the soft tissues have a lesser degree of flexibility, and the response to treatment is overall less favorable. In general the

---

Fig. 9-6. A pelvic film of a 4-month-old girl with arthrogryposis, principally on the right side, **A.** The right hip is dislocated, and the patient also had a congenital vertical talus on the right. Preliminary traction attempts at closed reduction were unsuccessful on two occasions. These efforts accompanied a two-stage vertical talus procedure. The hip remained dislocated at age 14 months, **B.** Note relatively good acetabular ossification. An open reduction was accomplished via the medial (adductor) approach by Dr. Albert B. Ferguson, Jr., **C,** and the follow-up pelvic films immediately after removal of the cast, **D,** and 3 years later, **E,** show a well-seated and normally developing hip. Although I do not usually favor the medial (adductor) approach for arthrogryposis, this patient seemed to be a good candidate.

"Teratologic" congenital dislocation 255

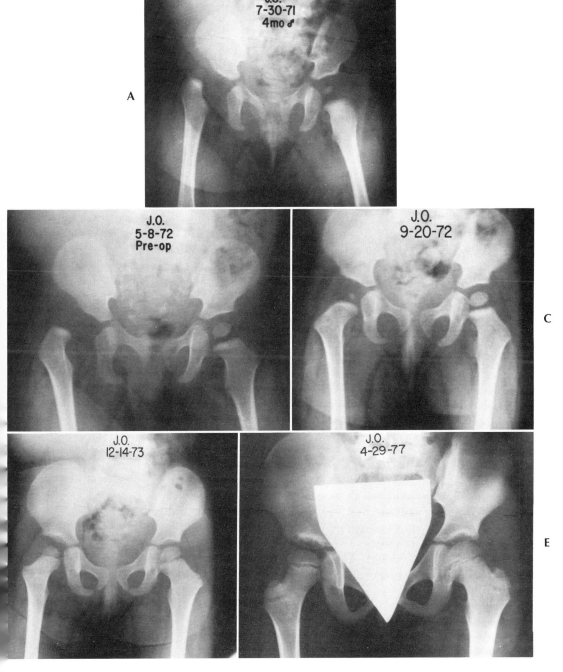

Fig. 9-6. For legend see opposite page.

upper age limit for attempting open reduction in children with arthrogryposis should be considerably lower than for otherwise normal children.

Operative approach

As previously discussed in Chapter 5, antenatal and teratologic hip dislocations are best operated on from the anterior (iliofemoral) approach, irrespective of age. In some rare instances of arthrogryotic hip dislocations where the acetabulum appears well developed, the hip is more mobile than usual, and the femoral head is not too high riding, a medial (adductor) approach might be very effective and therefore may be justified in children under 2 years of age (Fig. 9-6).

The follow-up care is basically no different from that in otherwise normal children, as discussed in earlier chapters. Because of the greater likelihood of significant acetabular dysplasia, however, these hips are more apt to require subsequent reconstructive surgery, such as innominate osteotomy (Fig. 9-4).

Summary

The approach to treatment of the prenatal dislocated hips in children with arthrogryposis or with multiple congenital anomalies clearly must be highly individualized. The factors governing the decision to operate are greatly different from considerations obtained in otherwise normal children with dislocated hips. All factors must especially be evaluated in the light of potential ambulation. Practically none of these hips can be reduced by closed methods. Furthermore, each of these children responds differently to open reduction of the hip, and the probability of surgically creating a stiff hip must weigh heavily in the decision to do an open reduction. When it is done, the anterior (more versatile) approach to the dislocation is usually preferred over the medial approach.

REFERENCES

1. Adams, R. D., Denny-Brown, D., and Pearson, C. M.: Diseases of muscle, a study in pathology, ed. 2, New York, 1967, Harper & Row, Publishers, p. 310.
2. Hass, J.: Congenital dislocation of the hip, Springfield, Ill., 1951, Charles C Thomas, Publisher.
3. Jacobs, L.: unpublished data.
4. Middleton, D. S.: Studies on prenatal lesions of striated muscle as a cause of congenital deformity, Edinburgh Med. J. **41**:401, 1934.
5. Sheldon, W.: Amyoplasia congenita, Arch. Dis. Child. **7**:117, 1932.
6. Stanisavljevic, S., and Mitchell, C. L.: Congenital dysplasia, subluxation, and dislocation of the hip in stillborn and newborn infants, J. Bone Joint Surg. **45A**:1147, 1963.
7. Stern, W. G.: Arthrogryposis multiplex congenita, J.A.M.A. **81**:1507, 1923.

CHAPTER 10

Implant hip reconstruction

General pathology and sequelae in the adult
   Dysplastic or subluxated hip with painful osteoarthritis
   Complete dislocation of the hip

In much of the foregoing text there has been frequent allusion to the eventual possibility or probability of the need for implant hip reconstruction. Indeed, the justification for undertaking certain operative procedures has been largely predicated on the assumption that certain salvage procedures, while rendering the patient temporarily more functional, are also being done in order to improve the facility with which total hip replacement might be accomplished later (see Chapter 8). It therefore is appropriate that the place of total hip replacement in congenital dislocation of the hip be thoroughly discussed.

It is not intended in this section to ignore the possible role of other implant arthroplasties, such as Vitallium cup or femoral head prosthetic arthroplasties, but I have gradually found that the indications for either the cup or the femoral head replacement arthroplasties in congenital dislocation of the hip have virtually become unacceptable to any patient who is presented with all of the facts and data supporting total hip arthroplasty versus cup and prosthetic arthroplasty. Recognizing the problems and prognostic uncertainties, as well as the duration of convalescent care in cup and femoral replacement arthroplasties, and comparing them to the similar parameters in total hip replacement, I find it difficult to perform or even recommend anything other than total hip replacement in adult patients having painful symptomatic arthritic sequelae of congenital dislocation of the hip. Therefore, the major thrust of this section will deal with the use of total hip replacement in this condition.

The development of total hip replacement is so well documented that little would be served by reviewing the historic evolution and the technical details of such a procedure.[1] As our experience and senses of values have grown, the indications and prerequisites for the operation have become more clear and the solutions to the many technical problems inherent in the procedure have become better standardized. It now appears that no patient having a painful hip or an ungainly limp resulting from congenital dislocation of the hip need tolerate such discomfort and disability if that individual is willing to undergo the surgical procedure and accept its attendant risks in order to achieve correction. This applies, provided that there has been no recent evidence of infection of the hip.

Recently there has been considerable interest in the subject of total hip replacement in congenital dislocation and its sequelae. There has been special emphasis on the technical details in-

258 *Congenital dysplasia and dislocation of the hip*

herent in treating the totally dislocated hip. Much of the discussion has also centered about the rather widely divergent pathology that is manifested in the adult in this complicated and highly challenging condition.

GENERAL PATHOLOGY AND SEQUELAE IN THE ADULT

Just as in the young infant and child, in an adult the anatomic abnormalities of this condition may vary from a mildly dysplastic acetabulum with secondary osteoarthritis to that of a completely dislocated hip. Therefore, at least two different pathologic problems present themselves for discussion in this section: (1) a dysplastic or subluxated hip with painful osteoarthritis (Fig. 10-1), and (2) a completely dislocated hip, with or without prior treatment, which may or may not have painful hip or back symptoms (Fig. 10-2). Since the hip is not articulated, the hip symptoms are not caused by hip arthritis but rather more likely by muscular, ligamentous, and postural factors. However, there may eventually be painful arthritic back symptoms as a result of the long-standing pelvic obliquity.

Each of these two conditions (dysplasia and dislocation) will be discussed separately because of the singular and highly individualized problems presented by each.

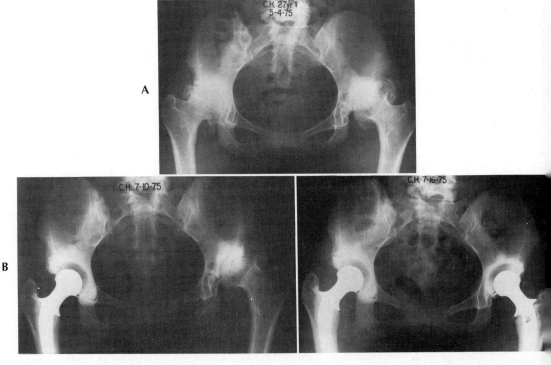

Fig. 10-1. Pelvic film of a 27-year-old woman who had undergone multiple operations for congenital dislocation during early childhood, **A.** Note upward displacement of femoral heads with severe degenerative changes. After the total hip arthroplasty on the right there was a 1½ inch increase in limb length on the operated side, **B.** This was of considerable distress to the patient until the left hip was operated, **C.** Observe the small, straight stem prosthesis and equalization of limb lengths.

Dysplastic or subluxated hip with painful osteoarthritis

In this particular section it is essential to assume that the arthritic changes in the hip are sufficiently well advanced and that the indications and prerequisites for more conservative measures are sufficiently lacking so as to serve as contraindications for a simpler reconstructive or salvage procedure such as a triple innominate osteotomy, a Chiari osteotomy, a proximal femoral osteotomy, or a shelf procedure (see Chapters 6 and 8). There are often certain anatomic features present in the dysplastic hip that may render the procedure more difficult to accomplish. These features also make it more essential that a thorough and critical advance analysis of the problem be made so that a careful and thoughtful solution can be generated in anticipation of the many problems that might occur. In most cases, however, the bony stock of the acetabulum and femur will be sufficiently well developed so as to receive a conventional cup and femoral component.

Unusual pathology. In nearly all dysplastic or subluxated hips the acetabula are shallow and sloping. When secondary osteoarthritis occurs it becomes necessary to ream the acetabulum superiorly and medially in order to gain sufficient depth of acetabulum as well as an appropriately shaped roof. This must be done carefully, because the more superiorly the socket is reamed, the thinner the wall of the ilium becomes (Fig. 10-3). Therefore, not only must one exercise judgment regarding the direction and shape in which the socket is reamed, but the surgeon must also have an assortment of available cups (Fig. 10-4) that will fit the newly created acetabulum. The newly reamed acetabular fossa will be higher than usual, and, if one utilizes retaining holes, it is *essential* to remember that the ischium and pubis will be in relatively different relationships to the newly reamed acetabulum than usual. Special care must, therefore, be taken in placing the retaining holes in the ischium and pubis.

The femur may also be abnormal in configuration, size, or both. The presence of angular or rotational deformities does not offer the magnitude of problem, how-

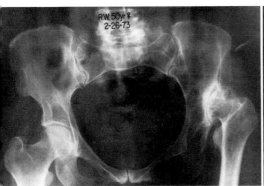
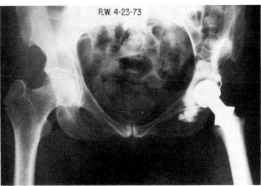

Fig. 10-2. Pelvic film of 50-year-old woman with a history of untreated congenital dislocation known since early infancy, **A.** The femoral head is in a false acetabulum, there was a 2½-inch limb length inequality, and she had a painful limp. Following total hip arthroplasty the limb lengths were equal and the hip pain was gone. However, the greater trochanter could not be reattached at the new level and, therefore, it was excised, **B.** She continued to have a slight gluteal lurch and mild hypesthesia of the skin over the dorsum of the foot.

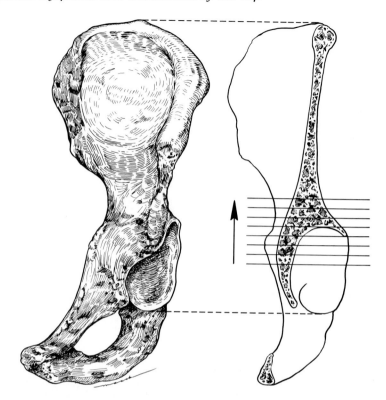

Fig. 10-3. Diagrammatic illustration demonstrating the progressive thinness of the acetabular wall as one reams the socket proximally in the area of the true acetabulum. Clearly, the closer that the level of the acetabulum can be established to the level of the original socket, the greater will be the bony stock suitable for placement and fixation of the polyethylene prosthetic cup. (Adapted from unpublished data of Dr. W. H. Harris.)

Fig. 10-4. A, Custom components for severe problems encountered in congenital dysplasia that require total hip replacement. Note that stems are straight and considerably smaller than standard femoral components. These femoral components have 26 mm heads and fit 50, 44, and 40 mm outside diameter acetabular components. **B,** Miniature and microminiature femoral components with 22 mm head. These are used for patients with very small medullary canals who also have very little acetabular bony stock. Use of 22 mm head makes it possible to use even smaller acetabular components such as 40, 36, and 34 mm outside diameter acetabular components illustrated. (Courtesy Harris, W. H., and Crothers, O. D.: Autogenous bone grafting using the femoral head to correct severe acetabular deficiency for total hip replacement. In The Hip Society: The hip, vol. IV, Proceedings of the fourth open scientific meeting of The Hip Society, St. Louis, 1976, The C. V. Mosby Co., p. 161.)

Implant hip reconstruction 261

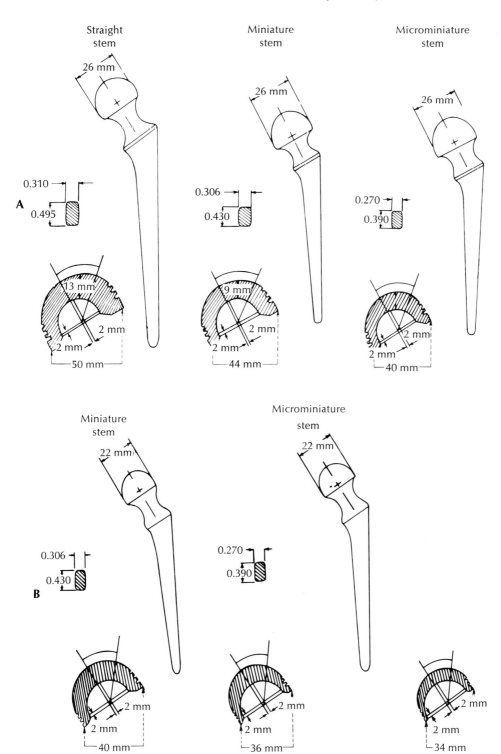

Fig. 10-4. For legend see opposite page.

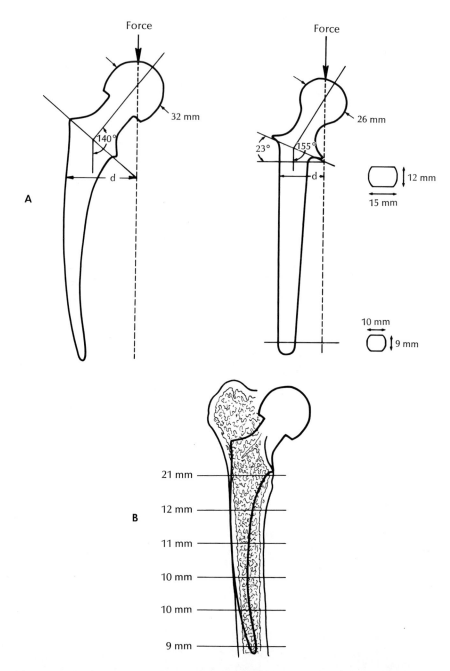

Fig. 10-5. Comparison view of Charnley-Mueller prosthesis and the custom-made prosthesis for patients with small medullary canals. The stem is straight and the neck-shaft angle is in more valgus than is customary, to reduce the bending movement on the smaller stem, **A.** The drawing, **B,** shows the average size and shape of the femoral canal of the patients treated by Dunn and Hess. It also shows that if a curved-stem prosthesis is used, the medullary canal actually must be larger than the prosthesis in order to accommodate it. (From Dunn, H. K., and Hess, W. E.: Total hip reconstruction in chronically dislocated hips, J. Bone Joint Surg. **58A:**838, 1976.)

ever, that the reduced caliber of the medullary cavity of the proximal femur potentially presents (Fig. 10-5). This diminutive medullary cavity may also make it impossible to use conventional femoral components; therefore, special sizes must not only be anticipated but must also be available. It is extremely important that a template be used preoperatively in order to gain some idea of the stem configuration of the femoral component that can be accepted by the femur. Often it will require a smaller and straighter stem than normal (Figs. 10-1 and 10-5).

It is almost never necessary to shorten the femur significantly when total hip replacement is being performed in cases of dysplasia or subluxation but potential alteration in limb lengths must be very carefully evaluated preoperatively because of the possible need for different combinations of components. This is especially true in cases of unilateral dysplasia and/or subluxation because of the many unusual aforementioned technical factors that must be dealt with.

Complete dislocation of the hip

The indications for performing total hip replacement in complete dislocation of the hip in adults are becoming increasingly better defined, reflective of the improvements in technology and the development of greater technical expertise. Past experiences have identified many of the problems and pitfalls that were responsible for the numerous complications and technical failures so often encountered as a result of treating the completely dislocated hip by means of total hip replacement. Numerous recent studies have served to accentuate the problems and complications unique to this condition.*

Problems unique to the dislocated hip. The facts that the femoral head is dislocated from the socket and that the femur is upwardly displaced are the most important problems one encounters in attempting total hip replacement in this condition. Because the hip is not articulated and has not been for nearly all of the patient's skeletal growth, a poorly developed, hypoplastic acetabulum results. This produces a reduction in acetabular bone stock, thus rendering prosthetic cup fixation more difficult. For the same reasons, the entire femur does not grow at the usual rate, and, therefore, the configuration of the proximal femur is often altered and the caliber of the entire femoral shaft, as well as the medullary canal is reduced. Upward displacement of the femur results in shortening of all soft tissues, including the important neurovascular structures. The muscles can usually be effectively lengthened in order to bring the femoral head down to the level of the acetabulum; however, the problems of stretching or elongating the neurovascular structures can sometimes be almost insurmountable. In summary, therefore, the three major technical problems that are peculiar to the dislocation are a shallow, deficient socket, a smaller, sometimes distorted proximal femur, and shortened soft tissues and neurovascular structures.

Acetabulum. It is essential that the cup be placed as close to the level of the original acetabulum as possible. This is necessary so that the cup can be supported by the maximum amount of bone. Previous efforts at placing the cup above the level of the original acetabulum or even on the iliac wing have almost invariably resulted in cup loosening, displacement, and failure (Fig. 10-6). Unless there is a good bony buttress superiorly, the stresses of weight bearing will gradually loosen and dislodge the cement and cup from the bone.

In a significant number of instances, even though the prosthetic femoral head

---

*See references 2, 3, 4, and 6.

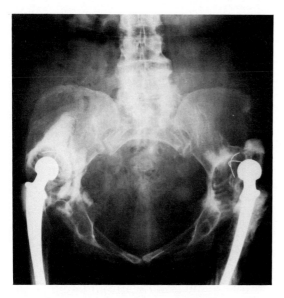

Fig. 10-6. Anteroposterior roentgenogram of hips and pelvis of patient who had bilateral total hip replacements inserted for treatment of bilateral total hip dislocation. Previous subtrochanteric osteotomy had been done on left hip. Cement has broken loose from bone on both sides because there is insufficient bony stock to support acetabular component against wing of ilium. Sockets should never be placed against wing of ilium for this reason. (From Harris, W. H., and Crothers, O. D.: Autogenous bone grafting using the femoral head to correct severe acetabular deficiency for total hip replacement. In The Hip Society: The hip, vol. IV, Proceedings of the fourth open scientific meeting of The Hip Society, St. Louis, 1976, The C. V. Mosby Co., p. 161.)

can be brought down to the level of the original socket, there will be insufficient bony stock to receive adequately the prosthetic cup. Tronzo[8] has described the original acetabulum as being a rudimentary "trough" obscured by a fibrous tissue membrane. In these instances several technical solutions have been devised to provide the necessary bony stock. Hess[5] has performed a stellate fracture of the medial wall of the acetabulum in order that the cup may be displaced further medially, thereby providing greater superior coverage (Fig. 10-7). Vitallium mesh may be utilized to reinforce the medial wall if necessary. Harris and Crothers[4] and Coventry[2] have utilized shelf techniques whereby a portion of the femoral head or a graft from the ilium is screwed or bolted onto the superior iliac portion of the rim of the acetabulum. This provides the necessary peripheral support required for adequate fixation of the cup. In these latter instances, however, since a bone graft is utilized, it is essential that weight bearing be restricted until adequate incorporation of the bone graft has taken place (Fig. 10-8). Harris and Crothers[4] have even recommended that nonweight-bearing or crutch-protected weight-bearing activities should continue for 1 full year postoperatively. This may be longer than essential, but the important thing to emphasize is the fact that incorporation of the graft and maturation of the bone in the graft must occur before full unrestricted weight bearing is permitted.

Proximal femur. As mentioned earlier, a template must be employed in all instances of congenital dislocation of the hip in order to determine the size of the prosthetic femoral stem that can be satisfactorily received by the proximal femur (Fig. 10-9). In this regard it is helpful to gain some approximation of the amount of femur that may need to be resected in order to achieve reduction safely. Fre-

Fig. 10-7. The "controlled" medial acetabular wall fracture is well demonstrated in this diagrammatic illustration. The frontal view shows the location of the bone grafts placed medially at the site of the medial acetabular osteotomy, **A.** The exact location of the osteotomy as viewed from the lateral side is seen in **B,** and the proposed location of the prosthetic cup is seen in **C,** which emphasizes the need for a displacement osteotomy or "fracture" of the medial acetabular wall. The preoperative x-ray film of an example patient shows completely dislocated hips with grossly deficient acetabula, **D.** The postoperative appearance is seen in **E.** (Courtesy Dr. W. E. Hess.)

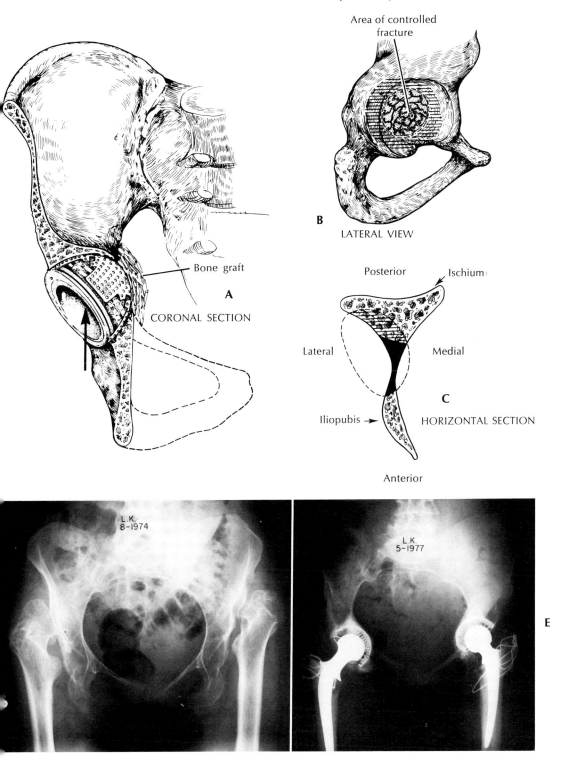

Fig. 10-7. For legend see opposite page.

266 *Congenital dysplasia and dislocation of the hip*

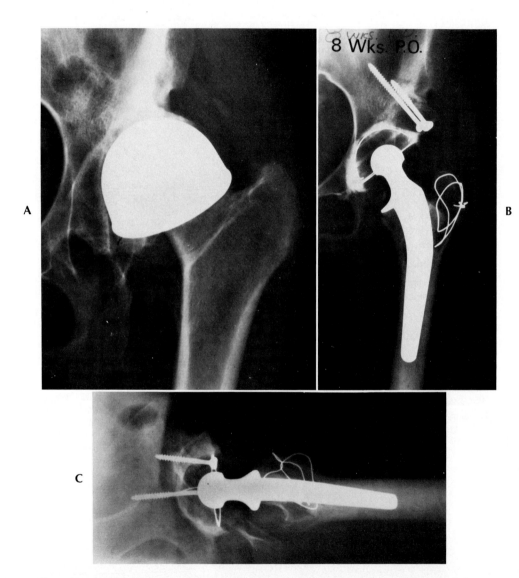

Fig. 10-8. An example of the use of autogenous bone grafting to support the prosthetic cup is illustrated in this 55-year-old patient who had undergone a previous shelf operation and then a subsequent cup arthroplasty for subluxation of the hip, **A.** The cup had not been placed in the original, deficient acetabulum, and this created a large defect in the superior aspect of the original socket. Total hip arthroplasty was successfully accomplished, utilizing a large bone graft taken from the excised femoral head and screwed onto the ilium in order to provide increased support for the polyethylene cup, **B** and **C.** (Courtesy Dr. M. B. Coventry.)

quently this may require femoral resection as far distally as the most inferior part of the lesser trochanter. When it becomes necessary to remove that portion of the femur containing the lesser trochanter, some effort at reattaching the lengthened iliopsoas tendon to the remaining femur must be made. In previously untreated patients only the distortion of angulation or rotation at the head and neck level typical of congenital dislocation of the hip will be present. Coventry has noted that the femoral head and neck may be anteverted as much as 90 degrees and that the greater trochanter is attached more posteriorly than usual. Even in these circumstances, however, no major technical problems should be encountered resulting from such abnormalities. On the other hand if prior treatment has been given, including angulation and displacement subtrochanteric osteotomies such as the Schanz and McMurray operations, then the existing deformity may require a totally different femoral component, even to the point of requiring special fabrication (Fig. 10-10). Clearly this determination *must* be made prior to embarking on the operation. More recent innovations in total hip reconstruction may make it possible to avoid such extensive reconstructive procedures when dealing with iatrogenic deformities in configuration of the proximal femur.[7] The newer "resurfacing" techniques that do not employ intramedullary stems can prove very useful in circumstances where the upper femur cannot accommodate a stem (Fig. 10-11).

Prior to surgery, not only must one determine the exact shape and size of the femoral component to be utilized, but the degree of upward displacement must also

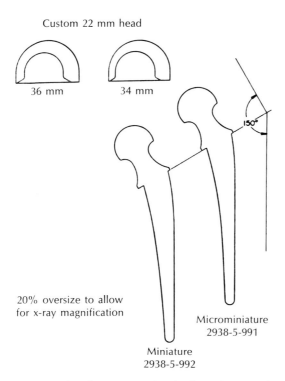

Fig. 10-9. Template that can be employed to ascertain what size femoral stem can be safely accommodated by the medullary canal. (Courtesy Howmedica, Inc.)

268 *Congenital dysplasia and dislocation of the hip*

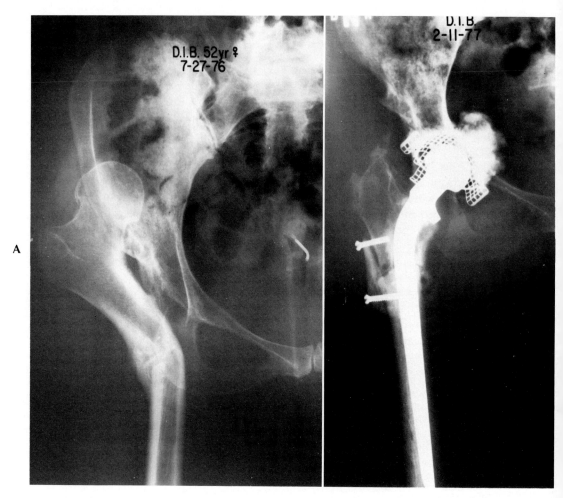

Fig. 10-10. Pelvic film of a 52-year-old woman who had undergone Schanz (pelvic-support) osteotomy during earlier adult life for instability of a dislocated right hip, **A.** This anatomic situation created a complex problem in performing total hip arthroplasty. Angulation osteotomy and femoral shortening were necessary, resulting in a satisfactory, painless hip, **B.** This illustrates the problems created by procedures that distort the anatomy of the hip joint and emphasizes the need for custom-made devices. (Courtesy Dr. H. K. Dunn.)

be assessed. As mentioned earlier, the femoral head must be brought down to the level of the original acetabulum. Preliminary traction, as noted by Lazansky,[6] is of no value in adults, because of the inelasticity of the soft tissues.

This procedure requires osteotomy of the greater trochanter in *all* instances. Not only does reflection of the greater trochanter provide better visualization and exposure, but this then permits resection of the femur sufficiently to allow a safe reduction of the prosthetic head. Also, the trochanter and its attached abductor muscles can thereafter be reattached to the upper end of the resected femur in order to enhance stability and future abductor muscle function. Occasionally the greater trochanter cannot be recessed far enough distally to permit

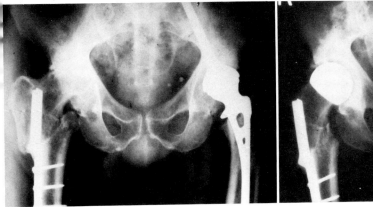

Fig. 10-11. In situations where an intramedullary stem is either difficult or impossible, as seen in **A**, a "resurfacing" total hip arthroplasty can best be employed, **B**. (Courtesy Mr. M. A. R. Freeman, London.)

firm bony fixation. Also, the trochanter may be very diminutive, having not been effectively used for many years. Any temptation to use wide abduction as an assist in reattaching the greater trochanter should be resisted, because a permanent abduction contracture may result, or the trochanter may be pulled off when the thigh is adducted.[2] In instances where the trochanter is very small or cannot be recessed far enough, I have simply excised the trochanter and reattached the abductor muscles to the still intact and redundant vastus lateralis and tensor fasciae latae muscles. This seems to provide the necessary stability, and adequate abductor strength is usually restored so that a very acceptable gait results. This technical maneuver is only recommended, however, when it appears inappropriate or impossible to reattach the trochanter directly to the upper femur (Fig. 10-2). It is not uncommon to find that the previously existing Trendelenburg gait is not reversed by the surgical procedure. Patients must, therefore, be warned in advance that they still may have a positive Trendelenburg gait and that a cane must be used periodically after surgery to assist them in gait.

These challenging technical problems on the proximal femur encountered in total hip replacement represent one of the major reasons why the salvage procedures outlined in Chapter 8 have assumed greater importance and why justification for the performance of such procedures in the older child and adolescent, especially in the completely dislocated hip, has become better accepted.

Soft tissues and neurovascular structures. As mentioned earlier, the musculotendinous structures about the totally dislocated hip offer a relatively minor problem during total hip replacement, as contrasted to the potential problems posed by the neurovascular elements. The muscles and tendons can easily be lengthened even though some minor loss of strength may result. However, the distal displacement of the limb required to achieve satisfactory reduction of the prosthetic femoral head may sometimes threaten to exceed the resilience and stretch capacities of the femoral artery and/or the femoral and sciatic nerves. This represents the most challenging and unpredictable part of the operation. There is no reliable mechanism by which the issue of downward displacement can be accurately resolved preoperatively, and there appears to be no proved means by which the surgeon can make this assessment at the time of surgery. Coventry[2] has shown that there is no statistical relationship between the amount of lengthening achieved and the incidence of nerve palsy, and he has been able to reduce the hip distally as far as 2½ inches without producing nerve paresis. Perhaps as our ability to monitor peripheral nerve function on the anesthetized patient becomes better developed, the intraoperative criteria governing the degree of maximum distal displacement of the lower limb can be more accurately assessed at the time of surgery. For, in the final analysis, the threat to sciatic nerve function limits the amount of downward displacement that can be effected.

While searching for a reliable mechanism to monitor nerve function, however, certain arbitrary guidelines have been established that are designed to govern the amount of distal displacement of the femur that can be safely accomplished. This figure varies from 4.0 to 9.0 cm, but these values seem to have been derived from observations that ostensibly are independent of the duration, rigidity, flexibility, or cause of the dislocation. Thus although they are helpful guidelines, Coventry believes that they are by no means rigid and at the present time are largely arbitrary.[2]

When postoperative nerve paralysis is encountered, it will nearly always be the result of nerve stretch (neuropraxia) and will most often involve portions or all of the sciatic nerve and occasionally the femoral nerve. In most instances gradual recovery will take place. However, there may be some minor residual hypoesthesia or paresis, and in rare cases permanent significant loss of function of either the femoral or sciatic nerve may persist. Dunn and Hess[3] have shown that paresis may occur as long as 2 or 3 days after surgery. They cited such a patient in their series, and it was believed that inappropriate postoperative positioning was a major causal factor. The patient should be positioned with the hip extended and the knee flexed in order to relax the sciatic nerve. Gradual correction of this position can be monitored accurately during the postoperative convalescence.

There are many factors that must be considered differently when total hip replacement in congenital dislocation of the hip is being performed in the adult, and it stands to reason that the postoperative treatment program must differ from the convalescent management in conventional total hip replacement. For example, in order to reduce the femoral head, the hip joint capsule must be completely excised, the iliopsoas muscle must be sectioned and/or lengthened, and the trochanter with its attached muscles must be reattached at a totally different level on the femur. Also, as indicated earlier, sometimes the trochanter must be excised in order to advance the abductor muscles to the femur by attachment to the vastus muscles. All of these factors tend to render the prosthetic hip joint potentially less stable than hip joints that follow conventional total hip replacement, and there is, therefore, greater likelihood of postoperative dislocation. Consequently postoperative positioning and range-of-motion activities must be carefully supervised. Furthermore active and resistive exercises must be prescribed on a highly individual basis, depending on the surgeon's appraisal of these issues, which are so variable from one case to another.

REFERENCES

1. Charnley, J., and Feagin, J. A.: Low-friction arthroplasty in congenital subluxation of the hip, Clin. Orthop. **91**:98, 1973.
2. Coventry, M. B.: Total hip arthroplasty in the adult with congenital dislocation. In The Hip Society: The hip, vol. IV, Proceedings of the fourth open scientific meeting of The Hip Society, St. Louis, 1976, The C. V. Mosby Co., p. 77.

3. Dunn, H. K., and Hess, W. E.: Total hip reconstruction in chronically dislocated hips, J. Bone Joint Surg. **58A**:838, 1976.
4. Harris, W. H., and Crothers, O. D.: Autogenous bone grafting using the femoral head to correct severe acetabular deficiency for total hip replacement. In The Hip Society: The hip, vol. IV, Proceedings of the fourth open scientific meeting of The Hip Society, St. Louis, 1976, The C. V. Mosby Co., p. 161.
5. Hess, W. E.: Unpublished data.
6. Lazansky, M. G.: Low friction arthroplasty for the sequelae of congenital and developmental hip dislocation. In AAOS Instructional Course Lectures: Volume XXIII, St. Louis, 1974, The C. V. Mosby Co., p. 194.
7. Samuelson, K. M.: Personal communication.
8. Tronzo, R. G., and Okin, E. M.: Anatomic restoration of congenital hip dysplasia in adulthood by total hip replacement, Clin. Orthop. **106**:94, 1975.

INDEX

A

Aarskog, D., 35
Abduction, severe restriction of, and instability of hip, 61
Abduction device
 metal-reinforced, semirigid, 80
 in treatment of dysplasia, 62
Abduction splint, plastic, 69
Abnormalities, congenital, associated with dislocation, 47, 66
Acetabular deficiencies, residual, correction of, 125-126
Acetabular dysplasia, primary; see Dysplasia, primary acetabular
Acetabular fossa, 13, 15
"Acetabular index," 54-56
Acetabular ligament, transverse, 15
Acetabular limbus in open reduction, anatomy and clinical significance of, 92-93
"Acetabular shelf," 53
 Wilson procedure of, 235-239
Acetabulum
 anatomy of, 14-18
 angle of inclination of 10, 53-54, 115
 articular cartilage of, 14-15
 capacity of, to remodel, 113
 changes of, in dislocation, 74
 character of, in anterior and posterior dislocations in arthrogryposis, 254
 in complete dislocation of hip, 263-264
 deficiencies of, correction of, 125-149
 depth of, during later months of intrauterine development, 8-10
 development of, following open reduction, 113
 dysplasia of
  primary; see Dysplasia, primary acetabular
  "redirectional" (Salter) osteotomy in treatment of, 137
  surgical procedures in treatment of, 162-173
  in teratologic hip dislocation, 254
 "horseshoe-shaped," articular surfaces of, 13
 interzone between femoral head and, at 8 weeks of gestation, 4
 normal relationship of, to proximal femur, 57
 obliquity of, 231

Acetabulum—cont'd
 operative procedures on, 162-172
 and pelvis, lateral view of, 13
 perichondrium of, at 7½ weeks of gestation, 3
 remodeling capacity of, 139, 140
 roof of
  slope of, as diagnostic aid, 53
  slope of, in dislocation, 74
  sloping oblique, 162
  at 13 weeks of gestation, 7
 rotation of
  combined with proximal femoral osteotomy, 173
  indications for, 165
 at 7 weeks of gestation, 2
 at 6 weeks of gestation, 2
 wall of
  "controlled" medial fracture of, 264-265
  progressive thinness of, 260
Adams, R.D., 249
Adductor approach to open reduction; see also Medial (adductor) approach to open reduction
 Ludloff, 88-91
 technique of, 87-91
Adolescent; see also Child
 diagnosis and treatment of residual dysplasia in, 155-174
 operative treatment of hip dysplasia in, 159-162
Africans, incidence of congenital dislocation in, 28
Age
 of fusion of each portion of triradiate cartilage, 12
 of patient in anterior and posterior dislocations in arthrogryposis, 254
Albee, F. H., 125
Ambulation
 following chondrolysis, 204-205
 potential of, in anterior and posterior dislocations in arthrogryposis, 252
Amyoplasia congenita, 249
Anatomy
 of acetabulum, 14-18
 and embryology of hip joint, 1-26
 of femoral head, 12-14

Anatomy—cont'd
  of hip joint, 18-22
    clinical correlations of, 25
    gross and functional, 11-25
Andrén, L., 34, 50
Angle
  of anteversion, 10, 114-115
  C-E, 156, 158, 160, 164
  of declination, 10, 114-115
  of femoral torsion, 114
  of inclination, 10, 53-54, 115
  neck-shaft, of femur, 10, 115, 196
  of retroversion, 114-115
  of torsion, 114-115
Angular osteotomy, 160
Angulation osteotomy, proximal femoral, 122
Anomalies, congenital, associated with congenital dysplasia and dislocation, 31-32
Anterior (iliofemoral) approach to open reduction, 84-86, 91
  vs medial (adductor) approach, 100
  technique of, 83-87
Anterior dislocation, primary, pelvic x-ray film of 18-month-old child with, 93
Anteroposterior view of hip and pelvis, 144-145
Anteversion
  angle of, 10, 114-115
  of femur, persistent, 121
Apaches, incidence of congenital dislocation in, 28-29
Apophyseal arrest of greater trochanter, technique of, 196-197
Apron, Frejka, 25, 60, 62
Arrest, apophyseal, of greater trochanter, technique of, 196-197
Artery
  femoral; see Femoral artery
  inferior gluteal, 22
  lateral circumflex femoral, 20, 24
  to ligamentum teres, 22-25
  medial circumflex femoral, 20-21, 24
  posterolateral epiphyseal, 25
  superior gluteal, 22
Arthritic sequelae, painful symptomatic, of congenital dislocation, 257
Arthrodesis, 247-248
Arthrography, 43-44, 160, 187-188
  in congenital dislocation, 111-113
  indications for, 112
Arthrogryposis, 249-256
Arthrogryposis multiplex congenita, 249, 252-253
Arthroplasty
  Colonna; see Colonna arthroplasty
  femoral head prosthetic, 257
  implant, 257
  "resurfacing" total hip, 269
  total hip, 266
  trochanteric, 243-247
  Vitallium cup, 257
Arthrotomy, 111, 148
Articular cartilage
  of acetabulum, 14-15
  hyaline; see Cartilage, hyaline
Aspirin in treatment of chondrolysis, 202-204

Autogenous bone grafting to support prosthetic cup, 266
Axial tomography, 115
"Axillary" position of hip spica cast, 79, 80; see also Position, cast

B

Badgley, C. E., 1, 6, 10, 36, 119
Bardeen, C. R., 1, 2, 3
Barlow, T. C., 28, 30
"Bifurcation" osteotomy, Lorenz, 241-242
Bigelow ligament, 12, 16-17
"Bilabial" femoral head, 117
"Bilabiation," 116
Bilateral dislocation; see Dislocation, congenital, bilateral
Bilateral dysplasia, 48, 56, 62-63
Bilateral knee extension contractures, congenital, 179
Bilateral limp, pelvic x-ray film of 5-year-old child with, 182
Bilateral subluxation, 62-63
Bilateral total hip replacement, 264
Biologic plasticity of acetabulum and femoral head, 133
Birth
  factors of, influence of, on congenital dysplasia and dislocation, 30-32
  order of, and incidence of congenital dysplasia and dislocation, 30
Bjerkreim, I., 29, 30, 31, 33
Blacks, incidence of congenital dislocation in, 28
Blastema
  innominatum, at 5 to 6 weeks of gestation, 2
  at 6 weeks of gestation, 3
Blood supply
  to femoral head, 22
  to hip joint, 22-25
Bone, heterotopic, about hip joint capsule, 215
Bone atrophy, 201
Bone grafting, autogenous, to support prosthetic cup, 266
Bone necrosis, femoral head; see Femoral head, necrosis of
Bone stages, fetal, at 6 weeks of gestation, 3
Breech births, incidence of congenital dislocation in, 10, 30-31, 36, 48
Burman, M. S., 54
Bursa, 19

C

Caffey, J., 54, 55
Calcaneovalgus, 32
Canadian Indians, incidence of congenital dislocation in, 28-29
Capsule of hip joint; see Hip joint, capsule of
Carter, C. O., 30, 36
Cartilage
  articular, of acetabulum, 14-15
  hyaline
    at 8 weeks of gestation, 4
    at 9 weeks of gestation, 5
  hyaline articular, 10
  at 6 weeks of gestation, 3

Cartilage—cont'd
  at 13 weeks of gestation, 7
  triradiate, age of fusion of each portion of, 12
Cartilage necrosis, 116, 205
  and chondrolysis, 200-205
  clinical manifestations of, 205
  pathology of, 205
Cartilage space, loss of, 201
Cast
  following open reduction, 87
  following closed reduction, 78
  position of; see Position, cast
  spica, 69, 79
Cavity, hip joint, anatomy of, 18-22
C-E angle, 156, 158, 160, 164
Central nervous system disease, absence of, and Colonna arthroplasty, 214-215
Chapchal, G. J., 121
Charnley-Mueller prosthesis, 262
Cheilectomy, 207
Chiari, K., 224
Chiari osteotomy, 224-234
  at age when there is remaining skeletal growth, 233
  complications and unique characteristics of, 229-234
  diagrammatic representation of, 225
  distal fragment of, 232
  high, 230
  indications for, 224, 225-226
  postoperative care of, 229
  prerequisites of, 226
  surgical technique of, 226-229
Child; see also Infant; Neonate; Newborn
  18-month-old
    pelvic x-ray film of dislocation in, 178
    pelvic x-ray film of primary anterior dislocation, 93
    roentgenogram of complete dislocation in, 74
  11-month-old, pelvic x-ray film of dislocation of left hip and subluxation of right hip in, 122-123
  11-year-old, pelvic x-ray film of, following arthroplasty, 101
  5-year-old, pelvic x-ray film of bilateral limp in, 182
  14-month-old
    with dislocation of right hip, pericapsular osteotomy in, 132
    pelvic x-ray film of dislocation of left hip in, 112
  14-old-old, pelvic x-ray film of bilateral dislocation in, 228
  4-year-old, pelvic x-ray film of untreated congenital dislocation in, 109-110
  4½-year-old, pelvic x-ray film of severe arthrogryposis in, 251
  9-year-old
    pelvic x-ray film of bilateral dislocation in, 157
    pelvic x-ray film of unilateral untreated dislocation in, 151
    pelvic x-ray film of untreated dislocation of left hip in, 190-191
  nonoperative treatment of dysplasia in, 157-159

Child—cont'd
  normal, femoral torsion in, 115
  older, diagnosis and treatment of residual dysplasia in, 155-174
  operative treatment of dysplasia in, 159-162
    general considerations of, 159-162
    indications for, 159-160
    physical examination in, 160-162
    radiographic evaluation in, 160
  over 18 months of age, treatment of congenital dislocation in, 98-119
  over 4 years of age, treatment of congenital dislocation in, 150-152
  6-month-old, pelvic x-ray film of bilateral dislocation in, 199
  16-month-old, pelvic x-ray film of dislocation of left hip in, 203
  10-year-old
    pelvic x-ray film of bilateral complete dislocation in, 150
  pelvic x-ray film of unilateral dislocation in, 223
  13-year-old, pelvic x-ray film of chondrolysis in, 201
  12-month-old, pelvic x-ray film of dislocation of left hip in, 76
  12-year-old
    pelvic x-ray film of bilateral dislocation in, 214
    pelvic x-ray film of unilateral dislocation of right hip in, 212
  21-month-old, pelvic x-ray film of bilateral dislocation in, 100
  28-month-old, pelvic x-ray film of bilateral dislocation in, 146
  2-month-old, pelvic x-ray film of dislocation of left hip in, 82
  2-year-old
    pelvic x-ray film of bilateral dislocation in, 156
    pelvic x-ray film of complete dislocation of left hip in, 143
    pelvic x-ray film of dislocation of left hip in, 147
  2½-year-old, pelvic x-ray film of bilateral dislocation in, 179
  under 18 months of age, diagnosis and treatment of congenital dislocation in, 72-94
  young, combined operative procedures in, 145-149
Chinese, incidence of congenital dislocation in, 28
Chondrolysis as complication during treatment of congenital dislocation, 200-205
  ambulation following, 204-205
  aspirin in treatment of, 202-204
  and cartilage necrosis, 200-205
  clinical manifestations of, 201-202
  etiology of, 200
  pathology of, 200-201
  pelvic x-ray film of 13-year-old child with, 201
  physical therapy in treatment of, 202
  traction in treatment of, 202
  treatment of, 202-205
Chondromalacia, 201
Chuinard, E. G., 36, 119, 121, 122, 172
Circumflex femoral artery
  lateral, 20, 22, 24
  medial, 20-21, 22, 24

Circumflex vessels
  femoral, relationship of, to adjacent musculature, 118
  lateral, 22
  medial, 22
Clark, C. H., 54
Closed reduction; see Reduction, closed
Closing wedge osteotomy of proximal femur, 240
Codivilla, A., 36
Collagen, 35
Colonna, P. C., 243
Colonna arthroplasty, 150, 192, 211-224
  and absence of central nervous system disease, 214-215
  and absence of infection, 214
  indications for, 211-212
  pelvic x-ray film of 11-year-old girl following, 101
  postoperative care of, 222-223
  prerequisites and contraindications of, 212-215
  special complications of, 223-224
  surgical technique of, 215-222
Combined operative procedures in young children, 145-149
Complete osteotomy; see Innominate (Salter) osteotomy
Complications during treatment of congenital dislocation, 186-208
  causes of, 181-186
  and problems, 175-208
Concentric reduction, 111-113, 146
Configuration and growth of proximal femur following open reduction, 113
Congenital abnormalities associated with congenital dislocation, 31-32, 66
Congenital bilateral knee extension contractures, 179
Congenital dysplasia; see Dysplasia, congenital
Congenital hyperthermia, 146
Contractures, congenital bilateral knee extension, 179
Contralateral distal femoral epiphysiodesis, 200
Coventry, M. B., 264, 267, 270
Coventry plates and screws, 124
Coxa plana, 116, 195
Coxa valga, 157, 231
Coxa vara, 195
Craig splint, modified, 58-59, 62
Creases, asymmetric thigh and inguinal skin, 47
Crego, C. H., 67, 75
Cross-table (groin) lateral view of hip, 43, 144-145
Crothers, O. D., 264
Curtis, B., 178
Czeizel, A., 28, 29, 30, 33, 35, 36

D

D (Hilgenreiner) distance, 50, 55, 56
Deformities, residual, treatment of, following reduction, 119-125
Dislocation, congenital; see also Dysplasia, congenital
  antenatal, 254
  arthrography in, 111-113
  bilateral, 51
    in arthrogryposis, 251-252

Dislocation, congenital—cont'd
  bilateral—cont'd
    pelvic x-ray film of 14-year-old child with, 228
    pelvic x-ray film of 12-year-old child with, 214
  diagnosis of, 72-75
    in child 18 months to 4 years of age, 95-154
    in child under 18 months of age, 72-94
    minimal number of x-ray films in, 144-145
    problems in, 175-176
  and dysplasia; see Dysplasia, congenital, and dislocation
  incidence of, 27-28
    in Apaches, 28-29
    in blacks, 28
    in Canadian Indians, 28-29
    in children of breech deliveries, 10, 30-31
    in firstborn infants, 30
    in Koreans, 28
    in Lapps, 28
    in Navajos, 28-29
    in North American Indians, 28-29
    and order of birth, 30
    in probands, 29
    and seasonal hormonal changes, 31
    and swaddling infants, 31
    in twins, 29-30
  irreducible, pelvic x-ray film of newborn with, 252
  of left hip
    complete, pelvic x-ray film of 2-year-old child with, 143
    pelvic x-ray film of 11-month-old child with, 122-123
    pelvic x-ray film of 14-month-old child with, 112
    pelvic x-ray film of 16-month-old child with, 203
    pelvic x-ray film of 12-month-old child with, 76, 112
    pelvic x-ray film of 2-month-old child with, 82
    pelvic x-ray film of 2-year-old child with, 147, 189
    untreated, pelvic x-ray film of 9-year-old child with, 190-191
  ligamentous laxity as cause of, 33-35
  mechanical factors as cause of, 35-36
  minimal number of x-ray films in diganosis of, 144-145
  neonatal, 33, 66-70
    "irreducible," 70
    pathology of, 66-67
    physical findings of, 67-68
    roentgenographic findings in, 68-69
    treatment of, 69-70
  painful symptomatic arthritic sequelae of, 257
  pathology of, 74-75
  physical findings of, 72-73
  posterior, 67
    in arthrogryposis, 252-254
  primary acetabular dysplasia as cause of, 32-33
  primary anterior, 75, 93
    pelvic x-ray film of 18-month-old child with, 93
    treatment of, 94
  problems in, 175-208
    caused by associated abnormalities, 177-179
    resulting from late diagnosis, 181

Dislocation, congenital—cont'd
  problems in—cont'd
    resulting from prior treatment in, 179-181
    unusual pathology in, 177
  racial and ethnic differences in response to, 152
  radiographic features of, 74
  relationship between dysplasia and, 40-41
  resulting from untreated newborn dysplasia or subluxation, 66
  of right hip, 68
    pelvic x-ray film of 14-month-old child with pericapsular osteotomy, 132
  slope of acetabular roof in, 74
  "teratologic," 249-256
    acetabular dysplasia in, 254
    pathology of, 66, 250-251
  treatment of
    causes of complications during, 181-186
    in child over 18 months of age, 98-119
    in child under 18 months of age, 75-94
      cast position in, 80
      open reduction in, 81-94
      traction and closed reduction in, 75-80
    complications during, 175-208
    and errors and technical failures in implementation, 186
    and failure to achieve and maintain concentric reduction, 181-184
    and failure to define problem accurately, 181
    and failure to implement appropriate operative procedure, 184-186
  "typical," pathology of, 66
  unilateral
    in arthrogryposis, 251-252
    diagnosis of, 95
    Galeazzi test in, 73
    and Trendelenburg sign, 96
    pelvic x-ray film of 10-year-old child with, 223
    physical findings in, 73, 95-96
    reduction of, 150
    in right hip, pelvic x-ray film of 12-year-old child with, 212
    untreated
      of left hip, pelvic x-ray film of 9-year-old Navajo child with, 151
      pelvic x-ray film of 50-year-old woman with, 259
Distal femoral epiphysiodesis, contralateral, 200
Distal femoral osteotomy, 125
Distance
  D (Hilgenreiner), 50, 55, 56
  H; see H (Hilgenreiner) distance
Dizygous twins, incidence of congenital dislocation in, 30
Double innominate osteotomy, 168-169, 170
Dunlap, K., 115
Dunn, P. M., 30, 262, 270
Dupuytren, J., 36
Dysplasia, congenital, 44-62, 176; see also Dislocation, congenital
  acetabular; see Acetabulum, dysplasia of
  bilateral, 48, 56, 62-63
  definition of, 41-42

Dysplasia, congenital—cont'd
  diagnosis of
    in high-risk infants, 47-50
    in newborn and neonate, 44-45
    physical features of, 45-47
  and dislocation
    congenital anomalies associated with, 31-32
    definition of terms of, 41-43
    diagnosis and treatment of, in newborn, neonate, and young infant, 40-71
    etiology and pathology of, 27-39
    influence of birth factors on, 30-32
    racial and ethnic influences on, 28-29
    seasonal influence on, 31
    sex and family influences of, 29-30
  incidence of, 27-28
  inherited, 32
  nonoperative treatment of, in infancy and childhood, 157-159
  operative treatment of, in childhood and adolescence, 159-162
    general considerations of, 159-162
    indications for, 159-160
    physical examination in, 160-162
    radiographic evaluation in, 160
  with painful osteoarthritis, 259-263
  pathology of, 44
  physical features of, 45-47
  primary acetabular, 32, 33-34, 64-66; see also Acetabulum, dysplasia of
    as cause of congenital dislocation, 32-33
    and ligamentous laxity, 32-36
  primary theory of, 32
  that proceeded to subluxation, 65
  relationship between dislocation and, 40-41
  residual, diagnosis and treatment of, in older child or adolescent, 155-174
  roentgenographic findings suggesting, 57-60
  and subluxation, hip roentgenograms illustrating difference between, 42
  treatment of, 60-62
  untreated
    in Navajo infants, 44-45
    in newborn that resulted in dislocation, 66
  x-ray changes in, 155-157

E

Edelstein, J., 28
Eisenstein, A., 200
Embryology and anatomy of hip joint, 1-26
Embryonic development of hip, 1-3
Epiphyseal artery, posterolateral, 25
Epiphyseal plate, 12-14
Epiphysiodesis, contralateral distal femoral, 200
Epiphysitis as complication during treatment of congenital dislocation, 192-200
Eppright, R. H., 126, 164, 169
Esterone, 34
Ethnic influences
  on congenital dysplasia and dislocation, 28-29
  in response to treatment of congenital dislocation, 152

Etiology and pathogenesis of congenital dysplasia and dislocation, 27-39
Examination, physical; *see* Physical examination
Extrapelvic protrusion, 231

F

Faber, A., 29, 32, 33
Family influences on congenital dysplasia and dislocation, 29-30
Farrell, B. P., 67
Fat pad, haversian, 15
Femoral artery
  lateral circumflex, 20, 22, 24
  medial circumflex, 20-21, 22, 24
Femoral components for total hip replacement, 260-261
Femoral epiphysiodesis, contralateral distal, 200
Femoral head; *see also* Femoral neck; Femur
  anatomy of, 12-14
  angle of declination of, 10, 114-115
  "bilabial," 117
  blood supply to, 22
  bone necrosis of; *see* Femoral head, necrosis of
  dislocated
    changes in, 74-75
    at 11 or 12 weeks of gestation, 6
    ossification of, 74
  earliest possible time of dislocation of, 11
  extrapelvic protrusion of, 169
  histologic section of capsule overlying, 210-211
  interzone between acetabulum and, at 8 weeks of gestation, 4
  and neck, angle of declination of, 114
  necrosis of, 25, 116
    roentgenographic diagnostic features of, 192-194
    treatment of, 195-196
  osteonecrosis of, 116
  perichondrium of, at 7½ weeks of gestation, 3
  prosthetic arthroplasty of, 257
  at 7 weeks of gestation, 2
  at 13 weeks of gestation, 7
  viability of, 115-119
Femoral metaphysis ("beak"), laterally disposed, 57
Femoral neck; *see also* Femoral head; Femur
  developing changes in anteversion of, 9
  and head, angle of declination of, 114
  posterior aspect of, 18
  shortening and valgus of, 194
  shortening and varus of, 194
Femoral nerve, 270
Femoral osteotomy
  distal, 125
  proximal, 119-125
Femoral stem, size of, for medullary canal, 267
Femoral torsion, angle of, 114-115
  in normal child, 115
Femoral vessels, circumflex, relationship of, to adjacent musculature, 118
Femur; *see also* Femoral head; Femoral neck
  growth and ossification of, diagrammatic representation of, 11
  head of; *see* Femoral head
  neck of; *see* Femoral neck

Femur—cont'd
  neck-shaft angle of, 10, 115, 196
  in neutral rotation, anteroposterior view of pelvis with, 144-145
  operative procedures on, 172-173
  persistent anteversion of, 121
  proximal
    anatomic dissection of, 20
    closing wedge osteotomy of, 240
    in complete dislocation, 264-269
    coronal section of, 23
    deformities of, 113-115, 194
    growth and configuration of, following open reduction, 113
    normal relationship of acetabulum to, 57
    posterior dissection of, 20-21
    reconstructive osteotomies of, 241-243
    reshaping of, by displacement of major trochanter, 242
  at 7 weeks of gestation, 2
  shortening of
    combined with pelvic osteotomy and open reduction, 148-149
    and open reduction, 100-109, 110-119, 183
  at 6 weeks of gestation, 2
  "stick," procedure of; *see* "stick femur" procedure
  upward displacement of, 162
Ferguson, A. B., 83, 254
Fetus
  bone stages in, at 6 weeks of gestation, 3
  development of hip in, 3-10
Fibers, retinacular, 16
Fibrous capsule of hip joint, 15-17; *see also* Hip joint, capsule of
Field, P., 205
Film, x-ray; *see* X-ray film, pelvic
Firstborn infants, incidence of congenital dislocation in, 30
Fixation, internal
  with flexible implants, 243
  utilizing plate and screws, 122
Flexible implant
  internal fixation with, 243
  in treatment of dysplasia, 62
Fossa, acetabular, 15
Fragment, inferior, failure to rotate, 184-185
Frejka apron, 25, 60, 62
"Frog-leg" cast position, 22, 116
Functional anatomy of hip joint, 11-25
Fusion of hip; *see* Arthrodesis

G

Gait, Trendelenburg, 165, 269
Galeazzi test in unilateral dislocation, 73, 96
Garceau, G., 207
Gardner, E., 1, 3, 7, 10
Gigli saw, 134-136
Gilbert, R. J., 231
Gland, haversian, 15
Gluteal artery, 22
Gluteus medius limp as indication for acetabular rotation, 165

Gonadal hormones, relationship of, to ligamentous laxity, 34-35
Gray, D. J., 1, 3, 7, 10
Greenfield, R., 126, 164, 168
Griffin, P. P., 205
Groin view of hip, 43
Growth
 and configuration of proximal femur following open reduction, 113
 and ossification of femur, 11

H

H (Hilgenreiner) distance
 in bilateral dysplasias or dislocations, 56
 foreshortened, value of, 55
H (Hilgenreiner) line, 50
Hagen, C. B., 29, 30, 31, 33
Harness, Pavlik, 60, 62, 69
Harris, W. H., 42, 264
Hart, V. L., 32-33
Hass, J., 33, 36, 44, 54, 67, 74, 241, 250
Haversian fat pad, 15
Haversian gland, 15
Head, femoral; see Femoral head
Hess, W. E., 262, 264, 270
Heterotopic bone about hip joint capsule, 215
Heublein, G. W., 54
Heusner, L., 33
Heyman, C. H., 125
High-risk infant; see Infant, high-risk
Hilgenreiner, H., 53-54, 55-56
Hilgenreiner distance, D and H, 50, 55, 56
Hip; see also Hip joint
 anterior aspect of, 19
 anteroposterior view of, with thighs in abduction and inward rotation, 144-145
 congenital dislocation of; see Dislocation, congenital
 congenital dysplasia of; see Dysplasia, congenital
 cross-table groin lateral view of, 144-145
 embryonic development of, 1-3
 fetal development of, 3-10
 fusion of; see Arthrodesis
 joint of; see Hip joint
 left, dislocation of; see Dislocation, congenital, of left hip
 newborn, method of examination of instability of, 46
 pain of, as indication for acetabular rotation, 165
 range of motion of, in anterior and posterior dislocation in arthrogryposis, 252-254
 reconstruction of, implant, 257-271
 replacement of
  bilateral total, 264
  femoral components of, 260-261
 right
  dislocation of, 68, 132, 212
  subluxation of, pelvic x-ray film of 11-month-old child with, 122-123
Hip joint; see also Hip
 anatomy of
  clinical correlations of, 25
  gross and functional, 11-25
 blood supply of, 22-25

Hip joint—cont'd
 capsule of, 17
  fibrous, 15-17
  heterotopic bone about, 215
  ligaments reinforcing, 16
 cavity of
  anatomy of, 18-22
  at 9 weeks of gestation, 5
 development of, clinical considerations relating to, 10-11
 diagrammatic coronal section of, 15
 at 8 weeks of gestation, 3
 at 11 weeks of gestation, 5-7
 embryology of, 1-11
  and anatomy of, 1-26
 at 4 weeks of gestation, 2
 nerve supply to, 25
 of newborn, roentgenographic findings of, 50
 penetration of, by pin, 184-185
 restriction of motion of, as complication of treatment of congenital dislocation, 205-207
 at 16 weeks of gestation, 7
 stiffness of, 231
 at 35 weeks of gestation, 8-10
 at 32 weeks of gestation, 8
 at 20 weeks of gestation, 7-8
 at 28 to 29 weeks of gestation, 8
 in 2-month-old infant, 14
Hisaw, F. L., 34
History and physical examination in diagnosis and treatment of congenital dysplasia and dislocation, 43-44
Hodgson, A. R., 28
Hormones
 changes in, seasonal, and incidence of congenital dislocation, 31
 gonadal, relationship of, to ligamentous laxity, 34-35
Howorth, M. B., 33-34, 36, 67
Hoyt, W. A., 92
Hubbard, D. D., 115
"Human" position of hip spica cast, 25, 79, 80, 116
Hummer, C. D., 31
Hyaline articular cartilage; see Cartilage, hyaline
Hyperthermia, congenital, 146

I

Idelberger, K., 29
Ilfeld splint, 58-59
Iliofemoral approach to open reduction; see Anterior (iliofemoral) approach to open reduction
Iliofemoral ligament, 16-17
Iliopectineal eminence, 14
Iliopsoas tendon, 92
Ilium, 12
Implant, flexible, internal fixation with, 243
Implant arthroplasty, 257
Implant hip reconstruction, 257-271
Incidence
 of congenital dislocation; see Dislocation, congenital, incidence of
 of congenital dysplasia, 27-28
Inclination, angle of, 10, 53-54, 115

Indians, Canadian and North American, incidence of congenital dislocation in, 28-29
Indications for open reduction, 81-82
Infant; *see also* Child; Neonate; Newborn
 firstborn, incidence of congenital dislocation in, 30
 high-risk
  diagnosis of congenital dysplasia in, 47-50
  subluxation in, 48
 Navajo, untreated dysplasia in, 44-45
 nonoperative treatment of dysplasia in, 157-159
 subluxation in, 62-66
 2-month-old, hip joint in, 14
 young, diagnosis and treatment of congenital dysplasia and dislocation in, 40-71
Infection, absence of, and hip operations, 243
Inferior gluteal artery, 22
Inguinal skin creases, asymmetric, 47, 73
Innominate (Salter) osteotomy, 113, 126, 133-138, 161, 162-164, 165, 186; *see also* Pericapsular (Pemberton) osteotomy
 advantages and disadvantages of, 133-138
 double, 168-169, 170
 and limb length inequality, 200
 and open reduction, 145-148
 and pericapsular (Pemberton) osteotomy, 138-145
 triple, 126, 164-168
Innominate (Steel) osteotomy, triple, 169
Innominatum blastema at 5 to 6 weeks of gestation, 2
Instability
 of newborn hip, method of examination of, 46
 and severe restriction of abduction of hip, 61
Internal fixation
 with flexible implants, 243
 utilizing plate and screws, 122
Intertrochanteric osteotomy; *see* Osteotomy, intertrochanteric
Interzone
 between femoral head and acetabulum at 8 weeks of gestation, 4
 at 6 to 7 weeks of gestation, 3
"Irreducible" neonatal dislocation, 70
Ischiofemoral ligament, 17
Ischiopubic synchondrosis, 14, 74
Ischium, 12

J

Jacobs, J. E., 31-32
"Jerk" of entry and exit of Ortolani, 44, 45, 68, 72
Joint, hip; *see* Hip joint
Joint space at 11 or 12 weeks of gestation, 6

K

Kawamura, B., 126, 169
Kirschner wires, 243
Kleinberg, S., 54
Knee
 extension contractures of, 178, 179
 level of, Galleazi test of, in unilateral dislocation, 73
 range of motion of, in anterior and posterior dislocations in arthrogryposis, 252-254
Koreans, incidence of congenital dislocation in, 28

L

Laage view of hip, 43
Labrum, 13, 15
Labrum glenoidale at 8 weeks of gestation, 4
Langenskiöld, A., 34, 119
Lapps, incidence of congenital dislocation in, 28
Larsen, L. J., 101, 243
Lateral circumflex femoral artery, 20, 22, 24
Lateral circumflex vessels, 22
Laurenson, R. D., 1, 55
Laxity, ligamentous; *see* Ligamentous laxity
Lazansky, M. G., 268
Le-Damany, P., 8-10, 36
Lengthening vs tenotomizing of iliopsoas tendon and muscle, 92
Lieberman, H. S., 54
Ligament
 Bigelow, 12, 16-17
 iliofemoral, 16-17
 ischiofemoral, 17
 pubofemoral, 16-17
 reinforcing hip joint capsule, 16
 transverse acetabular, 15
 Y (Bigelow), 12, 16-17
Ligamentous laxity
 as cause of congenital dislocation, 33-35
 persisting form of, 35
 and primary acetabular dysplasia, 32-36
 relationship of, to gonadal hormones, 34-35
 relationship of, to relaxin, 34-35
 temporary type of, 35
Ligamentous structures at 20 weeks of gestation, 8
Ligamentum teres, 12, 13, 15, 17-18
 artery to, 22-25
 at 9 weeks of gestation, 5
Limb length
 effect of osteotomies on, 161-162
 equalization of, 161
 inequality of, 200, 207, 228
  caused by stimulation following surgical treatment of congenital dislocation, 207-208
  and femoral osteotomy, 207
Limbus, 13
 acetabular, in open reduction, anatomy and clinical significance of, 92-93
 importance of, in open reduction, 92-93
 at 9 weeks of gestation, 5
Limp
 bilateral, pelvic x-ray film of 5-year-old child with, 182
 gluteus medius, as indication of acetabular rotation, 165
Line
 Perkins, 50, 56-57
 Shenton, 137, 139, 141-142, 143, 156, 162
Logan, N. D., 36
Longitudinal traction, 99
Lorenz, A., 33, 36, 119, 241
Lorenz "bifurcation" osteotomy, 241-242
Lovell, W. W., 69, 247
Ludloff, L., 36, 82
Ludloff approach to hip, 88-91

M

MacEwen, G. D., 30, 31, 47, 69, 146
MacKenzie, I. G., 119
McCarroll, H. R., 67, 75
McKibbin, B., 10, 35
Magilligan, D. J., 115
Massie, W. K., 34
Mau, H., 83
Mechanical factors as cause of congenital dislocation, 35-36
Medial (adductor) approach in open reduction, 91, 189
  vs anterior (iliofemoral) approach, 100
  technique of, 87-91
Medial circumflex femoral artery, 20-21, 22, 24
Medial circumflex vessels, 22
Medullary canal, size of femoral stem for, 267
Membrane, synovial, 3, 18-22
Mesh, Vitallium, 264
Metal-reinforced, semirigid plastic abduction device, 80
Metaphysis, laterally disposed ("beak"), 57
Microminiature femoral components for total hip replacement, 260-261
Middleton, D. S., 249
Miniature femoral components for total hip replacement, 260-261
Mitchell, C. L., 10, 92, 250
Monozygous twins, incidence of congenital dislocation in, 29-30
Monticelli, G., 121
Morville, P., 8
Muller, G. M., 31, 119
Muscle, iliopsoas, tenotomizing vs lengthening of, 92
Myositis ossificans, 214-215

N

Nailplate device, two-piece, 122
Navajos
  incidence of congenital dislocation in, 28-29
  pelvic x-ray examinations in, 55
  response of, to treatment of congenital dislocation, 152
  untreated dysplasia in, 44-45
Neck, femoral; see Femoral neck
Neck-shaft angle of femur, 10, 115, 196
Necrosis
  cartilage; see Cartilage necrosis
  of femoral head; see Femoral head, necrosis of
  osseous, deformities of proximal femur secondary to, 194
Nelson, M. A., 28
Neonatal dislocation; see Dislocation, congenital, neonatal
Neonate; see also Child; Infant; Newborn
  definition of, 28, 40
  diagnosis of congenital dysplasia in, 44-45
  diagnosis and treatment of congenital dysplasia and dislocation in, 40-71
  technique for taking pelvic x-ray film of, 52
Nerve, sciatic, 270
Nerve stretch, 270
Nerve supply of hip joint, 25

Neuropraxia, 270
Neurovascular structures and complete dislocation, 269-270
Newborn; see also Child; Infant; Neonate
  definition of, 28, 40
  diagnosis of congenital dysplasia in, 44-45
  diagnosis and treatment of congenital dysplasia and dislocation in, 40-71
  hip of, method of examination of instability of, 46
  hip joint of, roentgenographic findings of, 50
  pelvic x-ray film of irreducible dislocation in, 252
  pelvis of, 53
    radiographic techniques of evaluation of, 50
    roentgenographic determinants of, 50-60
  roentgenographic study of, 49
  untreated dysplasia or subluxation in, that resulted in dislocation, 66
Noel, S., 229
Nonoperative treatment of dysplasia in infancy and childhood, 157-159
North American Indians, incidence of congenital dislocation in, 28-29

O

Obliquity
  of acetabulum, 231
  pelvic, 178-179
Ogden, J. A., 116
Ombrédanne, L., 101
Open reduction; see Reduction, open
Operative procedure
  on acetabulum, 162-172
  appropriate, failure to implement, as cause of complication of treatment of congenital dislocation, 184-186
  for arthrogryposis, 254-256
  combined, in young children, 145-149
  on femur, 172-173
  in treatment of acetabular dysplasia, 162-173
Operative treatment
  of dysplasia in childhood and adolescence, 159-162
    general considerations of, 159-162
    indications for, 159-160
    physical examination in, 160-162
    radiographic evaluation in, 160
  of open reduction in congenital dislocation, 81
Orthoroentgenogram, 228
Ortolani, M., 44
  "jerks" of entry and exit of, 44, 45, 68, 72
Osseous necrosis, deformities of, proximal femur secondary to, 194
Ossification
  of dislocated femoral head, 74
  and growth of femur, 11
Osteoarthritis, 42, 116
  painful, 259-263
Osteochondritides, 14
Osteonecrosis
  as complication of treatment of congenital dislocation, 192-200
  of femoral head, 116
  roentgenographic changes diagnostic of, 193

Osteotomy
　angular, 160
　Chiari; see Chiari osteotomy
　closing wedge, of proximal femur, 240
　complete; see Innominate (Salter) osteotomy
　"decompression," 101
　derotational, 121
　"dial," 126, 164, 171, 172
　distal femoral, 125
　effects of, on limb length, 161-162
　femoral, and limb length inequality, 207
　innominate; see Innominate (Salter) osteotomy
　intertrochanteric, 119-125
　　contraindications and complications of, 125
　　evolution of, 119-124
　　preferred anatomic location of, 120
　　prerequisites of, 124-125
　　valgus, 196
　　varus, 121-122, 196
　Lorenz "bifurcation," 241-242
　pelvic; see Pelvic osteotomy
　Pemberton; see Pericapsular (Pemberton) osteotomy
　periacetabular "dial," 169-172
　periarticular, 171
　pericapsular; see Pericapsular (Pemberton) osteotomy
　proximal femoral, 119-125
　　angulation, 122
　　contraindications and complications of, 125
　　evolution of, 119-124
　　prerequisites for, 124-125
　　reconstructive, 241-243
　　rotational, 122, 187
　"redirectional" (Salter) in treatment of acetabular dysplasia, 137
　rotational, 160
　supracondylar, 125
　Salter; see Innominate (Salter) osteotomy
　Schanz "pelvic-support," 240, 241-242
　Steel, 169
　stellate, 222
　supracondylar, 125
　triplane, 173
　triple innominate (Steel), 126, 169
　varus intertrochanteric, 121-122
　varus rotational, 121, 159

P

Pathogenesis and etiology of congenital dysplasia and dislocation, 27-39
Pathology
　of congenital dislocation, 74-75
　of congenital dysplasia, 44
　of neonatal dislocation, 66-67
　of primary anterior dislocation, 75
　of subluxation, 62-64
　of "teratologic" congenital dislocation, 66, 250-251
　unusual, in treatment of congenital dislocation, 177
Pavlik harness, 25, 60, 62, 69
Pelvic obliquity, 178-179

Pelvic osteotomy, 184, 186, 227; see also Innominate (Salter) osteotomy; Pericapsular (Pemberton) osteotomy
　arthrotomy at time of, 148
　combined with femoral shortening and open reduction, 148-149
　and open reduction, 145-148
　pelvic x-ray film of 5-year-old child with, 183
　reconstructive, failure to gain reduction prior to, 184-185
Pelvic radiography in physical examination, 43-44
Pelvic-support osteotomy, Schanz, 240, 241-242
Pelvis
　and acetabulum, lateral view of, 13
　anteroposterior view of, with femora in neutral rotation, 144-145
　of newborn, 53
　　radiographic techniques for evaluation of, 50
　　roentgenographic determinants of, 50-60
　tomography of, 191
　x-ray film of; see X-ray film, pelvic
Pemberton, P. A., 125, 148
Pemberton osteotomy; see Pericapsular (Pemberton) osteotomy
Periacetabular "dial" osteotomy, 169-172
Periarticular osteotomy, 171
Pericapsular (Pemberton) osteotomy, 113, 125-133, 134-136, 164, 165; see also Innominate (Salter) osteotomy
　advantages and disadvantages of, 131-133
　in 14-month-old child with dislocation of right hip, 132
　and innominate (Salter) osteotomy, 138-145
　　complications of, 143-145
　　indications for, 138-145
　　prerequisites of, 141-143
　and open reduction, 145-148
　technique of, 127-130
Perichondrium of acetabulum and femoral head
　at 8 weeks of gestation, 4
　at 9 weeks of gestation, 5
　at 7½ weeks of gestation, 3
Perkins line, 50, 56-57
Persistent subluxation as complication during treatment of congenital dislocation, 186-188
Perthes disease, 25, 195
Pes planus, 32
Physical examination
　and history in diagnosis and treatment of congenital dysplasia and dislocation, 43-44
　in operative treatment of dysplasia in childhood and adolescence, 160-162
Physical findings
　in congenital dislocation, 72-73
　　in child 18 months to 4 years of age, 95-98
　　diagnostic, 45-47
　　neonatal, 67-68
　in subluxation, 64
Physical therapy in treatment of chondrolysis, 202
"Physiological" cast position, 116, 158
Physis, 12-14
Pin
　failure of, to transfix fragments, 184-185

Pin—cont'd
  penetration of hip joint by, 184-185
  Steinmann, 134-136
  transfixion, 122
Plastic abduction device, 69
  metal-reinforced, semirigid, 80
Plasticity, biologic, of acetabulum and femoral head, 133
Plate
  Coventry, 124
  epiphyseal, 12-14
  ordinary surgical steel, 124
  and screws, internal fixation utilizing, 122
Platou, E., 119
Position
  cast
    "axillary," 80
    following closed reduction, 78
    "frog-leg," 22, 116
    "human," 25, 80, 116
    "physiological," 116, 158
    in treatment of congenital dislocation in child under 18 months of age, 80
  in roentgenographic examination, 54
Posterior dislocation; see Dislocation, congenital, posterior
Posterolateral epiphyseal artery, 25
Precartilage at 6 weeks of gestation, 3
Preliminary traction in adults, 268
Price, C. T., 247
Primary acetabular dysplasia; see Dysplasia, primary acetabular
Primary anterior dislocation; see Dislocation, primary anterior
Primary dysplasia theory, 32
Probands, incidence of congenital dislocation in, 29
Problems
  in diagnosis of congenital dislocation, 175-176
  in treatment of congenital dislocation, 177-181
    and complications, 175-208
    unusual pathology of, 177
Progesterone, 34
Prosthesis, autogenous bone grafting to support, 266
Proximal femoral osteotomy, 172-173, 184-186
  angulation, 122
  combined with acetabular rotation, 173
  indications for, 172
  intertrochanteric, 119-125
  prerequisites of, 172-173
  rotational, 122, 187
  surgical technique of, 173
Proximal femur; see Femur, proximal
Pubis, 12
Pubofemoral ligament, 16-17
Pulvinar, 15
Putti, V., 32, 42, 53-54, 64, 67

R

Racial influences
  on congenital dysplasia and dislocation, 28-29
  on response and treatment of congenital dislocation, 152

Radiographic evaluation of operative treatment of dysplasia in childhood and adolescence, 160
Radiographic features of congenital dislocation, 74
Radiography, pelvic, in physical examination, 43-44; see also Roentgenogram; X-ray, pelvic
Ralis, Z., 10
Ramsey, P. L., 30, 47, 69
Reconstruction, implant hip, 257-271
Reconstructive pelvic osteotomy
  arthrotomy at time of, 148
  failure to gain reduction prior to, 184-185
Reconstructive proximal femoral osteotomies, 241-243
Redirectional (Salter) osteotomy, 137, 163, 164
Redislocation; see also Dislocation, congenital
  as complication during treatment of congenital dislocation, 188-192
  following closed reduction, 191
  following open reduction, 191
Reduction
  closed, 147, 156, 157, 189, 192
    cast postion following, 78
    of dislocation, 187
    and preliminary traction, bilateral dislocation treated by, 141-142
    redislocation following, 191
    and traction in treatment of congenital dislocation in child under 18 months of age, 75-80
    in treatment of congenital dislocation in child over 18 months of age, 99-100
  concentric, 146, 181-184
  case of achieving, 69
  failure to gain, prior to performing reconstructive pelvic osteotomy, 184-185
  guided, 69
  open, 144-145, 169, 177, 180
    acetabular limbus in, anatomy and clinical significance of, 92-93
    advantages and disadvantages of different methods of, 91-92
    cast following, 80
    and combined femoral shortening and pelvic osteotomy, 148-149
    concentricity of, 111-113
    development of acetabulum following, 113
    disadvantages and complications of, 93
    femoral shortening and, 100-109, 183
    growth and configuration of proximal femur following, 113
    importance of limbus in, 92-93
    indications for, 81-82
    by medial (adductor) approach to, 87-91, 189
    methods of, 82-93
    and pelvic (pericapsular or innominate) osteotomy, 145-148
    redislocation following, 191
    technique of, by anterior (iliofemoral) approach, 83-87
  in treatment of congenital dislocation
    in child over 18 months of age, 100-119
    in child under 18 months of age, 81-94
  stability of hip following, 69

Reduction—cont'd
  treatment of residual deformities following, 119-125
  of unilateral dislocation, 150
Relaxin, relationship of, to ligamentous laxity, 34-35
Replacement, total hip; see Hip, replacement of
Residual acetabular deficiencies, correction of, 125-126
Residual dysplasia, 155-174
Restriction of hip joint motion as complication of treatment of congenital dislocation, 205-207
Retinacular fibers, 16
Retroversion, angle of, 114-115
Rigid devices in treatment of dysplasia, 62
Roentgenogram; see also X-ray film, pelvic
  changes in, in osteonecrosis, 193
  changes in, in subluxation, 64
  of complete dislocation in 18-month-old child, 74
  in diagnosis of congenital dysplasia, 50-60
  diagnostic features of, of femoral head necrosis, 192-194
  illustrating difference between dysplasia and subluxation, 42
Roentgenographic examination, position of patient in, 54
Roentgenographic findings
  of congenital dislocation in child 18 months to 4 years of age, 98
  in neonatal dislocation, 68-69
  suggesting dysplasia, 57-60
Roentgenographic study of newborn, 49
Roser, K., 36
Rotation, acetabular
  combined with proximal femoral osteotomy, 173
  indications for, 165
Rotational osteotomy, 160
  proximal femoral, 122, 187
  supracondylar, 125
  varus, 121, 159
Rothschild, S., 200

S

Salter, R. B., 25, 30, 35, 36, 42, 80, 116, 125, 205
Salter osteotomy; see Innominate (Salter) osteotomy
Salvage procedures, 209-248
  introductions, purposes, and goals of, 209-211
  problems requiring, 211
Saw, Gigli, 133, 134-136
Schanz, A., 241
Schanz "pelvic-support" osteotomy, 240, 241-242, 268
Sciatic nerve, 270
Screw
  Coventry, 124
  and plate, internal fixation utilizing, 122
Seasonal hormonal changes and incidence of congenital dislocation, 31
Seasonal influence on congenital dysplasia and dislocation, 31
Seddon, H. J., 31, 119
Semirigid plastic metal-reinforced abduction device, 80

Severin, E., 50
Sex influences on congenital dysplasia and dislocation, 29-30
Shands, A. R., 115
Sheldon, W., 249
Shelf, "acetabular," 53
Shelf procedures, 125, 234-241
  indications for, 234
  surgical technique of, 234-241
  Wilson acetabular, technique of, 235-239
Shenton line, 137, 139, 141-142, 143, 156, 162
Shortening, femoral; see Femur, shortening of
Sign
  Ortolani, 44, 45, 68, 72
  Trendelenburg, 96
Skeletal traction, 75-80, 99-100, 121
Skin creases, thigh and inguinal, asymmetric, 47
Skin traction, 77
  preliminary, 192
  vs skeletal traction, 75-80
Smith, H. W., 67
Smith, W. S., 30, 34
Soft tissues in complete dislocation, 269-270
Somerville, E. W., 92, 119, 121
Southwick, W. O., 116
Spica cast, 69, 79
Splint
  Ilfeld, 58-59
  modified Craig, 58-59, 62
  plastic abduction, 69
  von Rosen, 58-59, 62
  weaning process from, 69
Spontaneous correction, 45
Staheli, L. T., 115
Stanisavljevic, S., 10, 44, 250
Steel, H. H., 126, 164
Steel osteotomy, 169
Steel plates, ordinary surgical, 124
Stein, W. G., 249
Steinmann pins, 134-136
Stellate osteotomy, 222
"Stick femur" procedure, 243-247
  results of, 246
  surgical technique of, 244-247
Strayer, L. M., 1, 2, 3-5, 10, 11
Subchondral irregularity, 201
Subluxation
  bilateral, 62-63
  definition of, 41
  and dysplasia, hip roentgenograms illustrating difference between, 42
  dysplasia that proceeded to, 65
  in early infancy, 62-66
  in high-risk infants, 48
  with painful osteoarthritis, 259-263
  pathology of, 62-64
  persistent, as complication during treatment of congenital dislocation, 186-188
  physical findings of, 64
  of right hip, pelvic x-ray film of 11-month-old child with, 122-123
  roentgenographic changes in, 64
  treatment of, 64-66

Subluxation—cont'd
  untreated, in newborn that resulted in dislocation, 66
Subluxation-provocation test, 45-47, 72
Superior gluteal artery, 22
Supracondylar osteotomy, 125
Surgical procedure; see Operative procedure
Surgical steel plates, ordinary, 124
Surgical technique; see Technique, surgical
Sutherland, D. H., 126, 148, 164, 168
Swaddling infants and incidence of congenital dislocation, 31
Synchondrosis
  ischiopubic, 14, 74
  triradiate, 12
Synovial membrane, 3, 18-22

T

Tachdjian, M. O., 146
Talipes equinovarus, 31
Technique
  of apophyseal arrest of greater trochanter, 196-197
  of femoral shortening and open reduction, 102-109
  of open reduction
    by anterior (iliofemoral) approach, 83-87
    and femoral shortening, 103-108
    by medial (adductor) approach, 87-91
  of Pemberton osteotomy, 127-130
  surgical
    of arthrodesis, 248
    of Chiari osteotomy, 226-229
    of Colonna arthroplasty, 215-222
    of pericapsular "dial" osteotomy, 169-172
    of proximal femoral osteotomy, 173
    of shelf procedures, 234-241
    of "stick femur" procedure, 244-247
    of triple innominate osteotomy, 165-168
    of trochanteric arthroplasty, 243-247
  for taking pelvic x-ray film in neonate, 52
  triple diaper, in treatment of dysplasia, 62
  of Wilson acetabular "shelf" procedure, 235-239
Tendon, iliopsoas, 92
Tenotomizing vs lengthening of iliopsoas tendon and muscle, 92
"Teratologic" dislocation; see Dislocation, congenital, "teratologic"
Thieme, W. T., 29, 35
Thigh segment, shortening of, in unilateral dislocation, 73
Thigh skin creases
  asymetric, 47
  and inguinal creases in unilateral dislocation, 73
Tissues, soft, in complete dislocation, 269-270
Tomography, 188
  axial, 115
  of pelvis, 191
Tönnis, D., 121
Torsion
  angle of, 114-115
  femoral; see Femoral torsion
Traction, 99
  and closed reduction in treatment of congenital dislocation in child under 18 months of age, 75-80

Traction—cont'd
  longitudinal, 99
  preliminary, and closed reduction, bilateral dislocation treated by, 141-142
  skeletal, 75-80, 99-100, 121
    vs skin traction, 75-80
  skin, 77
    preliminary, 192
  in treatment of chondrolysis, 202
Transfixion pins, 122
Transverse acetabular ligament, 15
Treatment
  of acetabular dysplasia
    "redirectional" (Salter) osteotomy in, 137
    surgical procedures in, 162-173
  of anterior primary dislocation, 94
  in arthrogryposis, 251-256
  of chondrolysis, 202-205
  of congenital dislocation; see Dislocation, congenital, treatment of
  of congenital dysplasia, 60-62
  and diagnosis
    of congenital dislocation
      in child under 18 months of age, 72-94
      in child 18 months to 4 years of age, 95-154
      and dysplasia in newborn, neonate, and young infant, 40-71
    of residual dysplasia in older child or adolescent, 155-174
  of dysplasia, 60-62
  of femoral head necrosis, 195-196
  of neonatal dislocation, 69-70
  nonoperative, of dysplasia in infancy and childhood, 157-159
  operative, of dysplasia in childhood and adolescence, 159-162
    general considerations for, 159-162
    indications for, 159-160
    physical examination in, 160-162
    radiographic evaluation in, 160
  of subluxation, 64-66
Trendelenburg gait, 165, 269
Trendelenburg sign in unilateral dislocation, 96
Triplane osteotomy, 173
Triple diaper technique in treatment of dysplasia, 62
Triple innominate osteotomy; see Innominate (Salter) osteotomy, triple
Triradiate cartilage, 12, 14
Triradiate synchondrosis, 12
Trochanter
  greater
    "overgrowth" of, 194, 195, 196-197
    technique of apophyseal arrest of, 196-197
    major, displacement of, reshaping of proximal femur by, 242
    at 13 weeks of gestation, 7
Trochanteric arthroplasty, 243-247
Tronzo, R. G., 264
Twins, incidence of congenital dislocation in, 29-30

U

Unilateral dislocation; see Dislocation, congenital, unilateral

V

Van Meerdervoort, H. F., 28
Van Neck disease, 14
Varus intertrochanteric osteotomy, 121-122, 196
Varus rotational osteotomy, 121, 159
Vasculature structures at 20 weeks of gestation, 8
Vitallium cup arthroplasty, 257
Vitallium mesh, 264
von Friedlander, F., 36
von Rosen, S., 29, 50
von Rosen splint, 58-59, 62
VonAmmon, 32

W

Wagner, H., 126, 164, 169, 172, 173, 242, 243
Watanabe, R. S., 1, 6-7, 10, 11, 36
Wedge osteotomy, closing, of proximal femur, 240
Weiner, D. S., 99
Weissman, S. L., 244
Wessell, A. B., 28
Westin, G. W., 99, 101, 243, 244
Wiberg, G., 158, 160, 165
Wilkinson, J. A., 30, 36
Wilkinson, J. S., 34, 35, 36
Wilson, J. C., 125
Wilson acetabular "shelf" procedure, technique of, 235-239
Wire, Kirschner, 243
Wynne-Davies, R., 29, 30, 33, 35, 36

X

X-ray film, pelvic, 50; *see also* Roentgenogram
  of bilateral dislocation
    in 18-month-old child, 178
    in 14-year-old child, 228
    in 9-year-old child, 157
    in 6-month-old child, 199
    in 10-year-old child, 150
    in 12-year-old child, 214
    in 28-month-old child, 146
    in 21-month-old child, 100

X-ray film, pelvic—cont'd
  of bilateral dislocation—cont'd
    in 2-year-old child, 156
    in 2½-year-old child, 179
  following Colonna arthroplasty in 11-year-old girl, 101
  of chondrolysis in 13-year-old child, 201
  of complete dislocation of left hip in 2-year-old child, 143
  of dislocation of left hip
    in 14-month-old child, 112
    in 16-month-old child, 203
    and subluxation of right hip in 11-month-old child, 122-123
  of 12-month-old child, 76
  in 2-month-old child, 82
  in 2-year-old child, 147, 189
  of irreducible dislocation in newborn, 252
  of limp, bilateral, in 5-year-old child, 182
  minimal number of, in diagnosis of congenital dislocation, 144-145
  in Navajo neonates, 55
  in neonate, technique of taking, 52
  of pelvic osteotomy in 5-year-old child, 183
  in physical examination, 43-44
  of primary anterior dislocation in 18-month-old child, 93
  of severe arthrogryposis in 4½-year-old child, 251
  of unilateral dislocation
    of right hip in 12-year-old child, 212
    in 10-year-old child, 223
  of untreated congenital dislocation
    in 50-year-old woman, 259
    in 4-year-old child, 109-110
    in 9-year-old child, 151, 190-191

Y

Y ligament of Bigelow, 12, 16-17

Z

Zona orbicularis, 17, 18